ARGUMENTS AND ANALYSIS IN BIOETHICS

VIBS

Volume 214

a volume in
Values in Bioethics
ViB
Matti Häyry and Tuija Takala, Editors

ARGUMENTS AND ANALYSIS IN BIOETHICS

Edited by
Matti Häyry, Tuija Takala,
Peter Herissone-Kelly and Gardar Árnason

Rodopi

Amsterdam - New York, NY 2010

Cover Photo: Morguefile.com

Cover Design: Studio Pollmann

The paper on which this book is printed meets the requirements of "ISO 9706:1994, Information and documentation - Paper for documents - Requirements for permanence".

ISBN: 978-90-420-2802-9
E-Book ISBN: 978-90-420-2803-6

Printed in the Netherlands

CONTENTS

FOREWORD

Walking down Broadway, the philosopher Arthur Danto once explained how he thought we can make progress on the most stubborn of philosophical conundrums. It was his experience that if he put enough analytical pressure on a philosophical problem and continued to apply that pressure, something would eventually "pop." I imagined my professor bearing down with all his might on a ball of granite and then gleefully smiling when he heard a "pop." If anyone had the power of mind to crack a philosophical ball of granite, Danto did.

While philosophers have not cornered the market in analysis and argument, it is our stock in trade. There is no substitute. As we wheel and deal, our wears are assessed by their consistency, plausibility, and power to make sense of our world. The articles in this collection, though not all written by philosophers, wheel and deal in analysis and argument. They address an eclectic batch of bioethical issues and bring a diversity of perspectives to bear on them. They are not cut from a common cloth. However, they do have a common thread: careful analysis and argumentation.

As such, they need to be reckoned with. The essays are provocative, indeed, some quite radical and disturbing, as they call into question many common methodological and substantive assumptions in bioethics. For example, we would normally assume that bioethics does not serve only the interests of the rich and powerful. However, Søren Holm argues that bioethical deliberations, for example about the sale of organs for transplantation, often assume a status quo of coercive social and economic inequalities. If these inequalities are not addressed, then the bioethical "solutions" are inherently biased against the poor and in favor of the rich and powerful. We would normally assume that we need bioethical principles to responsibly address bioethical problems. However, Simona Giordana challenges this common assumption, arguing that appeal to such principles does more harm than good. We would normally assume that it is not irrational and immoral to have children. However, Matti Häyry argues that it is.

Other articles raise critical methodological and conceptual issues for bioethics. What is the force of examples and counterexamples in bioethics? What are the relevance of moral intuition and the role of empirical evidence in bioethical argument? What notion of "function" underlies accounts of the distinction between normality and disease and between therapy and enhancement? Are such notions of function "value-neutral," as is commonly assumed? Is there an inherent conflict between research aimed at therapy and research aimed at gaining knowledge, such that the very notion of "therapeutic research" is an oxymoron?

Other essays address more particular substantive issues in bioethics. Again, they do so in a way that challenges common assumptions underlying most approaches to these issues and the analysis offers some surprising results. For example, is there any justification for the common practice of allocating expensive medical resources to rescue a few from rare diseases, when those resources could be used to treat devastating diseases that affect the many? Mark Sheehan suggests that there is none. Does commercial surrogacy violate the Kantian maxim never to treat people as mere means, as many have assumed? Stuart Oultram argues that this is a mistake. Does the use of Prozac and other anti-depressants make us inauthentic beings? John McMillan suggests that it does.

Socrates would be glad to see such a collection come into print. The essays in this volume are a swarm of gadflies, pestilent little fellows that disturb the comfort of how we commonly practice bioethics. They push the issues in new directions through critical reflection on what has been said and creative thinking about what needs to be said. In some cases, it is hard to think how we could responsibly consider these issues any longer without taking the authors' views into account. The literary theorist, Michelle Riffratere, once remarked that a text is never the same after it has been read by Jacques Derrida. It is safe to say that many of the issues addressed in this volume are no longer the same after they have been analyzed and worked over by their authors.

Dr John Lizza
Professor of Philosophy
Kutztown University
June 2008

PREFACE

This book continues the tradition of *Scratching the Surface of Bioethics*, edited by Matti Häyry and Tuija Takala (VIBS 144); and *Bioethics and Social Reality*, edited by Matti Häyry, Tuija Takala, and Peter Herissone-Kelly (VIBS 165). It is the third volume in our Special Series produced by a group of bioethicists in and around the universities of Central Lancashire, Keele, Lancaster, Liverpool, and Manchester, in the North West of England.

Most chapters in the following pages are based on presentations given in the Third North West Bioethics Roundtable (NorthWeb 3), organized by Dr Angus Dawson in Keele on 20 February 2004, and the Fourth North West Bioethics Roundtable (NorthWeb 4), organized by Dr Lucy Frith in Liverpool on 24 February 2005. Some additional thematically related chapters have been solicited from scholars who could not attend the meetings but whose work complements the original contributions.

The sponsors of NorthWeb 3 and 4, and the ensuing book project, included

- *Ethical and Social Aspects of Bioinformatics*, a project co-ordinated by Professor Matti Häyry and funded by the Academy of Finland research program Systems Biology and Bioinformatics;
- *Values in Bioethics*, a Special Series in Rodopi's *Value Inquiry Book Series*;
- *Centre for Professional Ethics*, Keele University;
- *Division of Primary Care*, University of Liverpool;
- *Centre for Professional Ethics*, University of Central Lancashire; and
- *Centre for Social Ethics and Policy*, University of Manchester.

The organizers, and the editors of this book, acknowledge this support with gratitude.

Matti Häyry, Tuija Takala, Peter Herissone-Kelly, Gardar Árnason
1 August 2008, Manchester and Preston, England

Introduction

ARGUING ABOUT ARGUMENTS, ANALYZING ANALYSIS

Matti Häyry, Tuija Takala, Gardar Árnason, and Peter Herissone-Kelly

1. The Place of Arguments and Analysis in Bioethics

Bioethics, in common with all philosophical endeavors, is centrally concerned with argument and analysis. First of all, it employs argument and analysis in addressing concrete questions about how healthcare professionals, life-scientists, legislators, and others ought to behave in particular situations, and with regard to particular problems. Ought we to allow human reproductive cloning? Ought we to create hybrid embryos? Ought we to endorse voluntary euthanasia? Where such questions have answers, those answers are to be arrived at through argument and analysis.

Sometimes, however, bioethics operates more reflectively than this. It does not simply *employ* argument and analysis, but instead *focuses* upon them. Is the Utilitarian (Kantian, virtue-theoretical) approach to bioethics the right one to use in answering a given question? Are the concepts employed in this piece of bioethical reasoning legitimate? Might there be different concepts and methods that can be pressed into service in bioethical analysis? In these sorts of questions, bioethical method is turned back upon itself.

This is a neat and useful theoretical distinction between what we might call first- and second-order bioethical inquiry. However, it is a distinction that in practice tends to become rather blurred. Books and articles that focus on particular first-order bioethical issues are apt at the same time, at least to some degree, to be critical analyses of the argumentative strategies brought to bear on those issues. And second-order investigations of bioethical methods and concepts tend to stress the sorts of outcomes that adoption of those methods and concepts will have for first-order issues. Consequently, whether we label a particular piece of bioethics first- or second-order is largely determined by its primary, rather than its exclusive, emphasis.

This volume contains twenty-one chapters, each of which has its primary emphasis on a different part of the first-order/second-order continuum. However, all of them have something important to say about the nature and place of argument and analysis in bioethics.

2. Bioethical Skepticism

The first three chapters of the book each display a certain skepticism about bioethics, or at least about some of the ways in which it is commonly practiced. In chapter one, Sirkku Hellsten focuses her attention on the use of false dichotomies and polarizations that she takes to be common in global bioethics (understood as a supposedly comprehensive, culturally neutral normative framework by means of which we can address bioethical issues). She argues that, if the enterprise of bioethics is to prove at all fruitful, what we really need to do is to understand ethical concerns solely in terms of the local, cultural contexts in which they arise. What is more, she urges that an awareness of common reasoning fallacies may teach us more valuable lessons than debates on common values or universal ethical frameworks.

In the second chapter, Søren Holm asks whether bioethics only serves the interests of the rich and powerful. Some may be shocked to learn that the answer is (a slightly qualified) "yes." The main focus of the chapter is on interpersonal coercion, in particular in the context of poverty and healthcare. Holm argues that poverty, at least at unjust levels, can provide conditions for coercion, with the implication that allowing poor people, say, to sell their organs would be morally wrong.

"Do we need (bio)ethical principles?" This is the question posed by Simona Giordano in chapter three. This time the answer is a completely unqualified "no." But Giordano goes even further, arguing that ethics based on principles causes harm by stifling authentic ethical thinking and debate. Given the preponderance of principle-based reasoning in the area of bioethics, this can be seen as a very radical conclusion.

3. Bioethical Methods

The next four chapters in the collection critically examine various tools that either regularly are or could be employed in bioethical inquiry.

Bioethics deals in arguments. It is, therefore, perhaps surprising that bioethicists—unlike lawyers, psychologists, linguists, and so on—have apparently paid no attention to the philosopher Stephen Toulmin's argumentation theory. In chapter four, Doris Schroeder and Peter Herissone-Kelly discuss the possible uses of that theory in bioethics. They argue that, while the approach might be useful for exposing deficiencies in existing bioethical arguments, it can hardly ever be used conclusively to justify claims. Its utility as an item in the bioethicist's toolbox is consequently severely restricted.

The first of Harry Lesser's two contributions to this volume concerns the functions of examples in bioethics. Lesser draws a distinction between pedagogical and what we might call argumentative uses of examples. As far as the former use is concerned, Lesser mounts a case for its pressing into service dramatic and real (or realistic) examples. When it comes to the argumentative use, he shows that examples, including counter-examples, are unable to settle arguments. They can, however, be legitimately and usefully employed to, as it were, move an argument along. In addition to their pedagogical and argumentative functions, examples can be used as thought experiments. In this guise, an example can be very helpful in introducing new concerns and ideas into an argument, but cannot determine that argument's outcome.

Lesser's second contribution addresses the question of the weight that ought to be given in ethical reasoning to our moral intuitions. It emerges that moral intuitions are of various kinds: some are mere reactions and have no place in ethical reasoning, some are conflicting and difficult to evaluate. Still others concern principles which are essential if we are to have any moral code at all. Those intuitions that turn out to be morally irrelevant are to be rejected, concludes Lesser, but any serious theory in bioethics should respect intuitions according to which particular policies or actions carry with them the risk of grave harm.

In chapter seven, Angus Dawson discusses the use of empirical evidence in ethical argumentation. In order to evaluate arguments that depend on such evidence, we first need to have in place criteria against which we can assess its quality. Dawson proposes four principles to guide the "fair use" of empirical evidence in ethical arguments, before anticipating and responding to four possible objections to his suggested approach. The usefulness of the approach is illustrated by reference to ethical arguments about the Mumps, Measles, and Rubella (MMR) combined vaccine.

4. Concepts and Distinctions

The next group of essays sets out to examine a selection of crucial bioethical concepts and distinctions.

Some significant attempts have been made to provide value-free accounts of the concepts of health and disease. One such account, which defines disease as an impairment of normal functional ability, serves as the basis of Norman Daniels's theory of just healthcare. In chapter eight, however, Cathleen Schulte urges that this model fails to analyze the theories of function that have been developed in the philosophy of biology. She argues that, in the absence of such analysis, the normal-function model, along with its concept of function, can be shown to have problematic implications for Daniels's theory. On the other hand, once that analysis is taken on board, the normal functional ability account of health turns out not to be value-free after all.

Stephen Wilkinson, in chapter nine, explores the distinction between positive and negative eugenics, asking how it relates to further distinctions between therapy and enhancement, and between disease and normality. Having analyzed the main accounts of the first distinction, Wilkinson concludes that they fail to show that it is morally significant.

Chapter ten represents the first of Niall Scott's two contributions to this volume. In it, Scott discusses the genetic fallacy in the context of behavioral genetics. He explains that we commit the genetic fallacy whenever we judge a claim or an object on the basis of its origin. In the arena of behavioral genetics, commission of the fallacy consists in our judging or explaining behavior in terms of its (alleged) genetic basis. Scott examines the relation of this fallacy to genetic determinism, illustrating his argument with the example of genetic "explanations" of homosexuality. He insists that an account of the genetic basis or origin of behavior is unable to supply us with an account of what that behavior *is*.

In Scott's second contribution, chapter eleven, we are brought back to the issue of eugenics. Wilkinson's discussion of positive and negative eugenics in chapter nine is related to the distinction between the "old" and the "new" eugenics, and to the more recent idea of liberal eugenics. Questions are raised about the meaning of enhancement and the nature of human flourishing. Scott concludes by pointing out that although liberal eugenics is ostensibly concerned with the enhancement of individuals, while the old eugenics is concerned with the enhancement of populations, in practice liberal eugenics would result in collective population enhancement.

5. General Approaches, Particular Issues

The next three contributions to the volume can be seen as explorations of the way in which various general approaches to bioethics mesh with very particular issues.

In chapter twelve, Anna Smajdor argues on Millian grounds that a ban on human reproductive cloning could only be justified if it could be shown that the practice would result in harm to those produced by means of it. It is often assumed that such harms would inevitably occur. Smajdor, however, regards that assumption with an intensely critical eye. She holds that the likelihood of harm to clones is typically overestimated, and that clones can certainly not be harmed simply by being brought into existence. Her conclusion is that although human reproductive cloning might still be unethical (a claim about which she is largely silent), that in itself, in the absence of proven harm, is not sufficient for its being outlawed.

Matti Häyry, in chapter thirteen, sets out to defend the position outlined in his controversial *Journal of Medical Ethics* paper "A Rational Cure for Pre-Reproductive Stress Syndrome" against criticisms from Søren Holm, Rebecca Bennett, and Sahin Aksoy. The central claim of that paper is that it is both irrational and immoral to produce children. It is irrational since—according to the "maximin" rule—deliberately allowing the worst outcome of our actions is irrational, and having children allows the worst outcome, in the shape of a life that for its subject is of a lower value than non-existence. And it is immoral since it is wrong to cause avoidable suffering, and bringing someone into existence invariably produces such suffering.

In chapter fourteen, Stuart Oultram aims to overturn claims that commercial surrogacy necessarily falls foul of the Kantian injunction always to treat others as ends in themselves, and never as mere means to our own ends. Oultram argues that the perspective on commercial surrogacy that gives rise to this conclusion is neither fair nor accurate. Neither the commissioning couple, nor the commercial surrogate mother, nor the agencies that arrange commercial surrogacy can automatically be assumed to possess the sorts of motives required to make the Kantian charge stick.

6. Perspectives on Well-Being

Chapters fifteen and sixteen are centrally concerned with the notion, surely of vital importance to bioethics, of well-being.

In chapter fifteen, guided by certain philosophical claims about what it is that makes a human life go well, John McMillan focuses attention on empirical data about personality changes in patients taking anti-depressants. He suggests that authenticity, understood as a state that exists when our reactions harmonize with our sense of who we are, is an essential ingredient in well-being. The state of being "better than well" said to be brought about by anti-depressants may, paradoxically, have a negative impact on our well-being, to the extent that it involves us in an inauthentic mode of being.

Floris Tomasini, in chapter sixteen, investigates the phenomenon of self-demand amputees: persons who have a felt need to have one or more healthy limbs or digits surgically removed. Tomasini argues that standard normative ethical theories (specifically, Kantianism and Utilitarianism) are inadequate tools with which to assess the ethics of a doctor's meeting or failing to meet a self-demand amputee's request for amputation. Both drastically fail to take into account the patient's own "lived experience," and with it her own sense of what it is that would constitute her well-being. In particular, Kantianism does not allow for the existence of diverse conceptions of embodiment, while Utilitarianism too falls short of a proper recognition of what it must be like to be a self-demand amputee, in so far as such a recognition clashes with the ethical justification that healthcare workers' professional identity demands.

7. Contested Concepts

The last five chapters of the volume all deal with certain controversial concepts that are often employed in bioethical argument and analysis.

In chapter seventeen, Mark Sheehan takes up the question of whether healthcare policy makers, in so far as they are involved in resource allocation, can be justified in providing very effective, but enormously expensive, enzyme replacement therapies to the sufferers of devastating and rare lysosomal storage disorders. Any plausible justification for such decisions would appear to be founded in a Rule of Rescue. That rule gives expression to the natural human tendency to want to rescue single endangered lives, regardless of cost, and despite the fact that doing so will reduce the amount of resources available elsewhere. If the rule is to have a normative dimension, instead of simply identifying a brute empirical fact about the human proclivity for saving identifiable individuals, then the most promising justification of it will appeal to agent-relative reasons. But these are precisely the sorts of reasons that we might think (wrongly, Sheehan argues) ought not to figure in the deliberations of policy makers.

Peter Lucas argues in chapter eighteen that the notion of therapeutic research, understood as a practice in which there is an essential link between the therapeutic goal and the goal of producing generalizable medical knowledge—is, in effect, a myth. There is, he insists, an ineliminable tension between the aim of conferring therapeutic advantage on the participant/patient, and the aim of gathering research data. Data-gathering in controlled trials, where it is ethically carried out, must to some extent undermine any therapeutic intent. On the other hand, in research that involves the testing of innovative treatments, the subject may gain a therapeutic benefit from participating. However, it is not strictly speaking in her interests to be involved in the research program. Lucas ends with the suggestion that we stop using the misleading label "therapeutic research," and opt instead for "medical research combined with medical care."

A pressing question in all areas of applied ethics concerns the legitimate scope of ethical concern. What sorts of beings are worthy of ethical consideration, or can be taken to possess basic rights? Lisa Bortolotti, in chapter nineteen, holds that "persons" is the wrong answer. However, she agrees with Tom Regan that a being's possessing sentience is not sufficient to render it worthy of moral concern. Even so, she believes that Regan's "subject-of-a-life" criterion—which demands that morally considerable beings have such characteristics as memory, a sense of their own future, and self-consciousness—sets the bar too high. She instead argues that basic rights can be accorded to any being that has intentional states.

In the volume's twentieth chapter, Jane Wilson examines the possibility, suggested by Tziporah Kasachkoff, that there may be forms of paternalism that are ethically justified. Kasachkoff's claims represent a critique of the dominant liberal rights-based conception of paternalism, which unrealistically assumes that all paternalistic action must be coercive in character. While Wilson agrees with Kasachkoff, her chapter concentrates on Mark S. Komrad's attempt to demonstrate a sphere of justified medical paternalism. Komrad's arguments are shown to have serious shortcomings, and to entail the legitimacy of unrestricted paternalism in the treatment of ill patients. Whatever the justification of medical paternalism—and Wilson assumes that there are contexts in which it can be justified—it is not the one offered by Komrad.

In the final chapter, Simo Vehmas discusses a group of issues surrounding our understanding of people with severe intellectual impairments, and with it the very notion of disability and various ways of conceptualizing it. Specifically, he examines four claims: that people with severe intellectual impairments are not persons; that they are burdensome, either to their families or to society as a whole; that they are members of an oppressed group; and that their disability is nothing but a social construct. He finds reason to question each of these assumptions, reaching some surprising and controversial conclusions along the way.

8. Pressing Onward

The twenty-one chapters in this volume strive, through the use of high quality argument and analysis, to get a good deal clearer concerning a range of issues *in* bioethics, and a range of issues *about* bioethics. They succeed in that aim. But perhaps their greatest success will involve something further: namely, their acting as a catalyst for future debate. The more arguments about bioethical argument, and the more analyses of bioethical analysis, the better.

One

GLOBAL BIOETHICS AND "ERRONEOUS REASON": FALLACIES ACROSS THE BORDERS

Sirkku Kristiina Hellsten

1. Introduction

The rapid developments in medical sciences and biotechnology in the globalized world have brought bioethical issues into the heart of the public and academic debates. International policy makers and healthcare professionals have disputed whether there should be a comprehensive, normative framework of "global bioethics," or whether we should settle with learning more about the differences between the various "local" bioethical norms.

In this chapter I want to focus particularly on the errors of reasoning in a global context. I claim that if we want to find a way toward any kind of global consensus on normative guidelines in bioethics, we need to be more aware of the common fallacies involved in bioethical argumentation across the borders. Recognizing these fallacies in our reasoning helps us to make a clear distinction between (1) actual moral value conflicts; (2) political views and rhetorical use of the main concepts; and (3) disagreements which appear to have moral foundations but actually are due to obstacles in our reasoning which prevent consistent and unbiased argumentation.

2. Opposites Attract: For and Against X

One way to defend a particular normative position in bioethics—as in any other philosophical and ethical argumentation—is to defend a preferred position against its rival. In early bioethics one of the most basic forms of argument was between opposite normative positions. One could, for instance, argue "for" or "against" euthanasia, abortion, population control, genetic engineering, and so on, by creating polarizations between the extreme, opposite views. One efficient way to do this is to set alternative or competing normative theoretical frameworks into combat against each other. For example, you can set your defense for an argument against marketing human body parts in a deontological framework, and then refute any views in favor by showing how morally suspicious is the willingness of utilitarian consequentialism to sacrifice innocent lives in the name of the common utility. Similarly, you could defend surrogate motherhood with a utilitarian argument of maximizing overall happiness, by highlighting the logical inconsistencies that attach to certain deontological arguments. The arguments in question claim that individual moral agents are to be treated as ends in themselves rather than as means to other ends, while simultaneously undermining that very moral agency in taking a paternalistic view toward those who have made the decision to try to have their own child by using any means available. Deontologists undermine the autonomy of those who have given their informed consent and have agreed to take upon themselves the burden of pregnancy in order to help others realize their dreams of producing genetically related offspring.

Such polarization is often more rhetorical than ethical. By setting one's own argument against any rival ones—and by rebutting the apparently incommensurable positions—we can easily create a "false dichotomy" that in turn provides a basis for rationalizations and polarizations: if I can prove that the opposite side is wrong, then my own view must be right.

3. Polarization Between the West and the Rest

Contemporary philosophical argumentation in bioethics within the Western framework has a lesser focus on competing theoretical frameworks and dichotomized positions. Instead, it attempts to show sensitivity to actual, practical ethical concerns and to be more responsive to public views as well as policy-making and legislative issues. The practical importance of bioethics has created a need to find arguments that look for the mean between the normative extremes, and that settle for a compromise position that most of us would (or could) agree upon at least to a degree (as the moral justification for various public policies and new laws). However, as inconsistent as it may seem, in the global dialogue in bioethics, we still have a long road to travel from falsely polarized cultural competition, to cross-cultural consensus and informed agreement.[1]

International debates in bioethics today are still often based on polarizations that result from false dichotomies and striking forms of "black-and-white" thinking (almost literally speaking). The main polarizations can be identified as follows: (1) a debate on the moral superiority/inferiority of a particular cultural tradition (namely, individualism versus collectivism); (2) a competition between two apparently opposite and incommensurable theoretical frameworks (namely liberal pluralism versus communitarian particularism); (3) the incomparability of two contrasting metaphysical worldviews (namely atomism versus holism); and (4) the plausibility of universalistic versus relativistic moral outlooks.

These various aspects of the debates tend to get tangled together resulting in a false dichotomy between supposedly opposing cultural moral traditions, namely Western universalistic individualism versus non-Western relativist collectivism.[2] The proponents of individualism from within the Western tradition argue against the non-Western collectivist frameworks by claiming that they lead to a suppression of the individual will and individual rights. This conclusion is drawn from premises that claim that in traditionally more collectivist cultures, the starting point for healthcare and medical treatment is not the individual—the patient himself or herself—but instead the community, and in particular the family.

To support these premises, empirical evidence is often given that in many Eastern and Southern countries such as Japan, China, the Philippines, and Indonesia, as well in Africa, people do not practice self-determination in the same explicit fashion as is required by the principles of individualistic, Western medical ethics. Decision-making is instead based on the values of social responsibility, solidarity, and egalitarianism. This means that a family or even a community as a social collective is expected to take part in making decisions with, and sometimes on behalf of, the patient. To proponents of individualism, such a "paternalistic" structure of decision-making suppresses individual freedom and violates people's moral agency. Since such a collectivistic cultural practice as communal support in decision making does not typically follow the universalistic demand for the value of individual autonomy and rights, Western individualists also see it as a form of cultural relativism.

The collectivist normative framework, however, has a logical defense for the values of social responsibility and solidarity. On the one hand, the family and community have special obligations to take care of the sick, not only in terms of material aid, but also in a psychological and social sense. They have a duty to help the patient make difficult decisions, in order to make everything work smoothly in his or her best interests. So, the community is there to protect a patient from further anxiety and difficult decisions that also affect those around him or her. From the collectivist point of view this is not an attempt to suppress an individual will. Instead, it is a caring and more democratic approach than the Western individualist one, which evidently leaves the entire burden of difficult decisions on individuals who are already suffering and worrying about those whom their decisions affect. The Western atomistic individual, detached from all social connections and networks, is seen as an illusion. From the perspective of more collectivist Eastern or Southern worldviews, the construction of a moral framework based on such a distorted view of our decision-making contexts merely promotes egoism. In practice, this easily precipitates the disintegration of family and communities, and creates a social context in which everybody cares merely for themselves, and not for anyone else.[3]

This polarization between Western individualism and non-Western collectivism seems to suggest that in a global context we are faced with fundamentally different cultural ethical positions, which lead into normatively incommensurable, practically opposed moral values and principles or ethical guidelines. The collectivist view criticizes the Western individualistic approach for its universalism. Collectivists maintain that attempts to justify certain moral rules and principles by socially "unembedded" reason leads to the enforcement of unwarranted Western cultural bias, which in practice further encourages imperialism and neo-colonialism. Using methodological, detached human reason as a justification for universal and absolute moral principles disregards the context of local belief and value systems.

1. Ethical "-isms":	
Individualism	Collectivism
a) Uniform (up to a degree) Western cultural tradition	b) Various non-Western (Eastern, Southern, and so on) cultural traditions
2. Theoretical frameworks:	
a) Liberal individualism —universalism —pluralism	b) Communitarian collectivism —relativism —particularism
3. Metaphysical worldviews:	
a) Atomism	b) Holism
4. Defined values/ideals (desired positive outcomes):	
a) Equal individual rights and freedom Reciprocal individual good	b) Social responsibility and egalitarianism, the common good
5. Actual/practical negative outcomes and related practices:	
a) Egoism, self-interest, social disintegration/competition.	b) Suppression of individual, paternalism/totalitarianism

Table 1.1 *Polarizations between individualism and collectivism*

The individualist view, for its part, tends to blame collectivism for fostering suppressive traditions and for disrespect of individual rights in practice. This false dichotomy sets different cultural traditions up in competition against each other, as if in themselves they present comprehensive normative theoretical frameworks. The individualist cultural tradition is taken to present a rights-based theory opposed to a collectivist communitarianism which is equated with the theory of collective social responsibility. Dialogue between such seemingly incompatible positions becomes futile.[4]

Table 1.1 maps out how the polarizations to which we subscribe can easily mislead us into seeing cultural frameworks as normatively incommensurable. In reality, however, we can actually find similar values in each framework. The reason for this is that the polarizations in question tend to combine different elements of the *-isms*. For example, in debates over conflicting values we tend to set the values of one framework against the actual practices of another: (4a) defined and pronounced values/ideals, set against (5b), the actual negative outcomes and related practices; and, *vice versa*, (5a) against (4b) and so on.

Table 1.2 shows how the descriptive elements of frameworks can be set against prescriptive ones, so creating false dichotomies: universalistic individualism (1a) against relativist collectivism (2b), and *vice versa*. We can also recognize here how both frameworks share the problem of relativism: individualism turning into relativist subjectivism and collectivism into cultural relativism.

	1. Universalism	**2. Relativism**
a) Individualism	Individual rights Value/goal: universal respect for human dignity, difference, and tolerance/freedom	Subjectivism Negative outcome: *Laissez-faire* ethics, moral indifference, and egoism
b) Collectivism	Collective/group rights Value/goal: universal respect for human dignity, difference, and tolerance/freedom	Relativism Negative outcome: Cultural relativism, tolerating intolerance, and group self-interest/competition

Table 1.2 *Polarizations, the naturalistic fallacy, and cultural generalizations.*

4. Descriptive versus Prescriptive Reasoning in Bioethics

Related to the false dichotomies between individualism, collectivism, universalism, and relativism is the problem of the *naturalistic fallacy*. Since bioethics is about normative guidelines for the biosciences and their everyday application in policy issues and medical practice, we need to engage in moral reasoning that is engaged in reflective value judgments. Arguments on bioethical issues may not originally, in many cases, provide for prescriptive value conclusions. However, our tendency to derive "ought" from "is" leads bioethics easily into the *naturalistic fallacy*. This fallacy is committed when we draw a normative conclusion from factual premises without any solid evaluative ethical support. Instead, we let our suppressed, implicit premises (*enthymema*) lead the way to a normative conclusion.[5]

In argumentation theory this tendency to derive prescriptive claims from descriptive reasoning is related to confusion between practical or pragmatic recommendations on the one hand, and moral judgments on the other. I can for instance give you the following advice: "If you want to live a long life, you should eat sensibly and get enough exercise." This, however, is a practical recommendation, and not a moral claim about the importance of a long life, or the good life, or life in general. Instead it might be based on my empirical observation or on scientific evidence that people who eat sensibly and exercise tend to die older than those who do not. On the policy level, this observation as such does not give (for example) the government any moral obligation to make sure that we, the citizens are getting sensible nutrition and plenty of exercise, nor does it oblige us to aim for a healthy and long life. Some other general principles or assumptions are needed in the premises to make it a moral recommendation, such as "long life increases human well-being and happiness; well-being and happiness are the intrinsic values/purpose of human life" (in a teleological sense).[6]

Similarly, we can reason that "mothers of new-born babies should be advised to breast-feed their babies, because most manufactured baby milks have been found to contain chemicals which can cause infertility," and here again—if we consider the should recommendation as a moral one—we need to agree with the principles that infertility or childlessness is somehow intrinsically morally undesirable.[7]

5. Rationalizing Hasty Generalizations

The reason why we should pay attention to false polarizations, hasty generalizations, and commissions of the naturalistic fallacy is that our argumentation, despite its potentially presenting itself as objective, is usually based on our earlier assumptions, learned values, and cultural background. If this goes unnoticed, we are liable to accept further presumptions, or to enforce our existing prejudices by justifying them with reason-substitutes instead of logically consistent, valid, and sound argumentation concerning the moral values involved. The result is "pseudo-morality," or argumentation that presents itself as making genuine moral judgments, while it is actually based on practical recommendations drawn from purely factual premises.

In order to show the fallibility of our reason, we need only consider a few evident examples from the history of Western philosophical argumentation, which has traditionally claimed superiority in the achievements of objective reason and logic in the universalistic and rationalistic approach to analytical and ethical argumentation. The main problem with Western philosophical argumentation has been its tendency to be blind to its own cultural biases. As a result, its argumentation remains arrogant enough to claim universality, and to disregard other cultures and their local wisdom. This is the case whether we talk about ethics, bioethics, or philosophical analysis in general. Excellent examples can be found throughout Western philosophical history from the Ancient Greek to the present day. In particular, the Enlightenment's philosophical tradition, which rhetorically preached the universality of individual rights and equality in human dignity, remained uncritical of its own logical inconsistencies based on culturally bound prejudices. In so doing, it directly undermined the very possibility of both the descriptive and normative universalism it claimed to pursue. Some of the greatest philosophical minds in the Western intellectual tradition—from John Locke to Immanuel Kant, and from David Hume to Friedrich Hegel—presented, in the name of universal reason, social and political views that are strikingly biased and culturally bound in their prejudiced, discriminatory, and repressive presumptions and communal values.

To enforce their own plausibility, these views effectively marginalized all non-Western views as primitive or pre-logical, and as based on irrational beliefs and emotions rather than on "Western" logic and "objective" reason. All in all, these culturally partial views denied the very existence of the reflective philosophical and ethical tradition anywhere outside the West—often also undermining the very humanity of non-Western people altogether, on a philosophical, intellectual, biological, and geographical basis.

We might think, for instance, of Locke's promotion of tolerance and individuals' natural rights to life, liberty, and property, which nonetheless conveniently excluded non-Western—namely non-Caucasian—people, from the scale of full humanity and denied them equal rights. Hume, the very person to warn us about the dangers of deducing "an ought" from an "is," saw no problems in classifying "the black person" (or as Hume put it "the Negro race") as naturally less civilized than the white European. And he used this fabricated, supposedly empirical generalization, as factual evidence to draw a normative conclusion that the exploitation of African and other colonies was justified. Kant, whose categorical imperative demanded that all human beings—as moral agents with moral duties—should be treated as ends in themselves and never solely as means, stated that "the Negro race" is inferior to the white race, and thus, not evidently deserving full human dignity and "moral autonomy."

Finally, Friedrich Hegel's Absolute Reason did not even recognize the existence of African or Asian cultural history. Hegel saw the end of the realization of Spirit as Absolute Reason in Enlightenment's Europe, and left no place for intellectual development outside that continent. Indeed, all places outside Europe were regarded as being without reason and, therefore, without history. They had no hope for civilization and no capacity for rational thought. Thus, in Hegel's reasoning slavery actually benefited the colonized because it provided them with at least some type of moral education. In his philosophy of history and more prominently in his *Philosophy Of Right*, the logic of reason that unfolds the Spirit is in capitalism, imperialism, and colonialism. The expansion of these is needed to universalize European ideals, and so to extend civilization to the rest of the world.[8]

From the point of view of logic and ethical reflection, these views from Western, supposedly universalistic philosophy, represent radical, culturally situated assumptions. They are also loaded with the most elementary formal and informal fallacies of reasoning, and particularly involve false generalizations concerning the issues of humanity, gender, and race. The lesson to be learned here is that when it comes to argumentation and the role of reason in their attempts to make plausible moral judgments, even philosophers of great intellectual capacity and rigor are as liable to culturally bound prejudices as anyone else. They categorize people who are less rational as less reasonable, and so as not reaching the expected standards of "intellectual capacity and moral autonomy." From such (pseudo-) "factual" categorizations, they derive normative ethical guidelines.

This is related in bioethics to Michel Foucault's discussion on "biopolitics," where "oughts" are derived from descriptive categorizations of people and their abilities. This leads to misguided moral justifications, which enforce global inequality. However, the difference between the prejudices of philosophers and those of non-philosophers is that philosophers can skillfully argue to support their cultural biases and use rhetorical means to persuade others to accept their ideas. Consequently, they have great influence on intellectual and social development, as well as on the legal and political arrangements based on their arguments. In bioethics this always creates the danger of eugenics. Seemingly objective scientific arguments are employed to justify normative judgments; facts about people's physical, mental, social, or genetic capacities are used to prove their "value of life," "their human worth," "their personhood," and so on.

For non-Western bioethics the bridge between universal reason and cultural connection is particularly relevant, since non-Western ethicists still today tend to be marginalized as cultural relativists due to their open interest in their own culture's heritage, their strong cultural identity, and their focus on culturally specific issues and cultural sets of values, in the place of attempts to find "universally" applicable guidelines to "global bioethics." Nevertheless, judging from the examples outlined above, the universalism in Western thought is still clearly a mere illusion, and philosophy in the West has never succeeded in liberating itself from its cultural and historical burdens. This it must do if it is to engage in balanced cultural dialogue on global bioethics.

6. Life and Death in a Vacuum?
Practical Context in Global Biomedical Ethics

Having looked at problems of logical inconsistency, I want next to discuss how socio-economic and cultural context may also encourage us to reconsider the validity of an argument. In other words, normative conclusions that might appear counter-intuitive to our moral sense may have unfailing logic in a different global and local setting. This is easiest to demonstrate by discussing professional medical ethics in an international context.

One of the central concerns of bioethics has been related to the interpretation of global and local values and normative guidelines, particularly when medical professionals are working across borders within different (cross-) cultural settings. The core principles of medical ethics are in general thought to have some universal applicability, so that they may protect patients' rights and maintain some shared standards of practice. These core principles are usually noted to be the following: respect for autonomy (including informed consent and confidentiality), beneficence (benefit), non-maleficence (avoidance of harm), and justice. Even if we agree with this theoretical set of fundamental bioethical principles, we are still bound to understand it within our particular cultural framework. As a result, we cannot always concur on which practical guidelines ought to determine our actions in various contexts. So, even if there were an apparent global agreement on normative principles (though with the cultural polarizations this is still a rather idealistic hypothesis), these principles themselves could not tell medical professionals what they should or should not do in certain situations, particularly without any wider understanding of culture, worldview, and local values.

Depending on our cultural backgrounds, we tend to give certain concepts different meanings. As a result, we have various interpretations of what particular values and norms may mean in various cultural as well as politico-economic settings. Even such basic concepts of bioethics as "health," "disease," and "sickness" tend to be social and cultural constructs. Their meaning may vary from one time to another, and from one place to another, according to different worldviews, belief systems, and values, and dependent on the resources available. Nevertheless, in the Western context, and in bioethics and medical ethics, it is commonly accepted that modern medicine is based upon scientific descriptions of nature and the human body. This links us back to the Foucauldian claim, discussed earlier, that Western "biopolitics" tends to use scientific knowledge to define "health" and "normality," and draws again from these descriptive premises a conclusion that presents a universal "normative" ideal of what kind of life everyone should live/have. This implies that there is universal or universalistic knowledge of health—that there is an accepted approach that applies to health problems the world over, because "objective" science delivers the objective truth.[9]

Rony Brauman, the former Director of Doctors Without Borders (Médecins Sans Frontières) has given illuminating examples of the thorny ethical dilemmas that the healthcare professional may face in an international or widely multicultural environment. These dilemmas are related to a conflict between the promotions of the best possible medical care available, while simultaneously considering the overall well-being of the patient in relation to his or her cultural beliefs. Brauman's first example comes from the war in Mogadishu, Somalia, where international medical experts were trying to help the casualties of the war, but found out that the decisions they made based on Western medical knowledge and technical diagnosis with their commitment to the four core principles of medical ethics mentioned earlier, as they are understood within the Western medical tradition, would lead to conflicts that might cause more suffering and harm to the patient. For instance, in cases in which the only solution to save a victim's life would call for an amputation (because of massive infections that could not locally be treated properly), many wounded young people would refuse the proposed procedure. They preferred to die with the body intact than to live with a visible mutation. This caused ethical dilemmas for the surgeons and other international medical team members, and indeed undermined their whole reason for being there in the first place. If a doctor cannot amputate in a war situation, his or her role as a healer is seriously diminished. The lives of some of the doctors were threatened because they were trying to convince the wounded that it was in their best interest to undergo amputation. From the point of view of Somali people, however, their best interest was not to receive such treatment. Their best interest was *not* to remain alive at any cost.

The interpretation of the meaning of the principles of respect for autonomy, beneficence, and non-maleficence were in such cases challenged by the local concepts of human dignity and well-being, and by the cultural understanding of health, injury, and "the good life." The foreign doctors could easily feel that is unethical, and so be reluctant, to respect autonomy, justifying this belief on the grounds that people in these conditions do not understand their own good, but are prisoners of some irrational cultural beliefs. This allows many to reason that since these patients are originally members of a collectivist culture with a holistic belief system, understandably they cannot be considered autonomous decision-makers in a sense that Western medical ethics requires. So, there are no real grounds to respect their wishes as manifestations of autonomous decisions, even if a principle of doing so applies in the Western context.[10]

The value of amputation in relation to health in a global context can be further discussed when we again set the issue in its Western pluralistic framework. In North America and Europe there are an increasing number of people who have now been diagnosed as suffering from a condition called Amputee Identity Disorder (AID). This is a "medical condition" in which a person voluntarily wants to receive amputation in order to feel "whole." AID sufferers can spend a lifetime wishing that a healthy arm or leg would be removed, and if they cannot find medical assistance for this problem, they may finally attempt a self-amputation or even suicide. So, for an AID sufferer to be cured, it is necessary that an otherwise physically healthy body be mutilated in order to give him or her a feeling of well-being and wholeness.

From the point of view of the medical practitioners working in Somalia—or practically anywhere—these requests for amputation would be "absurd." To many, they are basic violations of a doctor's duty to do his or her patients no harm. But the AID sufferers and their supporters argue that, for them, they are no less necessary or effective than any other amputation that is used to save a person's life. Some AID sufferers argue, for instance, that there is no difference between wanting a limb removed and wanting a shorter nose or smaller breasts. Others draw a parallel with extreme body piercing. But most say it has nothing to do with cosmetic preferences or subjective notions of beauty; instead, it is a question of identity. The analogy they draw is with gender reassignment. Sex-change patients claim that they were born in a body of the wrong gender. AID sufferers say they should have been born in the body of an amputee, and it is their right to get the treatment they need to feel "whole" and "healthy" again. Their autonomy should be respected based on their rational choice and informed consent.[11]

Another example that can shed light on the problems of cross-cultural understanding of "the principle of justice" is also taken from Brauman. The northeastern region of Karamoja in Uganda was suffering from a famine that affected about 50,000 people, but the food aid sent there was insufficient. International medical aid workers witnessed a terrible struggle for survival in the area, and established feeding stations according to the traditional approach, allocating food to the most malnourished—which were usually children under five and pregnant women. However, the food was, at the local level, taken away from the original target populations to be given to the elders of the villages. The moral value that Western medical professionals give to children and pregnant women—based not only on the fact that children and women are usually the most vulnerable, but also that children are innocent and that they are "the future"—was challenged by local customs and values. The Western doctors here again felt that the local people were uncivilized and cruel and that they did not have a proper understanding of the requirements of "the concept of justice." Logically speaking, however, there was no irrationality or inconsistency in the claim that the elders were of supreme importance because of the local values of social coherence, social authority, and decent social standards. After all, children do not yet know anything and can always be replaced, while there is no way to replace the elderly suffering from the famine.[12]

Healthcare professionals face similar situations in the cases of genital mutilation and various other practices that are in one culture considered important for a person's health and social status, and in another as dangerous and harmful. What is important in such cases is to go back to an evaluation of the facts and values involved. In the case of female genital mutilation, we need to take a wider look at the cultural arguments for the practice, the values presented in these arguments, and the actual practice and its persistence. When set in context and in relation not only to what we might think of as universal values (individual autonomy and rights) but also to local values (such as solidarity and egalitarianism in Africa, for example), we can easily find out that the practice might not promote even the local values it claims to promote. Also, we realize that such a practice, in one form or another, has in itself been quite universal and global. Many practices that Western individualists may think of as "non-Western," primitive traditions of as yet "uncivilized" cultures, are practices that have at one time or another existed in our own cultures, but with different justifications: for example, a medical rather than a social one. Various forms of genital mutilation have been defended on medical, aesthetic, hygienic, scientific, cultural, traditional, and religious grounds throughout history in most parts of the world. Different cultures just tend to rely on different justifications, thereby mixing up the issues of values and facts.[13]

That we do have different cultural understandings, interpretations, and applications of certain concepts as values need not be seen as cause for despair. While there may be no global set of bioethical values, the more we study the similarity and relevance of differing values, the better we learn to see the different situations in which we need to reconsider our own views and belief systems, and the easier it is to reach reciprocal, international understanding on the issues at stake. Such understanding addresses shared "concerns," instead of involving us in disputes over differences and conflicting values. If we return to the Ugandan example mentioned above, it is clear that had there been more resources available, the understanding of "the concept of justice" might have been very different to start with. Local circumstances and resources mold our views on what kind of ethics is most pragmatic and applicable. Not only our cultural beliefs but also changes in social, political, and economic circumstances, as well as the availability of resources, all affect our interpretations of particular values and norms. If we are looking for a global bioethics we need to examine all of these issues from their various sides, instead of settling with false polarizations and hasty generalizations. Only then will we be able to come up with more realistic and more applicable international agreements, which take into account not only the different worldviews and belief systems that people hold, but also the politico-economic realities related to the local and global distribution and allocation of resources.

7. Conclusion

Trying to understand the context of argumentation beyond our own cultural boundaries helps us to use logical analysis, as well as critical and self-critical inquiry, more efficiently. We can avoid fallacies by mapping out particular cultural presuppositions, biases, and other obstacles in our reasoning, and by recognize the inconsistencies that follow from these. Therefore, I suggest that rather than searching for "global and local bioethics," we should examine the global and local plausibility of ethical reflection. Instead of debating the universality or cultural confinement of our theoretical frameworks, we need to pay more attention to the universality of the mistakes of our reason, and to study how these errors of reasoning are related to our cultural presumptions and local beliefs. We also need to make a serious attempt to differentiate between values and facts when engaging in cross-cultural argumentation on bioethical issues.

NOTES

1. On contemporary bioethics see Matti Häyry and Tuija Takala, "What is Bioethics All About?" *Scratching the Surface of Bioethics*, eds. Matti Häyry and Tuija Takala (Amsterdam and New York: Rodopi, 2003), pp. 1–7.

2. See e.g. Seyla Benhabib. *The Claims of Culture, Equality and Diversity in the Global Era* (Princeton and Oxford: Princeton University Press 2002); Donna Dickenson, Sirkku Hellsten and Heather Widdows "Global Bioethics," *New Review in Bioethics* 1:1 (2003), Sirkku Hellsten, "Multicultural Issues and Human Rights in Maternal-Fetal Medicine," *Ethical Issues in Maternal-Fetal Medicine*, ed. Donna Dickenson (Cambridge: Cambridge University Press, 2002), pp. 39–60.

3. M. Cheng, K. K. Wong, and W. W. Yang, "Critical Care Ethics in Hong Kong: Cross-Cultural Conflicts as East Meets West," *Journal of Medicine and Philosophy*, 23:6 (1998), pp. 616–627 *Japanese and Western Bioethics: Studies in Moral Diversity*, ed. Kazumasa Hoshino (Dordrecht: Kluwer, 1997).

4. *Japanese and Western Bioethics*, ed. Hoshino; Godfrey B. Tangwa, "Genetic Information: Questions and Worries from an African Background," *Genetic*

Information: Acquisition, Access and Control, eds. Alison K. Thompson and Ruth Chadwick (New York: Kluwer Academic/Plenum Publishers, 1999); Hellsten, "Multicultural Issues and Human Rights in Maternal-Fetal Medicine."

5. *Enthymema* refers to implicit or unannounced premises as defined in Aristotle's argumentation theory. Aristotle, *Rhetoric*, *The Complete Works of Aristotle*, ed. Jonathan Barnes, (Princeton: Princeton University Press, 1985).

6. Anne Thomson, *Critical Reasoning in Ethics* (London and New York: Routledge 1999), pp. 5–8.

7. See *ibid.*, pp. 5–32; and Nina Rosenstand and Anita Silvers, "Moral, Legal and Aesthetic Reasoning," *Critical Thinking*, eds. Brooke Noel Moore and Richard Parker (London, Mayfield 1998), pp. 418–433.

8. *Race and Enlightenment: A Reader*, ed. Emmanuel Chukwudi Eze (Oxford: Blackwell 1997), pp. 3–9; Kant quoted in *ibid.*, pp. 38–69.

9. Michel Foucault, *Madness and Civilization: A History of Insanity in the Age of Reason* (New York: Vintage Books, 1965); and Michel Foucault, *The Birth of the Clinic: Archaeology of Medical Perception* (New York: Random House, 1973); Rony Brauman "Questioning Health and Human Rights," *Human Rights Dialogue*, 2:6 (2005), http:// www.cceia.org/resources/publications/dialogue/2_06/articles/643.html (accessed 8 January 2007); and Rony Brauman "Controversies within Health and Human Rights," Carnegie Council transcript (14 February 2001), http://www.cceia.org/resources/transcripts/93.html (accessed 8 January 2007).

10. See *ibid.* For the main "universal" principles of biomedical ethics see Tom Beauchamp and James Childress, *Principles of Biomedical Ethics* (New York: Oxford University Press, 5th ed., 2001).

11. Decca Aitkenhead, "And If Thy Hand Offend Thee, Cut it off," *The Sunday Telegraph Magazine*, 25 January 2004, pp. 30–35; Tim Bayne and Neil Levy, "Amputees By Choice: Body Integrity Identity Disorder and the Ethics of Amputation," *Journal of Applied Philosophy*, 22:1 (March 2005), pp. 75–81; Steven C. Schlozman, "Upper-extremity Self-amputation and Replantation: 2 Case Reports and a Review of the Literature," *Journal of Clinical Psychiatry*, 59:12 (December 1998), pp. 681–686.

12. Rony Brauman, "Controversies within Health and Human Rights."

13. See Hellsten, "Multicultural Issues and Human Rights," *Ethical Issues in Maternal-Fetal Medicine*, pp. 39–60; and Sirkku Hellsten, "Rationalizing Circumcision: From Tradition to Fashion, From Public Health to Individual Freedom," *Journal of Medical Ethics*, 30:3 (June 2004), pp. 248–253.

Two

IS BIOETHICS ONLY FOR THE RICH AND POWERFUL?

Søren Holm

The offer obviously hasn't been tempting enough, for Olga has turned it down. Perhaps if Amos had been able to suggest a meal he would have been more likely to succeed, for Sergio tells me he's spotted her pinching the greasy, tasteless cheese sandwiches left in the canteen each night in the vain hope that someone will be desperate enough to eat them. She's been slipping them into her bag to eat during the day. Presumably, she's surviving mainly on two o'clock chips and stew. Sergio's revelation doesn't surprise me, for Olga certainly isn't the first. I've been reading through the supervisor's notebook in the few idle moments I can catch alone in the cleaning store. This records any incident during the night, so the Casna managers can catch up on what's been going on. One entry from last year reads: "Ibrahim had his bag searched by security and they found a banana and some uncooked fish. He was told not to come back here again."[1]

1. Introduction

The question I have raised in the title is clearly much too large to answer in a single chapter, but I hope that it has caught your eye and that you are willing to read a little further to get a partial answer.

What I want to consider here is one aspect of how bioethics deals with the fact that wealth and power are unequally divided in the world, and in most if not all nation states. Is bioethics serving the interests of the rich or of the poor? This paper focuses mostly on the effects of wealth differentials, but it is crucial not to forget that wealth and power tend to go together both at the individual and at the group level, if for no other reason than because you can buy power with wealth in all societies, even those without direct corruption. In every society the rich and the poor live together in one sense, but in another sense they inhabit two very different worlds, as the initial quotation by the English journalist Fran Abrams illustrates. It is not only in low income countries that people struggle to find the money for their next meal, even when they have work.[2]

Being poor means that you are likely to accept offers that people who are not poor would not accept, and this raises the issue of whether being poor leaves you open to exploitation, whether we can say that poverty coerces and that this in general makes exchanges between the poor and the rich suspect. In bioethics the answer to this question has implications in research ethics, transplant ethics, reproductive ethics, and healthcare resource allocation.

In the first part of the chapter I will present a general analysis of coercion, whereas the second part will focus on the degree to which poverty can rightly be said to coerce.

The reason for choosing coercion and not exploitation as the central concept here is that there are people (ultra-libertarians) who deny that exploitation is wrong in itself, but who accept that some forms of coercion are wrong. To engage with their arguments I have to pursue the argument in terms of coercion. I believe that the same general line of argument works for exploitation as well, but will in the interest of brevity not pursue it here.

2. A General Analysis of Coercion

> The necessity is imposed by the agent when someone is forced by some agent, so that he is not able to do the contrary. This is called the necessity of coercion. Now this necessity of coercion is altogether repugnant to the will.[3]

One branch of the literature on the concept of coercion proceeds from a legal point of view because coercion, compulsion, or duress are recognized as legal defenses both in criminal and in civil law. The pertinent questions have therefore been:

> In what circumstances can somebody rightfully claim that he or she was coerced into doing a specific act, and thereby be excused from legal liability?

And:

> In what circumstances is it legal to exercise coercion against others?

Another branch of the literature has attacked the problem from the perspective of political theory and has asked grand questions like: Is the relationship between employer and employee necessarily coercive?

The purpose of this section of the chapter is more modest. I want first to sketch a general theory of inter-personal coercion, with specific reference to the field of healthcare. The analysis will therefore focus on the way in which coercion functions in relationships between persons. It will be neither a legal nor a sociological or political analysis, and it will not try to delimit the exact class of acts of coercion which ought to be legally forbidden or sanctioned. Moral wrongness and legal prohibition cannot always be matched precisely. There may be good reasons for not making laws against all acts which are morally wrong, but when this situation occurs it is important to remember that such acts are still wrong, they are just not illegal.

The theory developed here will be non-moralized in the sense that it will claim that calling some act an act of coercion is neither necessary nor sufficient to show that the act is morally wrong, all things considered. It only creates a *prima facie* assumption against the act.

The subject of coercion has a long philosophical history, as the quotation from St. Thomas Aquinas at the beginning of this section shows. It has been discussed by many of the great philosophers, and has been analyzed from many points of view. It is almost a platitude to say that the concept of coercion has fuzzy borders, since that is true of most important concepts in ethics, but in this case it is not an irrelevant platitude because the borders are fuzzier than most.

Coercion belongs to a cluster of overlapping concepts including compulsion, constraint, and duress. We could try to unravel the intricate differences within this cluster, but I think it would just be an unfruitful exercise in philosophical craftsmanship, so in the following I will use the word "coercion" to stand for this whole cluster of closely related concepts. Linguistically this will prevent me from conforming to the rule that a good writer will not use the same word for the same concept too often, since for clarity I think it is best to use only one word. A more serious philosophical problem is caused by the fact that we will have to make a distinction between coercion and other concepts like incentive, offer, and persuasion. We all know the mafia man in American movies who approaches the victim and says: "I'll give you an offer you cannot refuse." Is this coercion, incentive, or just persuasion?

The instances of coercion which are of interest here, are those instances where one person coerces another into performing or refraining from some act (interpersonal coercion). There is no doubt that nature can also coerce, for instance "the snowstorm left me no choice but to stay inside the house," but in the bioethics context interpersonal coercion is by far the most important type from the moral point of view, so my analysis will not include instances of coercion by nature.

The purpose of interpersonal coercion is, as stated above, to get somebody to do something he or she would not otherwise have done, but this is a feature which coercion shares with all of the other concepts mentioned above. When I offer you my extra ticket for the Saturday football game, it is because I want you to accompany me to the game, instead of doing what you had previously intended to do on Saturday afternoon. When I persuade you that a

Mercedes is really a better choice than a Lexus by showing you that the resale price of a Mercedes is much better than that of a Lexus, I also change your actions. And when I convince you that the act you are about to perform is morally wrong, I may also get you to act differently (if you do not suffer from weakness of will). If we want to distinguish coercion from offers, incentives, and persuasion we therefore need to look more closely at the way in which the coercer tries to change the action space of the coerced.

Let us look at the case of persuasion first, because it is in many ways the simplest. When I attempt to persuade people to do something, I usually point to some already existing features in the world which, if they were aware of them, would make them change their course of action. These features of the world may be in the external world (like the resale prices of cars), or in the internal mental world of the person in question (like an interest in football).

I might say, that given that you have a strong motivation of type X, you should be able to see that doing Y now is a contradiction of this motivation. Although I may very well want the person to do a specific thing, and although I may be very selective in the choice of facts to which I draw attention (that is, I may try to deceive the person), I do not try to change or alter the state of the external world, or the basic underlying motivations of the person I am persuading. This is, for instance, why moral persuasion generally only works with moral people. The question of incentives and offers is more difficult and is treated below.

Interpersonal coercion can take two different forms (here outlined for the prevention of acts, but similar definitions could be put forward for the induction of acts). The coercer C can physically prevent the coerced V from doing the act in question, for instance by putting V in a strait jacket. Let us call this physical coercion. Alternatively, C can coerce V by letting V know that C will perform some act CA, if V performs the act VA. Let us call this psychological coercion.

Whereas in physical coercion it is literally the case that I could not do otherwise, in psychological coercion there is always a possibility that I could act differently, and assessing a psychological coercion claim is therefore more difficult than assessing a physical coercion claim. Just pointing out that I chose to perform the act in question does not show that coercion was not present. In many circumstances it shows the reverse, that the coercion was successful.

In both types of case, coercion can only occur if there is some relationship and some communication between the coercer and the coerced, since C in both instances has either to interact physically with V or to communicate his or her intentions to V. If V is not aware that C wants to coerce him or her, psychological coercion cannot take place.

The act CA which C threatens to perform, must be an act which V perceives as threatening his or her welfare. In order for C to coerce V it is therefore necessary that C has, or at least is believed by V to have, some kind of power over things or circumstances that are of importance to V.

In physical coercion C has the power to control V's movements or physical environment, whereas in psychological coercion the power used could be of many different kinds. The power to control which C has, does not necessarily have to be used; often the mere threat of using the power may be sufficient. In the healthcare context it would often be a power to deprive V of something which has crucial importance for his fulfillment of basic biological, psychological, or social needs.

We have seen above that threats to deprive somebody of the means to attain the fulfillment of a basic need can be coercive, but what about offers? Can an offer to make somebody better off than he or she is now ever be coercive? Normally we do not take offers as coercive, even though they may change people's actions. If I offer you a job with twice your present salary, I have not coerced you if you accept the offer, although I have changed the way in which you would have acted, had I not presented the offer.

Our intuitions may however be different if we look at offers presented to persons in more difficult situations. What would we say, for instance, if I offered an Indian day laborer 5,000 British pounds for one of his or her kidneys, or perhaps even more problematically, 50,000 British pounds for his or her heart? In both situations it could be rational for him or her to accept, because he or she could secure the future well-being of his or her family with the money gained in the transaction. But would this not be a case of a coercive offer?

I think such an offer is coercive, and that its coercive nature stems from the combination of the offer and the condition of severe material deprivation in which the Indian day laborer finds him- or herself. What makes the offer coercive is, paradoxically, that it is an offer he or she ought to accept, but only because he or she is in a situation no human being ought to be in. Or to put it more formally, an offer is a coercive offer if

(1) the recipient of the offer is in a severely materially or socially deprived situation;
(2) this situation is not a situation in which the recipient ought to be on account of his or her own wrongdoing; and
(3) the giver of the offer is aware of (1) and intends to use the situation to his or her own advantage.

In the following I will assume that most poor people are not poor on account of their own wrongdoing, and will therefore not mention this qualification in the discussion. It is, however, important to note that those who are poor because of somebody else's wrongdoing cannot be held responsible for this, unless they are strongly implicated in giving those other people their power to do wrong. We cannot visit the sins of the parents on their children, or of dictators or despots on their citizens.

This would mean that an offer does not become coercive just because it has abnormal potency in a situation. If I offer a job to somebody, knowing that this is the job he or she has dreamt of all his or her life, I have not coerced him or her into taking the job, although the offer has an abnormal potency in this situation.

An alternative explanation of our different intuitions about the two offers could be that whereas accepting the job offer does not harm me, the Indian day laborer is harmed in some sense by accepting the offer because it involves physical harm to his body. That would imply that the offer is wrong, not by being coercive but by being harmful. But consider the following example. I offer the job, knowing (1) that your partner has a good job which he or she will not leave, and (2) that you will have to move if you accept the job. If you accept the job, as you probably will because it is the job you have always dreamt about, then you have been harmed, because you and your partner will have to live apart from each other. Does that make the offer wrong in some sense? Perhaps, but even if the psychological harm is of the same magnitude as the physical harm in the transplant case, few would think that the two offers are equally bad. This residue seems to be explicable only by the coercive element of the transplant case, and that can only be fully understood in terms of the background conditions of material deprivation.

A similar view on coercive offers is presented by Robert Nozick in his seminal article "Coercion,"[4] and has recently been defended in a modified form by Alan Wertheimer.[5] Nozick's basic idea is that the feature that makes some offers coercive is that the situation in which the person given the offer finds himself departs from what could normally be expected. The problem that Nozick recognizes is that "what could normally be expected" can be understood in two quite different ways. It can be understood either as an empirical statement about the normal development of a state of affairs in a given society, or as a normative statement describing what the person in question is morally justified in expecting. Nozick himself prefers the moral interpretation, but delivers a counter-example which he thinks shows that the empirical interpretation must be used from time to time. In Wertheimer's version this example runs as follows:

> *The Drug Case.* A is B's normal supplier of illegal drugs for \$20 per day. One day, A proposes to B that he will supply B's drugs if and only if B beats up C.[5]

Nozick believes that his idea of a moral baseline cannot show coercion to be present in this case, but since he believes that the situation is coercive he proposes to use the baseline which the person in question (B) would like to see used. Wertheimer rejects Nozick's claim that the choice of baseline is to be decided by the person receiving the offer and expands the number of possible baselines to 3:

- The statistical (what is normal in a given society)
- The moral (what morality requires)
- The phenomenological (what the person in question expects)

He further claims that there is no right answer to which baseline one ought to choose, and that each baseline gives rise to a coercion claim with a specific moral force. And he maintains that offers are only coercive if they involve a threat to make somebody worse off than he currently is in respect to one of these baselines.

I think that this is a mistake. In the Indian day laborer case discussed above, there is little doubt that he or she is actually not worse off with respect to any of these baselines after having received the offer. The offer is normal in the society in question (although the practice is illegal in India), he or she has no moral right to expect that this particular person is going to help him or her, and before the offer was given he or she could not expect any help, since he or she did not know the person giving the offer. Nevertheless, the offer must be considered as coercive. This can only be achieved by a theory which accepts that some cases of severe material or social deprivation may make any offer coercive, if the intention is to exploit the deprived condition of the person. Instead of looking at the interpersonal moral situation, we will have to cast our eyes wider and look at the systemic moral situation, where morality may well require that no one should ever be left in the situation that leaves them open to this kind of coercive offer.

The purpose of the analysis so far has been to reach an understanding of the concept of coercion and its defining components, but this still leaves one problem unsolved: namely, the question of whether the fact that an act is an act of coercion is sufficient in itself to show that the act is morally reprehensible.

I will assume that all acts of coercion are *prima facie* wrong since that is part of the normal connotation of the term "coercion," and that all acts of coercion therefore require a prior ethical analysis and justification. It is, however, obvious that not all acts of coercion are morally wrong, all things considered. A father who prevents his four year old son from running out on the main road during rush hour by grapping his arm is performing a paradigmatic act of physical coercion, but it is justified coercion, and we would actually hold the father morally culpable if he had refrained from using coercion. I also think that we would believe the father equally justified if he could have achieved the same aim by psychological coercion, for instance by shouting "If you do not stay here you will not get the ice-cream I promised you!"

The exact circumstances in which coercion can be justified in the case of competent persons are a subject of heated debate, and I will not try to present a solution to this question. It is however important to point out that it is generally accepted by almost all participants in this debate that a necessary, but not sufficient, component in the justification of coercion is that the action must either be beneficial for the person in question, or it must avert harm to others. Without this component coercion cannot be justified (for a thorough review of the literature and a defense of the view that beneficence is never a sufficient reason for coercion, see Heta Häyry, *The Limits of Medical Paternalism*[6]).

3. Can Poverty Coerce?

We can now return to the question of whether poverty can coerce. It is obvious that poverty in itself cannot coerce, because poverty as a state of material deprivation does not try to make people do anything specific, or impose any specific restrictions on them. But poverty means that some people are left in a state where some kinds of offers have added potency. This is especially true if the poverty is so severe that a person has difficulty in securing basic survival needs like food and shelter. If I am going to die, or if I am not going to eat today if I do not take up your offer, I am in a state where I am likely to accept offers I would not have accepted if I had other ways of fulfilling my basic needs.

This much is accepted on all sides of the debate, but it is often denied that it is enough to show that poverty coerces. In an op-ed piece for the British newspaper *The Guardian* on a market in organs, John Harris for instance writes:

> Some people say such a market would exploit the poor. First, it is hypocritical to think that denying poor people an opportunity to sell one of their few saleable assets is doing them any favours, at least so long as no attempt is made to alleviate their poverty in other ways. No one is exploited by an offer of money simply because they do something for pay which they would not otherwise do. I am sure I am not the only *Guardian* reader who would be unlikely to go to work if I was not paid for what I do![7]

Now, I would not for a moment want to claim that Manchester University exploits John Harris by employing him, and he is truly right that no one is exploited by an offer (that is, an offer that is not a coercive offer) simply because they do something for pay which they would not otherwise do. But I submit that Harris's analogy between his situation and the situation of the poor in regard to such offers is severely flawed.

If you are hungry, or will go hungry if you do not get work today, and I offer you a job at very low pay, knowing that that is your situation and that you will have to take it (and save me paying decent wages to someone who is not below the breadline), your choice situation is very different from the one Professor Harris is in when wondering whether to continue working for Manchester University, going somewhere else, or taking early retirement. Some of these choices would make him economically worse off, but none would leave him wondering where his next meal would come from. We have to keep in mind that the situation concerning dietary choice described in the following 1930s poem by Scottish socialist poet Joe Corrie still prevails for some in the so-called affluent West:

> "Eat more fruit!" the slogans say,
> "More fish, more beef, more bread!"
> But I'm on Unemployment pay
> My third year now, and wed.
>
> And so I wonder when I'll see
> The slogan when I pass,
> The only one that would suit me,—
> "Eat More Bloody Grass!"

But, could it not be claimed that as long as exchanges with the poor are mutually beneficial, they cannot be coercive? Again we have a situation where the fact that an exchange is mutually beneficial counts against it being coercive, but it does not rule out coercion. How can offers of a mutually beneficial exchange be coercive in this way (if we make sure that they are not re-described threats)? Well, they can if they exploit a vulnerability to accept such offers which is induced by an unjust social system, of which I who give the offer am a beneficiary. If you are in a situation you should not be in as a matter of justice, some of the offers you receive can rightly be labeled as unjust and coercive even if they are offers it would be rational for you to accept.

4. Serial Coercion and Extreme Poverty

Is there a further problem in focusing on one-off transactions between the rich and the poor, as much of the literature tends to do? Is it enough to be able to say that each transaction is mutually beneficial? Well, there might be a problem, because when we look at each transaction it is easy to forget that whereas it may leave the poor party to the exchange better off for the moment, in many cases this is only very temporarily. One of the common features of a life in poverty is that it is almost impossible to save and make yourself permanently better off. The poor are and remain poor, partly because their daily mutually beneficial exchanges with their employers do not add up to any other long-term benefit than being able to stay alive. It is, for instance, amply documented that it is impossible to live on the minimum wage in many parts of the UK and the USA, and totally impossible to save up for future contingencies or a better life.[8] This means that the poor can be serially exploited. I can exploit them today, and confidently expect them to be back in the same situation of exploitability tomorrow (through no fault of their own). It is also worth noting that when the poor have to borrow money, for instance when they are between two jobs, or if there is some emergency, they can usually only borrow money at rates far higher than the rates offered to the rich. This clearly adds to their serial exploitability.

The situation of the poor is therefore different from some of the analogies employed in the literature. You can, for instance, only serially exploit my desire for a better job by offering me better conditions each time you try to exploit this weakness in me. The employer, the buyer of blood plasma, or the contract research firm does not have to offer anything more each time they exploit the economic weakness of the poor, because the poor will be back at their *status quo ante* simply in virtue of having to buy necessities to stay alive. Only mutually beneficial exchanges of a size that give the poor a realistic chance of moving out of poverty can reasonably be analyzed in isolation as one-off transactions.

We are now in a situation where we can introduce a distinction between poverty and extreme poverty, where extreme poverty is characterized by two features in addition to the features of poverty itself: (1) an inability to satisfy basic needs for food and shelter on the income you have; and (2) an inability to save and thereby move out of poverty, because all income is used on basic needs or on servicing previously incurred debts.

We may deny that poverty coerces without denying that extreme poverty coerces. In extreme poverty it is not the case that you cannot get your wants satisfied; it is the case that you have no legitimate way of satisfying basic, organic survival needs. If you want to go on living you have to do something.

5. What Follows from a Denial of the Coercive Power of Poverty?

What are the philosophical consequences of denying that extreme poverty can coerce? Immediately the consequences may seem quite liberating and positive. By denying that extreme poverty can coerce we can remove one of the most powerful arguments in favor of prohibiting organ sales, commercial surrogacy, and economic incentives for research participation, and if we can have these prohibitions repealed, we can presumably save many lives through increased organ procurement and faster medical research.

But, unfortunately, there are also other consequences. If poverty does not coerce, and the poor therefore need no special protection against coercion, we also lose the best and most powerful arguments for a range of presumably beneficial legal rules, such as rules enforcing a minimum wage, minimum working standards, minimum building standards, compulsory education, and many other similar rules. For many of these it will be the case that they prevent some of the extremely poor from getting a job or a place to live, whereas they could get one in a free market and be allegedly "better off."

This is clearly a welcome result for the libertarian, but for those of us who think that there is more to morality than the maximization or protection of liberty, it should be an incredibly worrying result. If all we can establish in the welfare arena are negative rights, rights not to be directly harmed against your will (risk of harm that you accept as part of a mutually beneficial exchange cannot be regulated against on this line of argument), there is no way of preventing the poor, weak, and powerless from being comprehensively exploited "for their own benefit," and left to slide even deeper into poverty. Negative rights are simply not sufficient to protect them, and there is no reason to believe that charity will ever make up what we give up by abandoning positive welfare rights.

6. Can We Fall Back on Justice?

But can we not fall back on our theory of justice? Can we not say that what we should really do is remove the cause of poverty, the unequal and unfair distribution of wealth and power, instead of focusing on some of the effects of the current distribution (that is the potentially coercive exchanges)? I fully agree that we should strive to remove the causes of poverty, and the systemic injustice plaguing our society, but the argument put forward is that that is the only thing we should do, that we should not strive to remove the current local effects of poverty.

This is a popular argument in the debates about a market in organs and incentives in research. Michael Gill and Robert Sade for instance write:

> Moreover, if kidney sales are wrong because, like the other indignities poor people have to suffer, they are a symptom of a fundamentally immoral capitalist system, then it seems the appropriate response is to work for a redistribution of wealth and a change in the means of production. From the anti-capitalist perspective, opposing kidney sales (which could provide rapid financial opportunity for some poor people) while blithely

> acquiescing to the rest of the system appears to be unhelpful at best and hypocritical at worst.[9]

Is this a good argument, apart from its rather tendentious linking of resistance to kidney sales with anti-capitalism, and by implication that great American bugbear socialism? No, it is not. It sets up a false dichotomy between concerns about justice at the general level, and concerns about justice in specific practices. It is not impossible both to oppose unfair specific practices, and to oppose injustice in general. Now, if Gill and Sade had good reasons for the belief that justice is going to prevail imminently, and that the problem of poverty will be solved, then we could start talking about how to organize society in that radically new situation. But unfortunately they present us with no such reasons.

Julian Savulescu, also writing in the context of the sale of organs, is as usual more forthright:

> Secondly, people need to be fully informed and to give their consent freely. By "freely," I mean that they are not in a situation which is itself wrong or unacceptable. Poverty which is acceptable to a society should not be a circumstance which prevents a person taking on a risk or harm to escape that poverty. It is a double injustice to say to a poor person: "You can't have what most other people have and we are not going to let you do what you want to have those things."[10]

Here the level of poverty that is ethically acceptable quickly gets elided with the level of poverty that is acceptable to a society, and considerations of justice thereby into mere matters of convention and expediency (unless Savulescu has some normative construction of "acceptable to a society" to offer). But on most conceptions of justice, most affluent societies accept levels of poverty that are not ethically acceptable (I make this claim out in more detail in my forthcoming Oxford University Press book *Bioethics in an Unjust World*). What should we do in that situation? Should we continue to exploit the fact that some people are in a situation which is itself wrong and unacceptable, or should we try to stop the exploitation at the same time as we try to remove the injustice?

We might also note in passing that it is unclear whether sale of a kidney really generates enough money to allow a person to escape from poverty (see for instance Madhav Goyal *et al.*[11]). Those who sell vital organs will clearly escape from their poverty, but this is presumably not the sense of escape intended by Savulescu.

What Savulescu might have in mind is perhaps not an ethical argument, but a political consistency argument. If a society accepts or allows a specific level of poverty, and the attendant possibilities for exploitation of the poor, it would be politically inconsistent to single out some exploitative practices for prohibition while allowing others. This could possibly even be claimed to be unjust in a formal sense of not treating equal cases equally. However, if that is the correct understanding of Savulescu's argument, he owes us an explanation of why the formal concept of justice should be allowed to override a substantive concept of justice. Why should we allow (and philosophically justify) leveling down, when the ethically right thing to work for is leveling up? The society Savulescu describes is hypocritical in accepting levels of poverty that should not be accepted, but that hypocrisy is not resolved by his preferred solution. It is, to put it mildly, unclear how allowing the rich to exploit the poor more comprehensively can be said to contribute to a better and more just society. All it will do is to allow the rich to buy more services at prices below their fair price (the price they would have in a society with no more than ethically acceptable or just levels of poverty), and thereby allow them to be able to consume more than they would in a just society.

7. Is There any Hope for Bioethics?

At this point in the argument the non-philosophically trained reader may want to scream "Get real guys! Of course poverty coerces, and that is one of the bad things about being poor—you have to do more of the things you do not want to do than other people, and to do more of the things you really do not want to do." Before bioethics finds a way to accommodate that insight it will continue to be an occupation for the upper-middle-class academic, serving the interests of the really rich and powerful.

NOTES

1. Fran Abrams, *Below the Breadline: Living on the Minimum Wage* (London: Profile Books, 2002), p. 45.

2. *Ibid.*; Barbara Ehrenreich, *Nickeled and Dimed: Undercover in Low Wage USA* (New York: Granta, 2002); Polly Toynbee, *Hard Work: Life in Low-Pay Britain* (London: Bloomsbury, 2003).

3. St. Thomas Aquinas, "Summa Theologica, Question LXXXII," *Philosophy in the Middle Age*, eds. Arthur Hyman and James J. Walsh (Indianapolis, University of Indiana Press, 2nd ed., 1988), p. 547.

4. Robert Nozick, "Cocrcion," *Philosophy, Science, and Method: Essays in Honor of Ernest Nagel*, eds. Sidney Morgenbesser, Patrick Suppes, and Morton White (New York, St. Martins Press, 1969), pp. 440–472.

5. Alan Wertheimer, *Coercion* (Princeton, Princeton University Press, 1987), p. 209.

6. Heta Häyry, *The Limits of Medical Paternalism* (London, Routledge, 1991).

7. John Harris, "This Won't Hurt... Your Bank Balance. Short of Cash and in Possession of Two Kidneys? Philosopher John Harris Thinks You Should be Able to Sell One of them to the NHS—and the Medical Establishment is Taking him Seriously," *The Guardian*, 3 December 2003.

8. Abrams, *Below the Breadline*; and Ehrenreich, *Nickeled and Dimed.*

9. Michael M. Gill and Robert M. Sade, "Payment for Kidneys: The Case for Repealing Prohibition," *Kennedy Institute of Ethics Journal* 12:1 (2002), pp.17–46, at p. 22.

10. Julian Savulescu, "Is the Sale of Body Parts Wrong?" *Journal of Medical Ethics* 29 (2003), pp. 138–139, at p. 139.

11. Madhav Goyal, Ravindra L. Mehta, Lawrence J. Schneiderman, and Ashwini R. Sehgal, "Economic and Health Consequences of Selling a Kidney in India," *Journal of the American Medical Association* 288:13 (2002), pp. 1589–1593.

Three

DO WE NEED (BIO)ETHICAL PRINCIPLES?

Simona Giordano

1. Introduction

A large part of contemporary bioethics rotates around (bio)ethical principles, such as human dignity, promotion of equality, respect for autonomy, justice, freedom, integrity, and so on. As Joseph Raz notes, there is something inherently good and fashionable in ethical principles.[1] They attract wide consensus. They are often considered helpful instruments in the resolution of ethical dilemmas that arise in practice. Bioethicists generally employ them in support of their views. Public bodies, like the European parliament, also use them to decide on the ethical legitimacy of biotechnology and advances in medicine and science, and to set policies in response to developments in biotechnology. In addition to this, some may believe that (bio)ethical principles can remind us of the common substrate of ethical values that we apparently share.

In the first part of this chapter I argue that (bio)ethical principles are useless as instruments to direct practice; they do not create a common morality, they do not harmonize different views, and they do not express a common substrate of moral values. On the contrary, they express the variety of views and ethical conflicts. I will employ the example of cloning to illustrate the inability of ethical principles to contribute to the solutions of ethical dilemmas.

After having discussed this point, I will consider two other problems relating to the use of (bio)ethical principles:

- Ethicists and policy-makers sometimes present these principles as "intuitive truths" and self-evident concepts. However, they offer no explanation either for the principles themselves or for the way they are applied to individual cases. The result is that the general public is told what is right and wrong, without any explanation of why it is right or wrong. The risk is to leave the general public uninformed, and to reinforce common prejudices.
- (Bio)ethical principles are instruments of judgment, and leave no room for understanding and compassion. (Bio)ethical principles are supposed to promote "tolerance" but in fact they do not, as they do not tolerate exceptions to the rule. Because they do not admit consid-

> eration of the peculiar aspects of each individual situation, commitment to them may, and frequently does, harm people.

The next section shows the positive functions that are ascribed to (bio)ethical principles.

2. The Alleged Importance of (Bio)Ethical Principles

Contemporary bioethics values (bio)ethical principles very highly. (Bio)ethical principles are thought to discharge the following functions:

- Harmonization of different socio-cultural and religious traditions;
- creation of common values;
- solidarity;
- subsidiarity and tolerance;
- peaceful dialogue;
- respect for self-determination;
- consensus;
- derivation of solutions to ethically controversial cases.[2]

John Harris also argues that (bio)ethical principles can act as statements of commitment to some values, and provide ways in which a society can remind itself of its basic beliefs.[3] These principles also on occasion direct legislation. Cloning offers one example of how ethicists and jurists sometimes use (bio)ethical principles to resolve ethical dilemmas and to frame legislation.

3. Ethical Principles in Practice—The Case of Cloning

Immediately after the journal *Nature* released the news of the birth of Dolly the sheep (27 February 1997), the world's first cloned mammal, many institutions and organizations condemned any application of the procedure to human reproduction,[4] on the grounds that human cloning would violate fundamental human rights, such as human dignity, personal integrity, and identity.

Below, I report some pronouncements against cloning. The reason why cloning is prohibited is that it is thought to violate universal ethical principles and human rights.

4. Pronouncements Against Cloning

According to the European Parliament's Resolution on Cloning:

> Preamble, Paragraph B: ... the cloning of human beings, whether experimentally, in the context of fertility treatment, preimplantation diagnosis, tissue transplantation, or for any other purpose whatsoever, cannot under any circumstances be justified or tolerated by any society, because it is a *serious violation of fundamental human rights and is contrary to the principle of equality of human beings* as it permits a eugenic and racist selection of the human race, it *offends against human dignity* and it requires experimentation on humans [my emphases].
>
> Paragraph 8: ... the direct protection of the dignity and rights of individuals is of absolute priority as compared with any social or third-party interest.[5]

Here the implication seems to be that cloning would violate the dignity and rights of individuals. In several other points this document stresses or suggests that human cloning, in whatever form and for whatever purposes (presumably, also therapeutic purposes) is unethical because it violates human rights and ethical principles: namely, those of equality and dignity.

The Additional Protocol to the Convention for the Protection of Human Rights and Dignity of the Human Being with regard to the Application of Biology and Medicine, on the Prohibition of Cloning Human Beings (Paris, 12 January 1998) states:

> The member States of the Council of Europe, the other States and the European Community Signatories to this Additional Protocol to the Convention for the Protection of Human Rights and Dignity of the Human Being with regard to the Application of Biology and Medicine ....
>
> Considering ...that the *instrumentalisation of human beings through the deliberate creation of genetically identical human beings is contrary to human dignity and thus constitutes a misuse of biology and medicine*;
>
> Considering also the serious difficulties of a medical, psychological, and social nature that such a deliberate biomedical practice might imply for all the individuals involved;
>
> Considering the purpose of the Convention on Human Rights and Biomedicine, in particular the principle mentioned in Article 1 aiming to protect the dignity and identity of all human beings,

> Have agreed as follows:
>
> Article 1
>
> 1. Any intervention seeking to create a human being genetically identical to another human being, whether living or dead, is prohibited.[6]

And according to the Charter of Fundamental Rights of the European Union (2000):

> Article 3
>
> Right to the integrity of the person
>
> 2. In the fields of medicine and biology, the following must be respected in particular:
>
> ... the prohibition of the reproductive cloning of human beings.[7]

According to the Charter of Fundamental Rights of the EU, cloning involves a violation of an ethical principle: the individual's right to integrity, and this is why the European Parliament deems it unethical.

According to the Opinion of the Group of Advisers on the Ethical Implications of Biotechnology to the European Commission (No. 9), human cloning is ethically unacceptable for reasons relating to instrumentalization and eugenics (paragraph 2.6).[8]

The UNESCO Universal Declaration on the Human Genome and Human Rights (1997) states:

> Article 11
> Practices which are *contrary to human dignity, such as reproductive cloning* of human beings, shall not be permitted [my emphasis].[9]

UK legislation on cloning is coherent with the above declarations. The Government Response to the Recommendations Made in the Chief Medical Officer's Expert Group Report "Stem Cell Research: Medical Progress with Responsibility" reads:

> Recommendation 7. The transfer of an embryo created by cell nuclear replacement into the uterus of a woman (so called "reproductive cloning") should remain a criminal offence.

> 9. The Government has made its position on reproductive cloning absolutely clear on a number of occasions. On 26 June 1997, the then Minister for Public Health stated in response to a Question in Parliament:
>
> *"We regard the deliberate cloning of human beings as ethically unacceptable. Under United Kingdom law, cloning of individual humans cannot take place whatever the origin of the material and whatever technique is used."*[10]

The Human Reproductive Cloning Act 2001:

> (1) A person who places in a woman a human embryo which has been created otherwise than by fertilisation is guilty of an offence.

The case of cloning illustrates how (bio)ethical principles have been, and may be, used to judge the ethical legitimacy of practices. People value (bio)ethical principles because they assume that those principles can help to resolve moral dilemmas, as they should relate different positions to common values. However, (bio)ethical principles are unable to resolve ethical dilemmas or guarantee consensus on sensitive issues. In the case of cloning, despite the pronouncements and declarations in the name of ethical principles, a profound divide on the ethics of cloning still afflicts ethicists. Whereas many argue that cloning violates ethical principles, and therefore has to be prohibited, it may also be argued that such *a priori* prohibition of cloning violates ethical principles. As, for example, John Harris has stressed, to deny humans the possible benefits of cloning and to deny them the freedom to choose how to reproduce is a violation of fundamental human rights and ethical principles, such as respect for human dignity, equality, and autonomy.[11]

I do not wish in this chapter to take a position on cloning.[12] I only wish to point out that the agreement upon principles does not correspond to any agreement upon the ethics of the practice. We all seem to agree on values and principles, such as equality, dignity, integrity, and so on, but when it comes to the practice, this agreement is lost. Ethical principles, which should promote dialogue, consensus, and agreement on the practical matters, fail to promote any real consensus in practice. Why does this happen?

5. Abstract Principles Cannot Direct Practice

The disagreement on cloning in part hangs on how people interpret (bio)ethical principles. Most pronouncements declare that cloning violates dignity and other fundamental ethical principles, but people have different views on what these principles mean and how they should be understood. The concept of dignity, for example, appears in virtually all pronouncements on the topic. The Fifth General Assembly of the *Pontificia Accademia Pro Vita* understands dignity as integrity of the human body. The Assembly therefore will consider any act (including autonomous acts) of utilization or instrumentalization of the human body as contrary to human dignity (see the Final Declaration of the Vth General Assembly of the *Pontificia Accademia Pro Vita*, February 1999).[13] The Universal Declaration of Human Rights, instead, where the notion first appeared, associated the concept of dignity with those of equality and rights ("All human beings are equal in dignity and rights"). In this sense the concept of dignity means self-determination and freedom of choice, and to respect dignity means that everybody has a right to liberty, expression, and choice. To deny the exercise of such freedom is a violation of dignity (an interpretation that is diametrically opposed to the one that the *Pontificia Accademia Pro Vita* suggests).

The controversy on the meaning and scope of respect for dignity is not an isolated case. Other controversial concepts are those of equality (Ronald Dworkin, in his classic discussion of equality, writes that "equality is a popular but mysterious political ideal")[14] and justice, as Tuija Takala notes:

> In the spring of 1999 there was again in Finland the time for parliamentary elections. During the campaigns it became obvious that there was an overwhelming consensus among the rival parties that justice is important and that we should aim for a more just society. The only small difference between the parties was in the understanding of what justice is and what measures should be taken that justice would prevail. The right wing thought that by lowering the taxation of property and high salaries we would be able to do this. Meanwhile, the suggested solution from the left wing was to lower the taxation of the lower income groups and reaffirm the welfare rights, such as free education, free healthcare, and reasonable unemployment benefits. The political middle, representing the interests of agricultural Finland, reckoned that above all the government should fund the farmers. Same word, but different interpretations of what justly belongs to whom.[15]

It is an inherent property of (bio)ethical principles that they may be interpreted in different ways. (Bio)ethical principles are appealing, because they are solemn and noble declarations of ideals that we seem to share. They collect consensus *because* they are so abstract and general that they can be understood in different ways—and for this reason they can align different opinions. However, because (bio)ethical principles are so abstract and general, they are unable to help us understand what is good or right to do in individual cases. Henry Sidgwick, in his discussion of ethical principles—bioethical principles were beyond the horizon of speculation in the time in which he wrote—

pointed out that ethical principles are "of too abstract a nature, and too universal in their scope, to enable us to ascertain by immediate application of them what we ought to do in any particular case."[16] Since their meaning is not univocal, how should we interpret them? How should we apply them to the individual case? And if two or more principles conflict with each other, which one should we prefer?

Georg Wilhelm Friedrich Hegel also argued for the uselessness of ethical principles to direct practice, claiming that the morality that appeals to ethical principles is "empty formalism."[17] Dignity, equality, and integrity are abstract concepts devoid of any content. He wrote: "There is a period in the culture of an epoch as in the culture of the individual, when the primary concern is the acquisition and assertion of the principle in its undeveloped intensity."[18] For Hegel ethical principles were "abstract shadow[s]."[19] He pointed out that, being "divorced from all content,"[20] ethical principles are unable to exert any effect on reality.[21] Ideals are chimeras, mental fantasies, that are either too excellent to affect reality, or too weak to be able to edify it. They are empty simulacra that are impossible to concretize.

Some may fear that without (bio)ethical principles morality would collapse. People would have different opinions, and without principles they would not be able to decide which opinion is the most ethical. Hegel responded to this argument by holding that ethical principles exist precisely *because* different opinions exist. People have the impression that these principles may be able to pacify contrasts in views. However ethical principles do not "resolve" disagreement or "create" a common morality, because they are generated from that disagreement, and are an expression of it.

> Those who attach such importance to the ought of morality and fancy that morality is destroyed if the ought is not recognized as the ultimate truth, and those too who, reasoning from the level of the understanding, derive a perpetual satisfaction from being able to confront everything there is with an ought, that is, with a 'knowing better'—and for that very reason are just as loathe to be robbed of the ought—do not see that as regards the finitude of their sphere the ought receives full recognition .... The philosophy of Kant and Fichte sets up the ought as the highest point of the resolution of the contradiction of Reason; but *the truth is that the ought is only the standpoint which clings to finitude and thus to contradiction* [my emphasis].[22]

Ethical principles are abstract concepts that are born from differences in opinion, and only exist in virtue of these differences. Therefore, they (logically) cannot resolve these differences. If the ethical principles were able to make us agree on what is right or wrong they would become redundant and unnecessary. If people had only one ethical view and agreed on what is to be valued, they would not need ethical principles. Consensus obtained around these principles is therefore often fictitious—as the case of cloning shows.

Someone may object that (bio)ethical principles are valuable as they express common and fundamental ethical values that humans seem to share, and that it is important that people agree on these fundamental, though abstract, ideals. Dissent only concerns the scope and interpretation of these principles, a matter about which it is possible to discuss and find agreement.

However, dissent on the scope and interpretation of ethical principles is not "secondary to" dissent on the ethical principle itself. If parties dramatically disagree on what a concept means (dignity, for example, or justice, as Takala acutely illustrates) or to which cases we should apply them, then the agreement on an abstract concept, whose meaning is unknown or unclear to them, does not help them to harmonize their positions or to find uncontroversial solutions to practical dilemmas.

6. Philosophical Work is Marginalized

> High above the ship-wreck, from the belvedere of the light-house
> Looking down, from far away, at the disaster ....
> The Majority is ... peacefully tilling the horrible variety of its own prides[23]

The second problem has to do with the way that ethicists formulate (bio)ethical principles. These principles are collected in pronouncements that are the results of summits of experts. Nothing is wrong with this. The problem is that these pronouncements tend to present the principles as self-evident truths, which require no explanation. Instead of a critical analysis of the ethical issue, the pronouncements offer high-sounding and noble statements, with little or no philosophical argument in support of the resolutions. The most serious philosophical bioethical debate is thus marginalized.[24] The result of this is that the general public is told that a practice is "unethical" or that it is illegal "for ethical reasons," and who could disagree with that? Who could argue in favor of the unethical? But the public remains uninformed (and maybe in some cases prejudiced) about the topic and about the arguments for and against it.

7. To Die for Ideas...

> "To die for ideas," the idea is fascinating
> I was about to die, without similar ideas
> Since a crowd of people, fell on me
> shouting: "Long life to Death!!"[25]

With perspicacious foresight, Jean-Jacques Rousseau argued that in ethics, as well as in politics, the useless is also pernicious.[26] As I have shown at the beginning of this chapter, some people believe that (bio)ethical principles promote tolerance, dialogue, and peace. However, (bio)ethical principles are not as beneficial or innocuous as they appear, as literature, cinema, and music have often emphasized. Umberto Eco, in his *The Name of the Rose*, has sharply shown the harmful nature of ideals and principles. The book is set in 1327, in an abbey in the north of Italy. A murder has been committed and William, a brilliant monk, investigates. William notices that the tongues and three fingers of the right hands of the victims have black stains. He believes that the victims have been poisoned, and begins to suspect that the murders are related to the library. He discovers that the library is an impenetrable labyrinth. Only the librarian Jorge, a blind octogenarian, has access to its secret areas. He is the only person who has complete access to catalogues and texts. Eventually William penetrates the library, and understands the mystery of the deaths. The librarian, who was above any suspicion because of his blindness, was in fact the killer. He killed the monks because they had come into contact with a prohibited text, the second book of the *Poetics* by Aristotle. In this book, Aristotle talked about the importance of laughter as an instrument of dialogue and of the search for truth. This teaching contrasted with the doctrine of Christianity, as it was interpreted by the librarian. The ethos of Christianity involved a commitment to suffering and austerity, not lightness and laughter. Because Aristotle was an influential voice—"The Philosopher"—his ideas about laughter had to be hidden. Jorge therefore poisoned the pages of the book, so that everyone who came into contact with it would die. When William finds Jorge with the book, Jorge kills himself by swallowing the poisoned pages. Just prior to Jorge's death, he and William talk.

> Jorge: "I have killed no one. Each died according to his destiny because of his sins. I was only an instrument."
>
> William: "...Here [in the 2nd book of the *Poetics*] Aristotle sees the tendency to laughter as a force for good, which can also have an instructive value: through witty riddles and unexpected metaphors, though it tells us things differently from the way they are, as if it were lying, it actually obliges us to examine them more closely, and it makes us say: Ah, this is just how things are, and I didn't know it. Truth reached by depicting men and the world as worse than they are or than we believe them to be, worse in any case than the epics, the tragedies, lives of the saints have shown them to us .... But what frightened you in this discussion of laughter? You cannot eliminate laughter by eliminating the book."
>
> Jorge: "No, to be sure. But laughter is weakness, corruption, the foolishness of our flesh. It is the peasant's entertainment, the drunkard's

> license; even the church in her wisdom has granted the moment of feast, carnival, fair .... Still, laughter remains base, a defense for the simple, a mystery desecrated for the plebeians .... Here the function of laughter is reversed, it is elevated to art, the doors of the world of the learned are opened to it, it becomes the object of philosophy, and of perfidious theology .... Laughter frees the villain from fear of the Devil, because in the feast of fools the Devil also appears poor and foolish, and therefore controllable."

Jorge swallows the incriminating pages, and, in the spasms of dying, knocks over an oil lamp and sets fire to the library. William and his young novice Adso manage to escape. When they are finally safe, in the fields, watching the abbey in flames, William says to Adso:

> "Fear prophets, Adso, and those prepared to die for the truth, for as a rule they make many others die with them, often before them, at times instead of them. Jorge did a diabolical thing because he loved his truth so lewdly that he dared anything in order to destroy falsehood. Jorge feared the second book of Aristotle because it perhaps really did teach how to distort the face of every truth, so that we would not become slaves of our ghosts. Perhaps the mission of those who love mankind is to make people laugh at the truth, to make truth laugh, because the only truth lies in learning to free ourselves from insane passion for the truth."[27]

Part of the reason why (bio)ethical principles harm is because they are principles, and like all principles they do not tolerate compassion. (Bio)ethical principles are good for judging, as they make ethical judgment a relatively easy task (if a situation violates or threatens the principle, then that situation is wrong). However, they offer no instrument for understanding. Since (bio)ethical principles are *principles*, they are not generally conditional or relative to individual circumstances. Although they may certainly be used for important causes, for protecting vulnerable people and to guarantee respect for everybody's most fundamental rights, it is an inherent property of (bio)ethical principles that they offer scarce consideration, if any, of the circumstances and reasons that lead people to a decision. (Bio)ethical principles require coherence and respect, but not understanding, and therefore leave little room for compassion. The principle must be respected, however much it may cost to people. Before the principle, people's motivations, and often their suffering, are irrelevant or remain in the background.

8. Conclusion

Contemporary bioethics often rotates around (bio)ethical principles. Ethicists, policy-makers, and jurists often use them to judge the ethical legitimacy of practices that are ethically equivocal. I have argued against this method of assessing the ethical legitimacy of practices. (Bio)ethical principles necessarily fail to offer solutions for practical dilemmas; all they can create is a fictitious consensus.

This is, however, the minor inconvenience of ethical principles. The major problem is that ethical principles lead to people being harmed in the name of ethics. (Bio)ethical principles represent a new moral authority, a substitute for other sources of moral authority, such as religion. (Bio)ethical principles can silence moral reasoning and debate; people are not allowed to have their judgment, and different views and moral values are not tolerated within a society that subscribes to (bio)ethical principles.

(Bio)ethical principles are the result of a tradition of thought that in Europe has fought to free ethics from other sources of moral authority (mainly religion). Intellectuals such as Diderot, Voltaire, and in England, John Toland, Anthony Collins, and many others fought for individual thinking, autonomy, and responsibility, for a moral thought based on "evidence for and against," rather than "commandments" or prejudice. As Collins wrote in 1713, the only instrument I possess to distinguish the good and the bad is my mind and my thinking.[28] Morality should be based on free thinking and pondering, on *responsible* moral choices. For centuries intellectuals in Europe have fought to promote ethical debate and reasoning, and for the freedom of individuals to *think* about moral issues and come to their judgment. They argued not for a new authority, for a new truth, for an Institution that would tell people what is right or wrong (this being the Pope or the European Parliament) but for tolerance, reason, and skepticism (as the ability to question and doubt). This skepticism is often absent from modern (bio)ethical debate—religious authority has been replaced by a new authority, the authority of shared ideals and (bio)ethical principles.

NOTES

1. Joseph Raz, *The Morality of Freedom* (Oxford: Clarendon Press, 1988), pp. 227–229.

2. Martin Hans Sass, "European Bioethics on a Rocky Road," *The Journal of Medicine and Philosophy*, 26:3 (June 2001), pp. 215–224.

3. *Introduction to Bioethics*, ed. John Harris (Oxford: Oxford University Press, 2001).

4. Simona Giordano and John Harris, "Bioetica e tecnologia medica. Clonazione, ricerca sulle cellule staminali, statuto morale degli embrioni," *Bioetica, rivista interdisciplinare*, 11:3 (September 2003), pp. 427–441.

5. European Parliament, Resolution on Cloning, 1997 O.J. (C 115) 14.4/92 (12 March 1997).

6. Council of Europe, Additional Protocol to the Convention for the Protection of Human Rights and Dignity of the Human Being with regard to the Application of Biology and Medicine, on the Prohibition of Cloning Human Beings (Paris, 12 January 1998), ETS No. 168, http://conventions.coe.int/treaty/en/treaties/html/168.htm.

7. The Charter of Fundamental Rights of the European Union (Nice, 7 December 2000), http://www.europarl.europa.eu/charter/default_en.htm.

8. Anne McLaren, Opinion of the Group of Advisers on the Ethical Implications of Biotechnology to the European Commission, No. 9. (28 May 1997).

9. UNESCO, The Universal Declaration on the Human Genome and Human Rights (11 November 1997).

10. Government Response to the Recommendations made in the Chief Medical Officer's Expert Group Report (August 2000), The Stationary Office, Cm4833.

11. John Harris, "Goodbye Dolly? The Ethics of Human Cloning," *Journal of Medical Ethics*, 23:6 (December 1997), pp. 353–360; John Harris, "Cloning and Human Dignity," *Cambridge Quarterly of Healthcare Ethics*, 7:2 (spring 1998), pp. 163–167; Steven Malby, "Cloning Health and Human Rights," *Health and Human Rights*, 6:1 (2002), pp. 103–136.

12. John Harris and Simona Giordano, "On Cloning," *Routledge Encyclopedia of Philosophy Online*, ed. Edward Craig, http://www.rep.routledge.com.

13. Maria Grazia Giammarino, "Luci e ombre della Carta europea dei diritti," *Bioetica, rivista interdisciplinare*, 9:4 (December 2001), p. 712.

14. Ronald Dworkin, "What is Equality? Part 1, Equality of Welfare," *Philosophy and Public Affairs*, 10 (1981), pp. 185–246, at p. 185.

15. Tuija Takala, "What Is Wrong with Global Bioethics? On the Limitations of the Four Principles Approach," *Cambridge Quarterly of Healthcare Ethics*, 10:1 (January 2001), pp. 72–77.

16. J. B. Schneewind, *Sidgwick's Ethics and Victorian Moral Philosophy* (Oxford: Oxford University Press, 1997), p. 289.

17. Georg Wilhelm Friedrich Hegel, *Science of Logic*, transl. A. V. Miller (London: Humanities Press, 1969), p. 27.

18. *Ibid.*

19. *Ibid.*, p. 47.

20. *Ibid.*

21. *Ibid.*, p. 133.

22. *Ibid.*, p. 136.

23. "Alta sui naufragi dai belvedere delle torri, China e distante suigli elementi del disasastro … La maggior sta … Coltivando tranquilla l'orribile varieta` delle proprie superbie." Fabrizio De Andrè and Ivano Fossati, "Smisurata Preghiera", in *Anime Salve*, BMG Ricordi, Milano, 1996. My translation from Italian.

24. Giordano and Harris, "Bioetica e tecnologia medica."

25. George Brassens, *Mourir pour des idées* (France, 1960–62). My translation from French.

26. Jean-Jacques Rousseau, "The Discourse on Sciences and Arts," *The Discourses and Other Early Political Writings* (Cambridge: Cambridge University Press, 1997), p. 17.

27. Umberto Eco, *The Name of the Rose*, transl. William Weaver, (London: Vintage, 1998), pp. 468–492.

28. Giovanni Reale and Dorio Antiseri, *Il pensiero occidentale dalle origini ad oggi* (Milano: La Scuola, 1984), p. 586.

Four

BIOETHICS AND STEPHEN TOULMIN'S ARGUMENTATION THEORY

Doris Schroeder and Peter Herissone-Kelly

1. Argumentation Theory

> It is becoming quite common nowadays to see writers, whether popular or academic, speaking of a happy period which has just dawned, in which philosophers actually try to say something relevant to practical issues... I may perhaps be forgiven for finding this a little irritating.
> (R. M. Hare)

"Argumentation Theory" is the name of a set of approaches to the analysis of arguments that has, over recent decades, found significant favor amongst lawyers, psychologists, communication theorists, linguists, debaters, and others. However, it seemingly remains unused in the field of bioethics. There may be good reason for this—it may be that argumentation theory has been considered by bioethicists and has been found to be flawed, or for some reason specifically inapplicable to their discipline. We suspect, however, that it has simply not caught their attention. Our purpose in this paper, then, is to introduce argumentation theory for consideration, and to make at least a tentative evaluation of its merits as a tool for deconstructing bioethical arguments.

Modern argumentation theory begins with, and develops from, the version put forward by Stephen Toulmin in his *The Uses of Argument* in 1958.[1] Indeed, it was the publication of an updated edition of this book in August 2003 that ignited our interest. If a book is updated by an author almost half a century after its first publication, we can hope that it has something interesting to say (beyond revealing the secrets of a long life). Accordingly, it is Toulmin's influential variety of argumentation theory that will be our focus in what follows. In order to test it, we will use an example of a high-profile bioethical debate.

Our chapter has three parts. First, we will introduce the case we have chosen, and one possible response to the problems it poses. Second, we will briefly outline Toulmin's argumentation model. And third, we will establish how useful it is in the context of our case. We aim to make two points. First, we want to show that Toulmin's model is helpful in identifying incomplete or otherwise flawed arguments. Second, we want to argue that, if Toulmin's procedure is insisted upon, debates in bioethics almost inevitably run into cul-de-sacs, due to often insurmountable disagreement over normative ethical theories. The upshot is that if we accept the model, we can expose deficiencies in arguments and thereby defeat claims, but hardly ever justify them. Whether this is a flaw in Toulmin's argumentation model, or simply an intractable characteristic of ethical argumentation, remains to be seen.

2. The Case

The case on which we are focusing is a familiar one in the United Kingdom at the time of writing—that of the Whitaker family. Jayson and Michelle Whitaker are a British couple whose young son, Charlie, suffers from the life-threatening blood disorder, Diamond Blackfan Anemia. The only cure for the disease is a transplant of bone marrow or cord blood stem cells from a donor with the same immune system cells. Neither Charlie's parents, nor his existing sibling, are suitably matched. The chances of naturally conceiving a suitable sibling were one in four. However, these chances would be hugely increased—to around 98%—by a procedure that combined *in vitro* fertilization with tissue matching (IVF+TM). Having implanted a screened embryo produced in this way, stem cells for transplantation could be taken from the resulting baby's umbilical cord upon its birth.

The British Human Fertilisation and Embryology Authority (HFEA) refused permission for the Whitakers to have this procedure carried out in the United Kingdom, on the grounds that such procedures should only be performed for the benefit of the embryo (for instance, to screen for a serious genetic disease that would also affect the child conceived in this way).[2] The claim was that, in this case, the procedure would only benefit Charlie, and not the child whose stem cells would be used. Following this ruling, the Whitakers decided to undergo the procedure in the United States, and in June 2003, Michelle gave birth to Jamie, a suitable genetic match for Charlie.[3]

In "Is Conceiving a Child to Benefit Another Against the Interests of the New Child?" Merle Spriggs argues that IVF+TM "should be used to save a sick child and that it would be morally remiss for Jamie's parents not to consent to the use of his cord blood."[4] Her argument goes through several stages building up to the following: The only moral principles that count in IVF+TM are "individual welfare" and "autonomy," since that of "dignity" can be rejected.[5] Charlie's life should not be sacrificed for the rather vague conception of Jamie's dignity.[6] Parental consent is fully sufficient to satisfy the autonomy/informed consent criteria. Taking stem cells from cord blood poses no risk to the donor and the Whitakers have consented to the necessary procedures. So, as IVF+TM is compatible with Jamie's welfare[7] and the principle of autonomy has been respected, the Whitakers ought to be allowed embryo selection.

We are not going to challenge this argument, although several questions suggest themselves. Are "welfare," "dignity," and "autonomy" the only relevant moral principles? Why should the life of one person be more important than the dignity of another? Why should one accept Spriggs's claim that the argument from dignity is vague and religious?[8] And even if one were to accept this last point, why should the identification of an argument as "religious" supply sufficient grounds to reject it?

3. Argumentation Theory—Toulmin's Model

Toulmin's main aim in *The Uses of Argument* is to provide a model for the analysis of argumentation that does a better job than traditional logic of capturing the complexity of real-life arguments.[9] In so doing, he hopes to answer the question, "How ... should we lay an argument out, if we want to show the sources of its validity?"[10]

Two related points need to be made here. First, when Toulmin talks of validity, he rather confusingly does not have in mind the traditional notion associated with that word—that of formal validity. Instead he wants to move from "formal" to "procedural" validity.[11] What precisely he means by "procedural validity" is rather vague and hard to pin down, though it seems that, for him, a valid argument is any argument that it would be rational to accept. Thus, for example, inductively strong arguments, though formally invalid, will be valid in Toulmin's sense.[12] Let us call this sense "T-validity" (for "Toulmin-validity"). What it is important to realize is that an argument's being T-valid is not simply a matter of its being of a particular form.[13] A correlate of this point, and one of which Toulmin makes much, is that there are no universal norms that dictate when it is rational to accept an argument, regardless of its subject matter. What makes an argument good will differ significantly depending on the content of the argument: in Toulmin's words, what ultimately justifies an argument will be something "field-dependent."[14] It is worth noting as an aside that, while it might at first sight seem that T-validity is equivalent to the notion of soundness, this is not so, since a sound argument must be formally valid, whereas a T-valid argument need not be.

Second, in claiming that his model is able to "show the sources" of an argument's T-validity, Toulmin is not claiming that we can simply lay an argument out according to his model, and then "read off" its T-validity or T-invalidity. All that analyzing an argument using Toulmin's model can do is to show us the form of that argument, and T-validity, as we have seen, is not determined by form alone. So, once an argument has been analyzed using Toulmin's model, we still have to assess it. All that the analysis does is make the task of assessment easier, by breaking the argument down into its essential elements.

Toulmin models his theory of argumentation on the legal example of procedural reasoning. For him, "logic ... is generalised jurisprudence"[15] and patterns of argumentation correspond to the distinctions necessary for a fair legal process.[16] Using this procedural approach, arguments can be separated into six elements: claims, data, warrants, rebuttals, qualifiers, and backing.[17]

For Toulmin, arguments start with an asserted claim for which a potential challenger will demand justificatory evidence by asking "What have you got to go on?"[18] The first evidence given to respond to the challenge are the *data* or the *grounds*.[19] Data are facts one appeals to in order to provide a foundation for the claim.[20] For instance, if asked why we believe that student A has understood the content of the logic module, we reply "because she received a First in her coursework." A challenger who is not familiar with the British Higher Education system, might then ask: How do you get there?—a question that does not ask for more data, but for the relevance of the given data to the asserted claim. Perhaps in the challenger's country, a mark of "1" is the lowest possible mark. Challenged in this way, we will have to provide an inference license—a general, hypothetical statement—that can bridge the gap between claim and data. Such an inference license, which Toulmin calls a *warrant*, will usually be of the form: "For all x, one can assume y" or "Given D (data), one may take it that C (claim)."[21] In our case, the warrant would be something like this: "Within the British Education system, if somebody achieves a First when assessed, one may take it that she or he will have understood the topic under consideration."

A very persistent challenger may now ask: "But why do you think that?"[22] In other words: "Why do you think that a First will signify that the student has understood the material?" In this case, one can refer to university marking criteria, which specify, for instance, that a student who receives a First will have made "effective use of excellent knowledge and thorough understanding of a wide range of appropriate sources." Toulmin would call this move providing *backing* for one's warrants. In contrast to warrants, backings are expressed in categorical rather than hypothetical form.[23] Not all arguments have backing, as it is possible for a warrant to be self-justifying. An example of Toulmin's that would appear to be a self-justifying warrant is the following. We claim that "Harry's hair is not black." As datum we say: "We have seen that it is in fact red." The inference license in this case is rather trivial: namely, that "If anything is red, it will not also be black."

Importantly, Toulmin thinks, warrants in diverse fields of inquiry will require different kinds of backing. He says:

> the moment we start asking about the *backing* which a warrant relies on in each field, great differences begin to appear: the kind of backing we

> must point to if we are to establish its authority will change greatly as we move from one field of argument to another.[24]

This is what Toulmin means when he characterizes a warrant's backing as a "field-dependent" element of an argument.

As can be seen from our earlier argument, it is not normally necessary to make the warrant explicit.[25] Those familiar with the British Higher Education system will understand the datum's relevance to the claim without an explicit inference license. However, both local and overseas challengers could now produce further questions relating to the degree of force the data give the warrant.[26] Generically formulated, the question could be something like: "Are there any exceptions to the rule?" More specifically, the challenger could ask: "What about plagiarism?" or "What about bribed tutors?" If we have not already qualified our claim to make room for these rebuttals, we now have to grant these and other potential exceptions. Hence, we modify our claim by including a modal *qualifier* and possible conditions of exception or *rebuttals* to complete the argument.[27] In diagrammatic form, our argument would look as in figure 4.1.

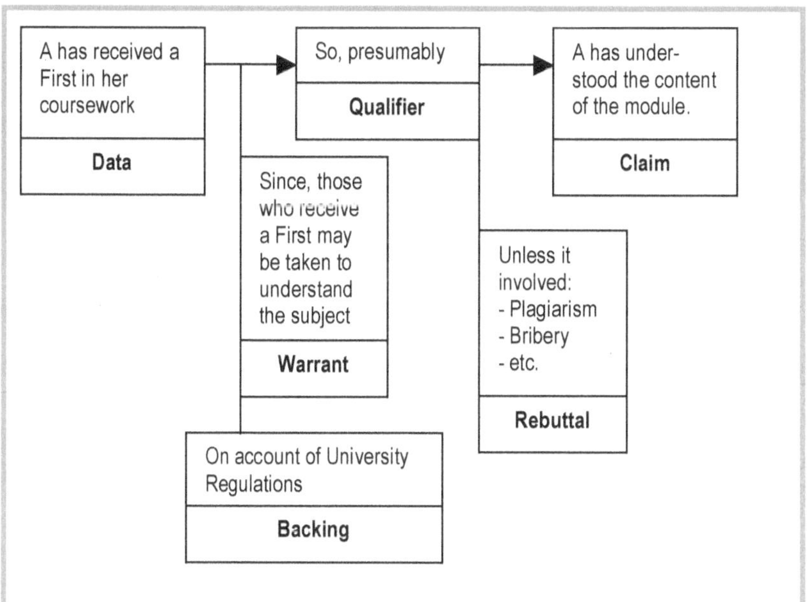

Figure 4.1 *An argument for "A has understood the content of the module"*

4. Applying Toulmin's Model—Particulars

Although Toulmin attacks traditional logic for allegedly rejecting ethical arguments as "incoherent, invalid, and improper,"[28] he himself does not use ethical debates in *The Uses of Argument* to test his model (though he does comment that they will need their own distinctive type of backing, without, however, expanding on what type of backing that will be).[29] This is not surprising, as we will argue later. Ethical debates are often built on intractably controversial backing, unlike the types of backing Toulmin uses in his own, non-ethical, examples (statutes, Acts of Parliament, statistical reports, experimental results, and references to taxonomical systems).[30] However, let us first consider whether Toulmin's model can be used to help analyze the merits of Merle Spriggs's argument in the Whitaker case.

Spriggs's main claim is twofold. She argues that IVF+TM "[first] should be used to save a sick child and [second] that it would be morally remiss for Jamie's parents not to consent to the use of his cord blood."[31] As IVF+TM involves an expensive procedure, which requires the full co-operation of both parents, the second of the two claims is not normally relevant to the debate. We can reasonably assume that all those who undergo the procedure do so without compulsion and would be willing for the donation of cord blood to go ahead. So, we will disregard the latter claim, as under the circumstances it states the obvious. Whether parental consent is appropriate in this case is a separate matter. According to Spriggs, "the lack of consent is not morally significant in this case."[32] We shall not argue this case. Likewise, we will disregard components of the debate which only refer to this claim and have no bearing on the first (for example, data supporting the claim), bearing in mind, though, that informed consent has been obtained from the Whitakers.

The factual information, or data, given by Spriggs to support her claim is: "taking stem cells from the umbilical cord poses no risk and no inconvenience to the new baby."[33] As in most cases of real-life argumentation, no warrant is made explicit, and consequently we have to reconstruct it. (David Hitchcock rightly argues that one has to be very careful when reconstructing implicit warrants, so as not to distort the text "in the light of our own prejudices."[34] However, we hope that our reconstruction is fair.) In the case at hand, the warrant is most likely going to be something like this: "If consent is present for a medical procedure, which does not cause any harm, we may carry it out." That being the case, the argument could be represented as in figure 4.2.

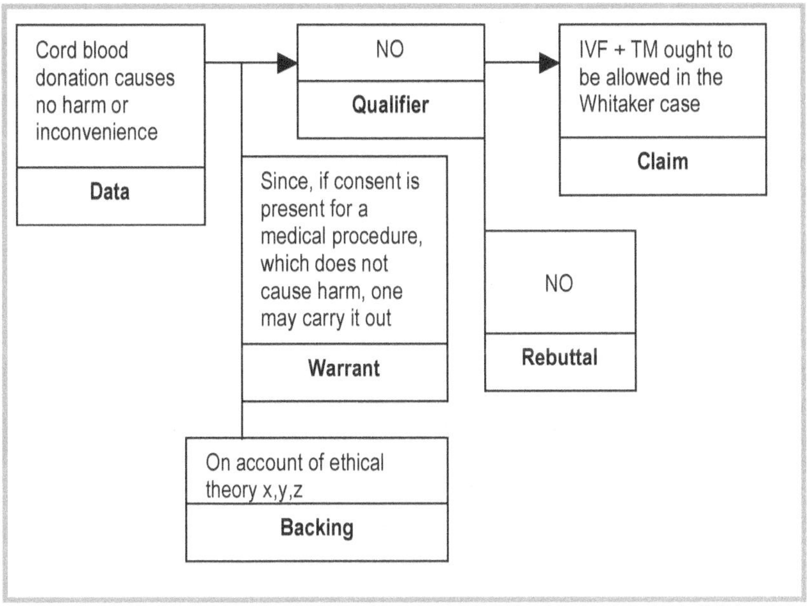

Figure 4.2 *An argument for "IVF+TM ought to be allowed..."*

Is anything wrong with this argument? Experienced healthcare personnel or ethicists would probably have noticed the problem without Toulmin's argumentation model, but with its useful dissection of the argument into various elements, the problem should now stare even unexperienced readers in the face. Two procedures are required potentially to cure Charlie: first IVF+TM, and second cord blood donation. Spriggs makes a claim about the former, while only providing data for the latter. Accepting our interpretation of Spriggs's warrant, we could infer that cord blood donation was justifiable, but this does not extend to IVF+TM, for which essential information is missing. Does IVF+TM cause harm or inconvenience? Martin Delatycki answers this question in his response to Spriggs. According to him, IVF and ICSI (intracytoplasmic sperm injection, required for prenatal genetic diagnosis)

> have been studied extensively and there are a number of negative outcomes that exceed rates seen in naturally conceived pregnancies. These include risks associated with multiple pregnancies, prematurity, in-utero growth retardation, and disorders of imprinting, particularly Beckwith-Weiderman syndrome.[35]

Assuming a typing error in Delatycki's article, Beckwith-Wiedemann syndrome is characterized by the following features: macroglossia (a large tongue which may cause breathing, feeding, or speech difficulties); umbilical hernia or exomphalos; overgrowth (children with the condition are bigger than their contemporaries); hemihypertrophy (one side of the body grows more than the other); hypoglycemia (low blood sugar) as babies; characteristic facial appearance; and indentations of the ears.

If we were interested in debating the case as such rather than the application of Toulmin's argumentation model, we would have to revisit the paradox of future individuals[36] or, as Derek Parfit calls it, the non-identity problem.[37] But this is not the case. Let us just remember that an essential piece of data is missing from Spriggs's article and that Toulmin's model helped us to identify this, as a mismatch between claim and data became apparent in a superficially plausible argument when dissecting it with the help of Toulmin's model. As it stands, Spriggs's argument has to be rejected on the grounds of—at least—incompleteness.

5. Applying Toulmin's Model—Generics

Let us imagine that IVF+TM does not have the above medical complications associated with it, and that it resembles natural conception in all relevant respects. Would the argument then be complete and convincing? To answer this question, let us assume the position of a challenger and try to defeat it. How can we reasonably defeat an argument using Toulmin's model? There seem to be four possibilities.

(1) The data can be shown to be incorrect.
(2) The backing for the warrant or a self-justifying warrant is indefensible.
(3) There is no backing or no self-justifying warrant.
(4) The rebuttal is stronger than admitted by the proponent of the claim.

(1) In our case, if one wanted to show that our new datum ("IVF+TM causes no harm") were incorrect, one could argue that, although there is no medically-induced harm in the procedure, the dignity of the child conceived in this way would be violated, and so the statement that the procedure does not incur harm would be incorrect. This would lead to a new argument, where the claim would be: "IVF+TM violates the dignity of a child conceived in this way," and then the challenger would become the proponent of the claim and have to offer data to support it. This is why Toulmin thinks that, when concentrating on any one argument, the data for that argument should be considered as already given. If they cannot be agreed upon, we must first shift

our attention to another argument to establish them. In this new argument, the datum should be factual and verifiable, as is standard in Toulmin's model. It could be something like: "A child has been created with the primary purpose of benefiting his elder brother."[38] The warrant for this argument could be: "If a human being is created primarily to benefit another human being, his or her dignity is being violated." And a Kantian-inspired ethical theory—drawing upon the second formulation of the categorical imperative—could provide the backing for such a warrant. It is worth noting at this stage that a disagreement over a datum has led to a new argument, for which the most likely point of contention is its backing.

(2) Moving to the second possibility of defeating a claim: if we wanted to argue that the backing or the self-justifying warrant were indefensible, we would first inquire about the status of the warrant and, second, if it were not self-justifying, we would ask for its backing. Is "If consent is present for a medical procedure, which does not cause any harm, we may carry it out" a self-justifying warrant? No. In this case, it seems perfectly reasonable to ask "why?" when in reply to: "If hair is naturally black, it cannot be naturally red" we would not think so. What sort of backing could be provided for our warrant? A categorical statement summarizing preference utilitarianism suggests itself, given the emphasis on individual liberty and welfare in the warrant, something like: "Moral goodness consists in the satisfaction of people's preferences, providing individual welfare is being respected." It seems safe to say that a backing of this type would not be left unchallenged, and that would leave us in the same sort of situation as (1) did.

(3) Where there is neither backing nor self-justifying warrant, it is likely that the argument's proponent has assumed that the warrant is self-justifying, or axiomatic, when in fact it is not. This case is unlikely to materialize in bioethical debates where variations of normative ethical theories always suggest themselves as backing.

(4) This leaves a fourth possibility of how an argument can be defeated, namely that the proponent miscalculates the probability of the claim being affected by rebuttals (to do this is to misapprehend the strength or inclusiveness of the warrant). When the claim was formulated the modal qualifier chosen was inappropriate. Instead of "perhaps," "almost certainly" was chosen. In the course of the discussion, however, it turns out that the likelihood of the claim going through is very low and the chance of a rebuttal defeating the claim very high. An example of this would be to argue that the success of transplantation with stem cells from cord blood is very high for anemia cases when accompanied by strong radiation and chemotherapy regimes to prevent graft-versus-host-disease. A rebuttal could be that the patient under consideration suffers from Fanconi Anemia (rather than aplastic anemia or Diamond Blackfan Anemia). Fanconi Anemia patients do not tolerate the high levels of radiation and chemotherapy commonly used to prepare them for transplanta-

tion, thereby complicating their treatment even if cord blood from a matched donor is available. Hence, the rebuttal about patient status will weaken the initial claim considerably.

We have already said that all Toulmin's model supposedly does is to make clear the various elements of an argument, in a way that makes it easier to evaluate its T-validity or T-invalidity. But it is vital to note that, while it does not *determine* T-validity, the form of an argument analyzed according to Toulmin's model does suggest that there is one way in which arguments will primarily be evaluated. Since, in any particular argument, the data are to be regarded as given, and the presence or absence of qualifier and rebuttal is dependent on the force of the warrant, it seems that our evaluative attention is inexorably directed toward the warrant. And since the vast majority of warrants will rely for their authority on their backings, it seems that it is the field-dependent backing that is the ultimate determinant of T-validity, and so the ultimate focus of assessment. Noting this brings us into agreement with a number of commentators on Toulmin's work. Thus, one prominent set of commentators can say that

> when talking about "validity" Toulmin is interested only in the backing … his only intention with his model is to show that it is the (field-dependent) backing for the warrant (whatever form it may take) which ultimately determines the validity or invalidity of an argument.[39]

This fits well with Toulmin's claim that there are no universal norms by which arguments can be judged as T-valid (or, for that matter, T-invalid). Instead, what makes an argument T-valid will ultimately be something "field-dependent," and the one field-dependent component in Toulmin's analysis of argument is the backing.[40]

But this means, somewhat unfortunately, that when considering whether we ought to accept any given bioethical argument, we will invariably be pushed toward considering whether we ought to accept the backing for its (ethical) warrant. And this backing, as we have seen, will always be a concise statement of, or perhaps a fragment of, some ethical theory or other. So, no matter what the bioethical argument is, when we come to assess it, we will be forced to avoid focusing on the particularities of the case, in favor of assessing whatever ethical theory underlies its warrant.

6. Conclusion

Despite questionable pronouncements about the limits of traditional logic, Stephen Toulmin's argumentation theory can be helpful in assessing arguments in bioethics. Laying out the different elements of an argument before coming to a judgment on the claim under consideration assists in finding potential flaws. In our case, a clear mismatch could be detected between the datum provided by Merle Spriggs to defend her claim, and the claim as such, namely that IVF+TM does not cause any harm or inconvenience.

However, except to eliminate claims that are incomplete or flawed, Toulmin's model cannot be used further in bioethics. Claims can be defeated, but not justified for the simple reason that Toulmin's model draws the analyst invariably to the backings of claims, and these will—almost always—consist of highly controversial normative ethical theories.

This leaves us with the following choice. Either we look elsewhere for a model of argumentation theory that will allow us to justify claims in bioethics, or we conclude that bioethicists ought to turn their attention toward moral theory rather than case-study-based analysis.

NOTES

1. Stephen Toulmin, *The Uses of Argument* (Cambridge: Cambridge University Press, 2003).

2. Human Fertilisation and Embryology Authority, "HFEA Confirms that HLA Tissue Typing May Only Take Place When Preimplantation Genetic Diagnosis is Required to Avoid a Serious Genetic Disorder," http://www.hfea.gov.uk/cps/rde/xchg/SID-3F57D79B9B86BBDB/hfea/hs.xsl/967.html.

3. "'Designer Baby' is Perfect Match," *BBC News*, 21 July 2003, http://news.bbc.co.uk/1/hi/health/3083239.stm.

4. Merle Spriggs, "Is Conceiving a Child to Benefit Another Against the Interests of the New Child?" *Journal of Medical Ethics*, 31:6 (June 2005), pp. 341–342, http://jme.bmj.com/cgi/content/full/31/6/341.

5. *Ibid.*

6. *Ibid.*

7. *Ibid.*

8. *Ibid.* See also Matti Häyry, "Another Look at Dignity," *Cambridge Quarterly of Healthcare Ethics*, 13:1 (January 2004), pp. 7–14.

9. Toulmin, *The Uses of Argument*, pp. 2, 8.

10. *Ibid.*, p. 88.

11. *Ibid.*, p. 40.

12. *Ibid.*, pp. 217–221.

13. *Ibid.*, p. 40.

14. *Ibid.*, p. 235.

15. *Ibid.*, p. 7.

16. *Ibid.*, p. 88ff.

17. *Ibid.*, pp. 90–96.

18. *Ibid.*, pp. 12, 90.

19. Stephen Toulmin, Richard Rieke, and Allan Janik, *An Introduction to Reasoning* (New York, NY: Macmillan, 2nd ed., 1984), p. 38.

20. Toulmin, *The Uses of Argument*, p. 90.
21. *Ibid.*, p. 91.
22. *Ibid.*, p. 96.
23. *Ibid.*, p. 98.
24. *Ibid.*, p. 96.
25. *Ibid.*, p. 92.
26. *Ibid.*, p. 93.
27. *Ibid.*, p. 93.
28. *Ibid.*, p. 161.
29. *Ibid.*, p. 109.
30. Bart Verheij, "Evaluating Arguments Based on Toulmin's Scheme," *Argumentation*, 19:3 (December 2005), pp. 347–371.
31. Spriggs, "Is Conceiving a Child…?"
32. *Ibid.*
33. *Ibid.*
34. David Hitchcock, "Toulmin's Warrants," *Proceedings of the Fifth Conference of the International Society for the Study of Argumentation*, eds. Frans H. van Eemeren, J. Anthony Blair, Charles A. Willard, and A. Francisca Snoeck Henkemans (Amsterdam: SicSat, 2003), pp. 485–490, http://www.humanities.mcmaster.ca/~hitchckd/ToulminsWarrants.pdf.
35. Martin Delatycki, "Response to Spriggs—Is Conceiving a Cild to Benefit Another Against the Interest of the New Child?" *Journal of Medical Ethics*, 31:6 (June 2005), p. 343, http://jme.bmj.com/cgi/content/full/31/6/366.
36. Gregory Kavka, "The Paradox of Future Individuals," *Philosophy and Public Affairs*, 11:2 (1982), pp. 93–122.
37. Derek Parfit, *Reasons and Persons* (Oxford: Clarendon Press, 1984).
38. John Smeaton, quoted in "'Designer Baby' Born to UK Couple," *BBC News*, 19 June 2003, http://news.bbc.co.uk/1/hi/health/3002610.stm.
39. Frans H. van Eemeren, Rob Grootendorst, and Tjark Kruiger, *Handbook of Argumentation Theory* (Dordrecht: Foris Publications, 1987), p. 201.
40. See Toulmin, *The Uses of Argument*, p. 96.

Five

THE USE OF EXAMPLES IN BIOETHICS

Harry Lesser

1. The Pedagogic Function of Examples

This chapter has two aims. One is to consider some of the different functions of examples in philosophical argument, and especially in bioethics. The other is to consider how far these functions are, or can be, fulfilled in practice. Examples have either one or both of two purposes: to help an audience or readership to understand a particular position or theory, or a particular problem and why it is a problem, and to advance the argument in a particular way. It is fairly clear that the first, the pedagogic, purpose is often achieved; but whether, and how, the second aim can succeed is a much more complex question.

But even within pedagogy there are several aims to be distinguished: to make things clearer, because for most people the concrete is easier to understand than the abstract; to bring things alive and arouse the interest of the hearer/reader; to demonstrate that the issue is a real one and concerns things which actually happen, and are significant. This raises two questions about the nature of the examples. The first is whether they should be mundane or dramatic.

Mundane examples were much favored by English, and some American, philosophers of a generation ago, who would consider the force of "good" in "this is a good thumb-tack," and the moral implications of not returning borrowed books and taking too large a helping at dinner. They have the advantage of illustrating a very important principle in a manner that enables it to be considered without the distortions of emotion and prejudice, and also without getting sidetracked onto any irrelevant details that may feature in the example; and so they fulfill the task of making things clearer. But there is evidence that they have the serious drawback of trivializing the issue, rather than arousing interest and showing its significance: in theory, a minor instance of an important moral principle illustrates it just as well as a major one, but in practice students—and even academics who should know better, such as Ernest Gellner in various places in *Words and Things*—tend to conclude either that the principle itself is trivial or that the lecturer/writer is not treating it seriously.[1] The dramatic example consequently seems preferable, as better serving both to establish that the issue is a genuine one and to fix it firmly in the mind of the hearer. Generations of students have come to realize that there is a real practical problem with inductive inferences by reading or hearing Russell's story of the turkey who concluded that, because the man had come every morning to feed him, he would always come every morning to feed him, but found on Christmas Eve that he was wrong!

But an example may be dramatic while being, unlike this one, totally unrealistic, or even impossible. We will consider this later from the point of view of the development of the argument. From the point of view of pedagogy, unrealistic examples, if they are dramatic, succeed in many ways; but they do fail to show that the issue is a real one. They can be used to illustrate how things are by focusing attention on what we would be inclined to say if they were different. But on the whole, from the pedagogic point of view, what is wanted is an example which is both striking and realistic; and the risk that the audience will get too involved in the argument is worth taking.

2. The Use of Counter-Examples

However, the pedagogic functions of examples are often not their only or prime function, and may not be their function at all. Examples are also used to further an argument, primarily, as we shall see, in two ways, though no doubt there are others. One is to defeat a theory, or at least show that it needs modifying, by giving a counter-example. So, the suggestion that one should treat a patient only with their express consent, so that to treat them without this consent is always a violation of their rights, may be challenged by giving the entirely realistic example of a patient who is unconscious, and so, while urgently needing treatment, cannot give consent. More generally, the moral theory of act-utilitarianism, which asserts that the right thing to do in any situation is what will maximize happiness or minimize suffering, is challenged by examples of situations in which the maximum happiness/minimum suffering overall could be achieved only at the cost of grave injustice to an individual. So the most efficient way of ending a crime wave might be to frame an innocent person, if one cannot catch a guilty one, and punish them extremely severely as a warning.

The interesting question is: how much can a supposed counter-example, even if well-chosen and relevant, actually prove? Even in the "hard" sciences many people have argued that they cannot destroy a theory, but show only that it must be modified. To this, though, it might be replied that even a modification may be an advance and an improvement, bringing the theory more in line with reality. Sometimes the stronger point can be made that the modification needed requires one to posit something too wildly implausible to contemplate, even if one is unable to prove that it is impossible. For example one can maintain the "phlogiston" theory (the theory, popular in the eighteenth century, that burning involved the loss of a posited substance called "phlogiston") in the face of the evidence that burning results in an increase in weight; but only if one holds that phlogiston has "negative weight." It may be physically possible that a substance should have negative weight, but it is certainly unlikely.

Often, though, we have a problem of what exactly the counter-example establishes. And when we move from science to ethics we find a number of new problems. First of all, the counter-examples in ethics typically involve judgments about what is obviously right or wrong—"moral intuitions." So, it seems obviously wrong, indeed absurd, to delay treating a person who is seriously injured and unconscious, on the ground that they have not given permission. But the exact relation between moral theories and moral intuitions is hard to define: whereas a scientific theory must be consistent with the observations, it is not obvious that a moral theory must be consistent with our moral intuitions. In this case of the unconscious patient, most people might well feel that it is more certain that the seriously ill or injured person should receive treatment than that the theory that leads to the conclusion that they should not could be a correct one. But in other cases, such as the status of act-utilitarian theory, things are more finely balanced. Many people would hold that it is more certain that one should not act unjustly to individuals than that one is obliged always to do what would be best overall; but the alternative position, that the rational thing to do is always what does the most good or the least harm, and excessive concern for abstract justice is an unreasonable prejudice, has its adherents and is not self-evidently absurd.

In a third type of case, it seems clear that application of a rational moral theory shows that apparent moral intuitions—for example that interracial sex is wicked and "unnatural," or that people should be punished by the law for private sexual behavior—are nothing more than emotional prejudices. So, at any particular time and in a particular society, there might in practice be a great deal of agreement over when one has a genuine counter-example to a moral theory and when one does not. "The patient may be unconscious" is conclusive against "One may never treat a patient without their permission"; "homosexuality makes me feel sick" is irrelevant against "private sexual behavior is not the law's business"; when "minimizing overall suffering would involve injustice to individuals" is set against "one ought to minimize overall suffering" the argument continues. But it is unclear on what basis these distinctions are being made. We must now try to see whether it is possible to give criteria for the genuineness of a proposed counter-example.

Perhaps the crucial point here is that the production of the counter-example does not end the matter: one has to examine whether there is any rational reason for its being a counter-example and how strong this reason is. Simply to produce the supposed intuition, and to say "it makes me sick" or "it's what we do," and refuse to take the matter further, or to provide any justification, is a move that need not be taken seriously. It is a version of what is traditionally called the appeal *ad verecundiam* (to shame or modesty), the attempt to make the opponent embarrassed to continue the argument by implying that asking why such a cruel or disgusting practice is wrong is already to show that one is not a healthy, "right-thinking" person.

But if one is to maintain that counter-examples must be backed up by argument or evidence, and may legitimately be ignored when they are not, one must meet the challenge posed by those followers of Wittgenstein who claim that "moral bedrock," or the basis of ethics, is provided not by beliefs which can be expressed in propositions, but by our actual practices. Thus Anne Maclean argues in *The Elimination of Morality* that we do not have a belief that it is wrong to kill babies, which she thinks would imply that we had actually thought over that proposition in our minds, but we simply treat babies in a way that excludes the idea that their lives are at our disposal, and this way of behaving cannot be further justified.[2]

This suggestion is very important; and it raises the whole question of the status of examples in ethical argument, not only when they are used as counter-examples. For if it is actual practice that is what ultimately counts, then the working out of general principles is impossible; and the function of the philosopher is precisely to assemble examples as reminders of what we actually do, in order to cure the problems we have got into by forgetting this. So we have a crucial question: must examples be backed up by arguments showing their supposed significance, or are they, so to speak, themselves the argument?

There are a number of problems with the position that a universal moral practice is its own justification. Sometimes the practices that are appealed to are not in fact universal: there have, for example, been societies which have considered that it is the responsibility of the parents to decide whether their new-born children live or die. But the argument is plausible only when one is dealing with a universal practice, as otherwise one will have to endorse every practice generally accepted in every society, including racism, sexism, and mutilations of many sorts. But even when a practice is universal, and for the most part followed without most people feeling any need to reflect on why it should be followed, it still presupposes certain beliefs. The Wittgensteinians (who perhaps would not like this title) make two mistakes here. First, they assume that it is only correct to say that someone believes a proposition if that person has actually formulated the proposition and mentally assented to it. But many beliefs are expressed simply in behaving in a way that makes sense only if the belief is true, as I have believed for some time that the chair I am sitting on will bear my weight, even though I thought of it only when reaching this sentence and looking for an example! Second, it is assumed that because it would be odd to utter a statement, the statement itself must be senseless or meaningless. It is true that "it is wrong to kill babies" is a weird statement, partly because it is obvious and partly because it is inadequate: a word of much stronger moral condemnation is needed. But it is nonetheless both intelligible and true. One cannot treat a practice, even a universal one, as "bedrock" if that practice makes sense only if certain things are true. This is so even if those operating the practice do not themselves consider the question of its truth. For example, Anne Maclean considers the termination of the pregnancy of "a frightened fourteen-year-old who lacks the support both of the child's father and of her own family" and says "what is held to justify the abortion is an inability to cope: the child's entitlement to life, or lack of it, does not enter into the matter."[3] But it does: if the doctor does not consider it, this is because she has already decided, whether she knows it or not, that the unborn child has no right to life. There are people who are, rightly or wrongly, so convinced to the contrary that they would not even consider the question whether an abortion was justified.

One reply to this would be to say that some of these assumptions are themselves "bedrock": they require no further justification and none can be provided, because they are more certain than any supposed justification. This is something specifically rejected by Anne Maclean,[4] since, as we have seen, she denies that the "bedrock" is propositional. But we have also seen that this claim does not hold up. If people hold that a practice is justified, and if it can only be justified given a certain assumption, then it is perfectly legitimate to consider the merits of this assumption, even if the people themselves have not considered it. Even if no one had considered the question whether an unborn child has a right to life, it would be perfectly in order to raise it. And if this is so, it is equally the case, though more disturbing, that one may raise the question whether a neonate does have the right to life.

But are any of these assumptions beyond further discussion? It is true that one might well wish to argue that there are some propositions which cannot be denied if one is going to be moral at all. Thus there are many different views of what behavior should be punished and how, but everyone agrees that it is not right to punish the innocent, that, regardless of what the rules say, if a person has not broken any rule they should not be punished. Again, Anne Maclean is surely right to say that babies are not there to be at our disposal, for us to treat as we choose. So may not the Wittgensteinians maintain that some examples do simply have the function of reminding us of what is unquestionable in ethics? They may concede, however reluctantly, that moral practices are not unquestionable and that it makes sense to ask what they presuppose; but they may still want to maintain that some of these presuppositions are unquestionable in the sense that it makes no sense to suppose that one could have morality (as opposed, for example, to the mere pursuit of enlightened self-interest) without them. And some, though not all, examples used in bioethics will be used only to remind us of this.

It seems to me that this is true, but of very limited application, and not a great deal follows. To see this, consider the example mentioned above, that it is not compatible with morality to have a system of punishment in which the innocent are standardly or habitually punished as well as the guilty. This may well be true; and there could be a stage in a moral argument in which a reminder of it was needed. But it is much more likely that the question will be not whether habitual punishment of the innocent is right or wrong but whether such punishment is justifiable on a particular occasion. Here the examples do not settle anything on their own but require analysis: we may be confident that a particular course of action would be both unjust to an individual and beneficial to society at large, but this does not in itself determine whether it is right or wrong. Another example, more relevant to bioethics, is that of neonates. It is true that the lives of neonates are not simply at our disposal, and there are times when we should be reminded of this. But that will not settle the question of whether the parents of very severely disabled neonates should be allowed to decide whether they should be kept alive.

The conclusion of all this should be, I think, that examples, whether used as counter-examples or more generally, cannot in themselves decide anything, but have to be used to promote further discussion. They move the argument along, so to speak, but they do not settle it, or even determine the direction in which it must go. No doubt, as I suggested at the beginning, the example is often introduced with this aim; but what is typically achieved is simply the introduction of a new factor, itself based on a principle, assumed or explicitly stated, which may be responded to in more than one way. This is true whether the attempt to bring things to an end is relatively crude or relatively sophisticated. It is fairly obvious that "it makes me sick" settles nothing, but requires further discussion to see whether the activity is merely physically disgusting, which is of no moral relevance, or whether there is a ground for moral disgust as well (compare homosexuality and pedophilia). But the same is true, as I hope I have shown, of "this is what we do": a practice makes sense only given certain presuppositions (of which those who follow the practice may or may not be conscious); and we may always discuss the truth of these presuppositions. For example, although people who have to decide when an abortion is justified may not concern themselves with the right to life of unborn children, this does not mean that we cannot or should not consider whether unborn children have a right to life. Finally, there is the most radical and most sophisticated version of this use of examples, in which the example is designed to demonstrate a principle that must be part of ethics and that we cannot intelligibly reject. Even here the example will not end the argument, for one of two reasons: either it may be a matter for debate as to whether the principle must be part of ethics (as in the debate over whether ethics must use some concept of rights), or this may be agreed, but the question remains whether it is an absolute principle or admits of exceptions (as in the question whether it is ever right to punish the innocent). Examples, it would seem, especially when introduced as counter-examples, introduce new and useful issues into an argument or into the discussion of whether a particular theory is correct, but cannot in themselves settle an issue or close a discussion.

3. "What Would We Say If..."

There is, though, another important use of examples in bioethics, and in philosophy in general. This is to raise the question of what we would say under certain conditions, to perform a "thought experiment": the conditions in question may be possible or impossible, or currently impossible but maybe possible in the future. From what they allege we would say about an imagined situation if it happened, about how we might describe it metaphysically (those who discuss the nature of personal identity often bring in stories of brain bisection or people apparently switching bodies), or how we might judge it morally, or what we think a person ought to do in that situation, people draw inferences about what we should say about some actual type of situation. But how reliable are these inferences?

As an example, we may consider one of the most famous of them. Judith Jarvis Thomson, in a widely discussed article, argued that, even if an unborn child is a person, that person has no actual right to occupy the mother's womb; and therefore a woman commits no injustice by having an abortion, although she has no right to kill the child once it can survive outside her body, and although to have an abortion for a trivial reason would be cruel and unreasonable.[5] Part of her argument involved the thought experiment of imagining that in order to save a person's life, his friends had kidnapped you and plugged your bodies together, and you woke up to be told that if you unplugged yourself at any time in the next nine months you would kill him, so that you must remain as you are for nine months to come. She takes it as obvious that you would nevertheless commit no injustice by unplugging yourself; and therefore if you remain plugged it is an act of charity rather than a strict duty. And from this she infers that similarly a mother has no strict duty to allow her unborn child to remain inside her.

But is this so obvious? First, what ought we to say about the thought experiment? The claim that you have no strict duty to refrain from unplugging yourself is derived from the supposed moral principle that you have an obligation only if you take it on voluntarily. But this is a very dubious principle: two plausible exceptions are the obligations to your parents and siblings, even though you did not ask to be born, and the obligations that arise purely because you happen to be in a certain place at a certain time, such as the obligation to rescue a drowning person if you are a strong swimmer and the only person around. Second, how alike are the two cases? Ways in which it has been suggested that they crucially differ include (1) that you are not the mother of the person you have been joined to; (2) that getting pregnant, except in the special case of rape, is a voluntary act (Judith Jarvis Thomson discusses this herself); and (3) that the commitment to a child is not for nine months but for twenty years, and in some respects until the death of one party, if not beyond.

The issue is rather like the problem of precedent in law. No two cases are exactly identical: the question is whether the later case is relevantly similar to the earlier case, and therefore should be decided in the same way, or whether there is a relevant difference. For example, the law of libel, relating to written material, is different from the law of slander, relating to spoken material. At one time it was uncertain whether recorded spoken material should come under slander because it was spoken or under libel because it was recorded: libel was the eventual decision. Similarly in ethics: even if we agree over what we would say in case X (and we may well not), there is still the problem of whether case X and case Y are relevantly alike. To give one more example of this, unfortunately not a mere thought experiment, those who oppose legalized euthanasia sometimes use the example of the Nazis, and point to the fact that the extermination program began with the "euthanasia" of the "unfit." Those who reject the analogy point out that even what the Nazis started with differed from anything proposed regarding euthanasia, (1) in being involuntary and (2) in having as its aim not the relief of suffering but the elimination of the "socially undesirable." And so the debates continue.

But to return to thought experiments. There is a contrasting use of them, in which the point is not the resemblance between the thought experiment and the actual situation, but precisely the difference. For example, writers sometimes consider what might or should be done if people were not liable to be corrupt, precisely in order to point out that as things are we need to do something different. This, though, is really a pedagogic use of the example: the point, that in devising structures and codes we have to remember human corruptibility, could be made without it, but gains some force from a comparison with how uncorrupt beings might do things.

More subtle is the use of examples somewhat in the manner of Mill's method of difference, in which the imagining of a society without some major feature of our own may help to show the ethical importance of that feature. Or the process may be reversed: there have been attempts to get at what is essential in human personhood by asking what animals or machines would have to be able to do, in addition to what they do already, for us to grant that they are persons. Here we have something more than the pedagogic: we do have a way of getting suggestions as to what skills, if any, are conclusive evidence of personhood. But once again, anything we come up with is controversial: there is room for disagreement both over what we would say and how much it proves. We know that chimpanzees can develop some linguistic skills: we still have the question whether this can ever amount to a language and the question, supposing it can, of how this should affect our ethical attitude to this species. So, once again, the example introduces new ideas into the argument but does not determine the outcome.

One final general point remains, especially with regard to the use of thought experiments. If the experiment requires us to posit something radically different from our actual situation, is it legitimate to refuse to accept it at all, on the ground either that we simply do not know what we would say under those conditions or that it is so different from actual conditions as to be irrelevant? It would seem that much depends on the use that the writer or lecturer wants to make of the thought experiment, and the inference that he or she wants to draw. But we can make the general point, that when someone invokes "what we would say if…" one response may be, on occasion, that because what follows the "if" is totally different from anything we have experienced we are not in a position to know what we would say: we would, as it were, be different people! And even when we feel that we know what we would say, there is still the question of how it is to be applied.

The conclusion of all this seems to be as follows. Examples have an important pedagogic role in bringing an issue alive. They also have an important role in introducing new relevant considerations into an argument, especially, but not only, by being used as counter-examples and thought experiments. But it is never, or hardly ever, beyond dispute (1) in what terms, above all in what moral terms, the example should be described, (2) whether it is relevant at all to the issue in hand, and (3) how it is relevant, if it is. Consequently, one should normally not expect an example to succeed in establishing a point once and for all, or even in determining the progress of the argument for the hearers or readers, even though this may well be the aim of the person who has introduced it. What examples are able to do, in addition to their pedagogic function, is to introduce something new into the argument, and especially to draw attention to a relevant principle that is getting overlooked or even that has not previously been considered. Finally, to return to pedagogic considerations, we should note that this is often most effective if the example is important rather than trivial and is taken from fact rather than fiction. With regard to the validity of the argument these considerations do not matter, but with regard to effective presentation they do!

NOTES

1. Ernest Gellner, *Words and Things* (Harmondsworth: Penguin, 1959).

2. Anne Maclean, *The Elimination of Morality: Reflections on Utilitarianism and Bioethics* (London: Routledge, 1993), pp. 35–36.

3. *Ibid.*, p. 30.

4. *Ibid.*, pp. 35–36.

5. Judith Jarvis Thomson, "A Defense of Abortion," *Philosophy and Public Affairs*, 1:1 (1971), pp. 47–66.

Six

MORAL INTUITIONS IN BIOETHICS

Harry Lesser

1. Introduction

In the methodology of philosophical ethics, and perhaps especially bioethics, the relation between ethical theories and specific moral convictions, often called "intuitions," about what is right or wrong, good or bad, raises an important theoretical and practical problem. Should the intuitions give way to the theory or the theory give way to the intuitions, and if it should be sometimes the one and sometimes the other, on what grounds should this be decided? As a first move, let us consider the suggestion, quite often either made explicitly or else presupposed, that intuitions are in this area epistemologically superior to theories, however rationally based, so that it is a requirement of an ethical theory that it be consistent with our ordinary moral intuitions, just as a scientific theory must be consistent with the observations. Admittedly, in both cases what is meant by "consistency" is a complex matter. In science, this sometimes refers to observations that are nearly universal (for example, any account of the real movements of the heavenly bodies must explain their apparent movements), more often to observations which require complex apparatus and training both to make and to interpret. In ethics the "intuitions" are sometimes ones very widely accepted, such as the wrongness of punishing the innocent, sometimes the intuitions of people thought to be specially qualified because of their particular experience or moral seriousness or sensibility. But that there should be this consistency has been often held, especially by the classical ethicists.

Aristotle, Kant, and Bentham all imply, to put it no more strongly, that they see themselves as providing a more explicit and rationally argued account of the basis and the implications of what most people believe already, and as going beyond this only at a later stage, if at all. Aristotle refers several times to what is "generally agreed";[1] Kant starts explicitly with "ordinary rational knowledge" of morality;[2] Bentham argues explicitly that everyone is in practice a utilitarian.[3] With the support of these great names, can we not therefore agree that consistency with ordinary moral intuitions must be a requirement for any ethical theory? We should not argue from authority, but with these authorities behind us may we not expect to find good arguments for proceeding in this way?

2. Are Intuitions Superior to Theories?

There are indeed three possible arguments for giving the priority to moral intuitions. The first is that intuitions are a very much more powerful motivating force than are conclusions from theories, however rationally based; and ethics is above all about motivating and guiding action. A firm conviction that an action is wrong, however arrived at, is more effective in preventing a person from doing it than is the same conclusion merely logically derived from a plausible premise. An example, which I used also in a previous volume in this series, is C. S. Lewis's rhetorical question whether you would rather play cards with a man who knew all the rational arguments against cheating or a man who had been brought up from childhood to believe that a gentleman just does not cheat.[4] Now this does indeed show that it is not easy for intuitions to be altered; and also, arguably, that sometimes, maybe often, it would be better not only not to try to alter them but also not even to try to reinforce them with rational arguments, which could have the unfortunate effect of raising unnecessary doubts. But it does not show that it is never right to challenge these intuitions. In this example, the intuition appears on reflection to be obviously a rational one, and it coincides with the conclusions of all serious ethical theories. But sometimes there are serious grounds for holding that the intuition is irrational, for example, if it is a passionate belief in the moral wrongness of "inter-racial" sex; and then the mere strength of the conviction gives not the slightest ground for preferring it, as a guide to morality, over the rational conclusion that the skin color of the participants has no possible relevance to whether a sexual act is right or wrong. (These prejudices may have to be taken into account, like it or not, when considering how to behave in a particular society, and whether it is necessary to let ill alone; but that is another matter altogether.)

The second argument may have more force. In Book I of the *Nicomachean Ethics* Aristotle points out, in effect, that intuitions in ethics necessarily precede theories.[5] The exact point he makes is that people cannot benefit from the study of philosophical ethics—and since ethics is always a practical branch of knowledge, cannot make themselves better—unless they already have both experience of life and a good moral training. This implies that learning that specific types of action are right or wrong has to precede the construction of any general moral theory: it is not just that we have to be taught to behave properly at an age when we cannot theorize, but that we could not form theories at any time unless we already had the practical experience. In turn, this implies that any theory will be necessarily influenced by the prior training of the theorist and the specific convictions which it has produced. No doubt this is true; but it does not follow that the theory will be totally determined by what has been previously believed and that the theorist cannot reach any conclusions which differ from what they were taught in childhood.

Aristotle himself in Book X of the *Ethics* reached conclusions about the supreme value of contemplation that most people of his time would, as he knew, find very surprising;[6] his teacher Plato had earlier come up with some startling ideas about the appropriate role of women in society.[7] Specific intuitions must contribute to the forming of theories, and any theory will show their influence; but this does not show that the theory must or should be consistent with all, or any specific one, of them. An ethical theory could presumably not be inconsistent with all of them and still be intelligible, just as a scientific theory could not be inconsistent with all of our pre-scientific beliefs and still be intelligible. But no single belief, of either sort, should be immune from change if rationality and the evidence require it. What after all is more apparently obvious than that the sun goes round the earth?

So these two arguments give us grounds for taking intuitions very seriously, but not for preferring them to the results of a rationally worked out ethical theory. But the third argument is stronger. This is the argument that intuitions have a better epistemological basis than do theories. Intuitions are often based on direct experience of how you have reacted to situations or actions, whether your own or other people's, and whether actual or considered; otherwise, they are based on your training, which, it might be argued, passes on the experience of previous generations. In contrast, theories are based on reasoning; and the likelihood of making mistakes in reasoning, however skilled you become, is always extremely high: if this were not the case, many philosophical problems would by now have been solved, or at least we would be agreed as to the nature of the problem and the kind of solution required. So, it might be said, a strong conviction that something is right or wrong is always more reliable than a philosophical argument leading to the opposite conclusion, just as G. E. Moore and others have claimed that they were more sure that the physical world existed than they were of the soundness of the arguments for saying it does not.[8] This is the strongest argument for giving the preference to intuitions.

3. The Problem

By the same token, this is where the problem begins. We do indeed have these moral convictions. Sometimes it is entirely appropriate to treat them like experimental results in science, and require a theory incompatible with them to be rejected or modified; at other times, in contrast, it is appropriate to prefer the dictates of reason to what seems to be arbitrary prejudice. Thus, to repeat an example from my earlier chapter, a common objection to utilitarianism as a moral theory is that a utilitarian code would require us on occasion to act very unjustly, for example to frame an innocent person for a crime or to use torture to get information, since sometimes the good to society would outweigh the harm to the individual. This objection presupposes that the wrongness of the actions is more certain than the soundness of the arguments for utilitarianism: otherwise the utilitarian could simply reply that the intuitions are understandable but mistaken. A few utilitarians have taken this line; but the more usual response is to accept the intuition as valid and then argue that an appropriately modified utilitarian theory, that pays proper attention to long-term consequences and not just immediate ones, does not yield these results, because the acceptance of these practices, even as ones to be very rarely adopted, would in the long run do far more harm than good. Thus in the development of modern utilitarianism, for example in R.M. Hare's *Moral Thinking*, the intuition has functioned like a deviant experimental result that produces a modification of a theory to make it more accurate.[9]

In contrast to this, consider the view, still held by a few, that homosexuality is proved to be wrong because the thought of it makes them feel sick. There is quite rightly a rejection of this kind of argument, on the ground that the so-called "yuk factor" is simply morally irrelevant. The mere existence of the emotion of disgust as such, which can be elicited, for example by a type of food or the sight of mud and slime, proves nothing at all about the moral status of an activity, unless there are grounds for saying that the disgust itself is a moral response, for example to the bullying or deceiving of the helpless. In itself the fact that some, or many, people are physically disgusted by an activity is relevant to whether it may be performed or simulated in public, but proves nothing at all about whether it is right or wrong. There may be grounds for saying that homosexuality is wrong, though this is far from obvious; but the fact that we in the heterosexual majority find it physically disgusting cannot be one of them.

Hence the problem. What distinguishes the case of homosexuality from the case of punishing the innocent? What is the difference between those cases when we should rely on the intuition and those when we should rely on the theory, and what justifies making this distinction? Talk of a "reflective equilibrium," found for example in discussions of Rawls's work, acknowledges the problem but does not solve it.[10] One cannot solve the problem by constructing a more elaborate theory, because the issue is precisely the relation between intuitions and theory. One also cannot realistically solve it by always relying on theory: even if we deny, on metaphysical or epistemic grounds, that there really are moral intuitions in the full sense of the word, we shall have to admit, as the example of punishing the innocent shows, that sometimes we are more sure that an action is right or is wrong than we are of the validity of any argument to the contrary. Yet one cannot solve it purely by appealing to intuition, because, as the example of inter-racial sex shows, we still have to find a way of distinguishing genuine moral intuitions from mere cultural prejudice. So how should we proceed?

4. Tackling the Problem

I suggest that as a first move we should distinguish between moral and non-moral reactions, positive and negative. As an example, I will try to spell out in more detail what I said above about disgust. Disgust may be stimulated by either physical or moral conditions, by the smell of a sewer or by blatant hypocrisy. It could be argued that we have here two different emotions, called by the same name, and that, though in either situation a person might say "I feel sick," they would mean it literally in one case and metaphorically in the other. Nothing hangs on this: we can take either view, but we must recognize that physical and moral disgust are different but can be confused. There is such a thing as morally disgusting sexual behavior, such as using physical or psychological pressure to obtain sexual favors, as by an adult on a child or near-child. But the disgust produced in (probably) the majority by homosexuality or (probably) a minority by some heterosexual variations is a purely physical disgust, and to base a moral judgment on it is a category-mistake: moral and physical are different categories.

What happens psychologically here is analogous to what happens when someone dislikes a person or a group. That person begins with the dislike, and pretends to herself that it is directed at the bad qualities of the individual or the group, usually bad qualities they do not in fact possess, when in fact the object of dislike is simply the person or group as such. Much racism is of this type; it was well analyzed many years ago in an article by C.D. Broad.[11] So here: one dislikes the activity on purely physical grounds and pretends that one dislikes it because it is wicked. In other cases the basis for the dislike may be psychological or cultural, rather than physical, as with the aversion of some people to inter-racial sex. Again, what is disturbing is confused with what is wrong.

A similar thing happens at the other end of the pleasure-pain scale, when what is simply pleasant may be confused with what is virtuous or creditable. One example of this happily belongs in our society largely to the past. It is the satisfaction over severe punishment, especially corporal or capital punishment, which would now often be seen as sadism or self-righteousness, but which was taken previously as moral endorsement. There are very strong arguments for punishing some types of behavior very severely (though probably not physically in this way), but the fact that people find it satisfying is not one of them.

A different kind of example is the assumption made by some people that because a certain way of life, or a certain way of conducting part of their lives, such as work, or family life, or religion, suits them and their circle, it not only suits everyone else but is morally what they ought to aim at. What they recommend may indeed have merits, but the mere fact that they like it and it suits them does not in any way show that people with quite different needs, tastes, and abilities are obliged to follow them.

Finally, a more subtle example. Some activities may appear, especially to those performing them, to be the discharge of a moral duty, and in that way give satisfaction to their agent, but turn out on examination to be neutral or even harmful, the harm arising precisely because the attention of the agent is on their own feelings and not on the actual effect of their actions. One fictional example is in a story in Gogol's *Mirgorod*, in which a certain Ivan, a relatively wealthy man, makes a point of always talking pleasantly to beggars after church on Sunday but fails to give them any money.[12] He feels he has acted well by making himself agreeable; and he is totally oblivious to the pain he has caused by raising expectations and not fulfilling them.

We thus have a variety of examples of the confusion of the non-moral with the moral. This gives us the first step, though only the first, in dealing with the problem: we have to make sure that we are dealing with a true moral intuition and not merely a feeling that something is physically or psychologically nice or nasty. We also have to acknowledge that the point is practical and not merely academic, because this confusion is often made.

But one objection could be made at this point. Granted the distinction, it might be said, what we find pleasant or unpleasant is a reliable guide to what is in fact good or bad. Disgusting things, like dirt, ordure, and rotten food, are also unhealthy, while the foods that we like and want are also those we need. Similarly hunger, thirst, wanting to excrete, and wanting to sleep are all desires that correlate with the body's needs. The exceptions to this, such as addiction, are the result either of illness, as in the desire of the diabetic for sugar when they need insulin, or of a perverted physical or psychological palate. So, it could be urged, the disgust of a healthy person is, in the appropriate context, a reliable sign of something morally wrong, and the relish of a healthy person a sign of moral worth.

There are two problems with this. One is the difficulty of defining "healthy" in a way that is not circular. The other is that even physically it is not always true: even healthy people often enjoy eating more sweet things than is good for them. Still less is it always true morally: even healthy people do not necessarily enjoy hard work or dislike idleness or are able always to be well-behaved to other people without effort! So the point seems to stand: we need to be clear whether we are dealing with a moral intuition or a feeling of mere attraction or repulsion. The second of these should perhaps on occasion encourage us to try to work out the moral position, but it cannot by itself ever tell us what it is.

5. Moral and Non-Moral Reactions

If the above is more or less correct, we have some idea of what a moral intuition is not, but less idea so far of what it is. As a first move we may agree with Hume that the moral attitude is by definition disinterested, that is, concerned with the general effects of an action rather than with its effect on oneself: thus a criminal might consider his sentence to imprisonment unpleasant but in no way unjust. Indeed, some of the above examples relate essentially to the difference between what is pleasant or unpleasant for the individual and what can appropriately arouse moral approval or disapproval.[13]

But this is not enough. The attitude to homosexuality that I have argued is physical rather than moral may still be a kind of disinterested disgust, a disgust that this should take place at all rather than that one might ever oneself have to witness it. Yet it is at best aesthetic rather than moral. Morality is not only a matter of disinterested reactions, but, one may suggest, of responses to what affects human welfare in general and its distribution.

Now as soon as one says this, one must make some modifications, or it will be plainly untrue. Many people now would extend morality to include the welfare of animals, or even of the environment in general. In contrast, in the past many people have seen their duty as extending to only part of the human race: this may well be the wrong moral position to adopt, but it is still a moral position. Second, "welfare" can be interpreted in more than one way, in particular either as involving the satisfaction of desires or as involving human development and fulfillment—the line favored, in different ways and not always explicitly, by Aristotle, Kant, and Mill.[14] But it remains true that to count as "moral," a claim or intuition must relate to some conception of welfare. Thus, to say that homosexuality is wrong because it is disgusting is to fail to make a moral claim at all. To say, in contrast, that it is wrong because it is a form of sexuality which stunts human development rather than enhancing it is to make a genuine moral claim—though one which requires further evidence and may well turn out to be false.

If this conclusion is correct, there are some interesting consequences for bioethics. These consequences do not settle any issue, but show something about what kinds of appeals are relevant. Appeals to the disgusting or aesthetically unpleasing nature of a proposed procedure, though often made, are irrelevant to whether it is right or wrong, though they may be relevant to whether it should be introduced into a particular society at a particular time. Various other kinds of irrelevant appeal are also sometimes made. For example, one is sometimes told that the high number of abortions in our society is "unacceptable." Now there are various moral views of abortion; and on some of these all, and on some part, of the abortions performed ought not to be performed; and these views should be considered. But numbers are relevant only when one is dealing with an activity which does good, or at least no harm, if practiced to a limited extent but becomes harmful when this limit is passed: and abortion is surely either right or wrong from the start. A final example would be, in contrast to these, the attempt to justify a change of procedure precisely on the ground that it is startling and repellent: "we must think the unthinkable." A policy might be right despite being startling but hardly *because* it is startling. Indeed this particular appeal is, as far as I know, never made explicitly; but it is made at the level of implication and innuendo, as a way of making people feel brave and good for supporting it!

So we can, I think, identify the genuine moral intuitions, which are those which are disinterested and which relate to some conception of welfare, human or animal. But we now have another problem: it is notorious that these "intuitions" differ over time, between societies and between individuals. This is true, but some seem to be universal. Thus there are many different views about punishment, both at the social level and in homes and schools. There is disagreement about whether it should be used at all, about the forms it should take, about what kinds of behavior should be punished and with what severity. But there is no disagreement on the point that, whatever the rules of a particular system are or should be, the "innocent" should not be punished. This point, if obvious once pointed out, is not trivial: there are still many countries where, even if the law is oppressive, people would be very grateful for a system under which they could be reasonably sure of being unmolested as long as they obeyed it.

Some people have argued that principles of this sort are actually innate. There is an interesting example in Truffaut's film *L'enfant sauvage* and the eighteenth-century account on which it is based. There was a boy of about twelve found in the woods in southern France, having been lost or abandoned many years previously and having somehow learned to survive. A doctor took him in and taught him to live in human society, and also studied his behavior. He disciplined the boy by making him sit in a cupboard when he misbehaved; and the boy accepted the discipline. To see if the boy had a sense of justice, despite never having been in human society since infancy, he tried to put him in the cupboard when he had not misbehaved. The boy fought back and struggled violently, whereupon the doctor released him and embraced him, delighted with this proof, as he thought, that the sense of justice is innate. Whether or not it establishes this much, it seems at least to establish that the existence of rules is sufficient to create the expectation that one should be punished only if one has broken them. It also suggests that awareness of a moral principle does not require that it be verbalized or even conscious, since it can be demonstrated by a person's behavior, or as here by the contrast between how the boy behaved on this occasion and how he behaved when the punishment was fair or legitimate.

Intuitions of this sort are more numerous than one might at first think. That the "innocent" (as defined by the rules) should not be punished is only one of a number of intuitive principles of justice. Others are the principles that no one should be a judge in his or her own case, and that both sides should be heard. These are primarily legal maxims, but operate also in moral contexts. A more complex example is the keeping of promises and contracts. It is more complex because many, maybe most, people would hold that, although a promise creates a *prima facie* duty, the duty can be overridden—for example, if the promise was exacted by force or if to keep it would do great harm—but there is also disagreement as to exactly when breaking a promise becomes permissible. Yet the intuition that making a promise creates a duty to keep it, other things being equal, seems to be universal: what else could be the point of promising? There may indeed also be bizarre circumstances under which it becomes right to punish the innocent, but in principle and under normal conditions it is unjust.

All this raises the question of the content of these intuitions, once one grants that people who hold them are not always able to put them into words. This suggests that they are clear about their basic content but may not have worked out the details. Thus we may all be clear that one should keep promises, but some of us may simply never have had occasion to reflect on whether this is always the case or whether there are exceptions, and others may be clear that there can be exceptions but be unclear as to what they are and perhaps feel that one can worry about that if and when the time comes. So even when something is a *prima facie* duty that admits of exceptions—and maybe Aristotle was right to think that all duties are of this type[15]—it can still be the object of a general intuition that it is a duty: perhaps indeed, if one excludes young children and the mentally ill, a universal intuition.

What these moral intuitions, which include not only principles of justice but also, very importantly, basic duties such as not to murder or steal or lie, have in common is not only that they are very widely held but also that their total denial, as opposed to their admitting of principled exceptions for which reasons can be given, involves a kind of unintelligibility. So if the penalties for breaking the rules landed as often, or more often, on those who kept them as on those who broke them, there would be no system of rules. One cannot have contracts without a duty to keep them, or property without the prohibition of theft, or communication without a presumption that people speak the truth, or society without the outlawing of murder. This feature, that the total removal of these principles is actually unintelligible, shows, I think, that the intuitions of which they are the content are intuitions with which any moral theory must be consistent.

But this claim is not actually as strong as it looks at first sight. All these principles seem to admit of exceptions, sometimes indeed of quite frequent, though principled, exceptions: murder may be an exception, in that "murder" and its equivalents in other languages are defined as "wrongful killing," but the problem will then re-emerge in that there can be disputes as to what morally constitutes murder. So the intuitions can be consistent with a variety of overlapping but different theories, which may recognize different kinds of exceptions or indeed may recognize none. What is excluded is a theory leading to the conclusion that one of these principles was not a moral principle at all or could be regularly and easily overridden.

One such theory is act-utilitarianism in its crude form, the view that in each situation one should perform the action likely to do the most good or the least harm, that is, produce the most pleasure or the least pain. It follows from this that one ought to break promises not only when keeping them would do great harm but whenever it would do more good or less harm than keeping them. This conclusion is absurd: one cannot simultaneously have people making and exacting promises and at the same time breaking them whenever it is better on the whole! So the intuition must be preferred to the theory. Indeed no one now holds this crude version of utilitarianism, and partly because of this argument, which has been made many times already, and which first appears, though in a different context, in the examples of moral duties in Part II of Kant's *Groundwork for the Metaphysics of Morals*.[16]

So at one end of the spectrum we have moral principles which cannot be totally denied without absurdity, such as the principle that promises must be kept, and with these any theory of ethics must conform. At the other end we have psychological reactions "masquerading" as moral principles. These not merely may but positively ought to be ignored, as guides to general right and wrong, by the ethical theorist, though they may affect decisions as to what it is politically necessary to take into account. But what about the middle of the spectrum, the intuitions which are clearly moral but lack this logical or quasi-logical backing? In particular what is to be done when intuitions conflict, as they seem to do in the case of abortion? Even when there is now agreement, we have to acknowledge that this was not always so. The use of torture to extract information is now prohibited in the UN Universal Declaration of Human Rights and the EU Charter of Fundamental Rights and officially condemned very widely—though it often takes place and some have argued for its legalization. But past ages accepted it as necessary; and only a few legal systems tried to do without it. In the light of this, can any intuitions of this sort be used to test theories, given the absence of universal support?

A possible suggestion is this. In the case of torture, one thing is not in dispute, namely that if it is wrong it is very gravely wrong: it not only causes pain but also violates human dignity. It is also the case that even supposing it to be justifiable, to forbid it would do little if any harm, given that other methods of obtaining information are probably more efficient as well as more humane. Hence to allow torture is to run the risk of doing a grave wrong, for little if any gain; and this is incompatible with a serious ethical approach. In short, an intuition that something, if it is wrong, is a grave wrong is still the kind of intuition that can be used to test a theory. A theory that justified torture under extreme circumstances is a possible moral theory (whether or not a correct one); but a theory that treats it as a normal practice cannot be—despite the fact that earlier ages failed to recognize this, and we are in general not obviously better than them. Similar things could be said about the intuition against slavery.

But, it might be asked, how is the case of abortion different? In the case of torture, or of slavery, it is not in dispute that great harm is done by the practice: the defense can be only that this *might* be outweighed by the subsequent good, and this is a defense that lacks what may be called moral seriousness. It is also not in dispute that little or no harm is done by not allowing torture as a general practice (as opposed to under some extreme conditions). But in the case of abortion the degree of harm done is disputed, since people dispute the moral status of the fetus/unborn child, the degree of harm done by not allowing it is also disputed, and that not allowing abortion does much harm (even though some would say less harm than allowing it does) is generally agreed. It seems therefore that here intuitions will not help us. But it may be that there is more to be said.

6. Conclusion

We may sum up as follows. Some apparent moral intuitions are in fact merely physical or psychological reactions, and there is no requirement for an ethical theory to be consistent with them. With regard to genuine moral intuitions, there are three kinds of case. There are issues such as abortion and animal rights where the "intuitions" conflict and seem to offer no help: one reason for this is that the whole moral status of unborn children and animals is very difficult to determine. There are issues where the intuition that something is wrong has not been universal, as with torture and slavery, but where the intuition that if it is wrong it is a grave wrong is enough to show that no serious moral theory can endorse the practice, since even to run the risk of such grave wrong is incompatible with moral seriousness. Finally there are intuitions about principles which cannot be totally abandoned if we are to have a moral code at all, such as the principles that promises should be kept and that the innocent should not be punished. With regard to bioethics the most relevant part of this conclusion, assuming it to be correct, is the negative part, the suggestion that "intuitions" which are in fact disputed or which turn out to be non-moral should be rejected. But there are also the intuitions that particular policies or actions may involve the risk, even if not the certainty, of grave harm: and these should be respected by any serious theory in bioethics.

NOTES

1. Aristotle, *Nicomachean Ethics* (Oxford: OUP World's Classics, 1998).

2. Immanuel Kant, *Groundwork for the Metaphysics of Morals,* ed. Lara Denis (Plymouth: Broadview, 2005).

3. Jeremy Bentham, *An Introduction to the Principles of Morals and Legislation* (Oxford: Blackwell, 1960).

4. C. S. Lewis, *Present Concerns* (Glasgow: Collins, 1986), pp.105–106.

5. Aristotle, *Ethics,* pp. 4–6.

6. Aristotle, *Ethics,* bk. 10.

7. Plato, *Republic* (Harmondsworth: Penguin, 1987), bk. 5.

8. G. E. Moore, "A Defence of Common Sense," *Philosophical Papers* (New York: Collier, 1966), pp. 32–59.

9. R. M. Hare, *Moral Thinking* (Oxford: Oxford University Press, 1981).

10. *E.g.*, Ronald Dworkin, "The Original Position", *Reading Rawls*, ed. Norman Daniels (Oxford: Blackwell, 1978), pp. 16–52.

11. C. D. Broad, "Various Uses of the Term 'Unconscious,'" *Proceedings of the Aristotelean Society,* 23 (1922–1923), pp. 173–198.

12. Nikolai Gogol, "The Story of How Ivan Ivanovich Quarrelled with Ivan Nikiforovich," *Village Evenings near Dikanka* and *Mirgorod* (Oxford: Oxford University Press World's Classics, 1994), pp. 406–452.

13. David Hume, *Enquiry Concerning the Principles of Morals* (Oxford: OUP, 2004), pp. 104–118.

14. Aristotle, *Ethics,* esp. bks. 1 and 10; Kant, *Groundwork,* esp. section 2; John Stuart Mill, *On Liberty* (Oxford: Oxford University Press, 1998), esp. ch. 3.

15. Aristotle, *Ethics*, pp. 2–3.

16. Kant, *Groundwork*, p. 82. See also John Searle, "How to Derive 'Ought' from 'Is,'" *The Is/Ought Question*, ed. W. D. Hudson (London: Macmillan, 1972), pp. 120–134; and John Rawls, "Two Concepts of Rules," *Contemporary Utilitarianism*, ed. Michael D. Bayles (New York: Doubleday, 1968).

Seven

TOWARD THE "FAIR USE" OF EMPIRICAL EVIDENCE IN ETHICAL ARGUMENTS: VACCINATION, MMR, AND DISAGREEMENT

Angus Dawson

1. Introduction

Some ethical arguments use premises that (explicitly or implicitly) contain an appeal to empirical evidence (either quantitative or qualitative in nature). Such arguments, therefore, rely upon empirical evidence to support the argument's conclusion. Let us call such arguments "evidence-dependent" ethical arguments. One problem with such arguments is that they are potentially vulnerable if the empirical evidence itself is contested or controversial. Given the nature of empirical evidence, this will often be the case. The result is that it is very common for different ethical views to emerge on an issue in bioethics because authors make different assessments of the same evidence or, alternatively, appeal to different (and often contradictory) evidence. As a result ethical disagreement persists because of a dispute about the supporting empirical evidence. Good examples of issues in healthcare ethics where this kind of gridlock exists are arguments about the use of drugs in psychiatry and the harms and benefits of reproductive technologies such as surrogacy and *in vitro* fertilization (IVF).[1] Some progress might be made in assessing the evidence-dependent ethical arguments related to such topics once we have a set of criteria in place to establish what might count as "fair use" of empirical evidence in such arguments.

The relationship between empirical evidence and ethical arguments has long been a source of discussion in the ethics literature. However, in this chapter I am not concerned, at least directly, with the well-worn issue of whether or not it is legitimate to move from empirical factual matters to normative conclusions (the so-called is-ought problem).[2] Here I will assume that there are at least some ways of being able validly to make this type of move within the context of an argument.[3] However, even if this turns out to be false, the appeal to empirical evidence in the premises of ethical arguments is so common that it seems appropriate to explore this issue independently of any conclusion to the is-ought debate.

Evidence-dependent ethical arguments are perhaps more common in the bioethics literature than might be expected. They involve an appeal to empirical evidence relating to the particular ethical issue under discussion. For example, many consequentialist arguments will involve a judgment about the actual or likely balance between the harms and benefits following from an action (or inaction). In such arguments a claim is made that we should perform a particular action (or continue with an inaction) because the best possible outcome will result. Of course, this type of calculation can only be made if the relevant empirical evidence is either available or could in principle become available. However, it is not just consequentialists who will be concerned with how empirical evidence is used in ethical arguments. Other moral traditions, such as deontology (at least in some forms) will have similar concerns. For example, if a deontologist wants to argue that surrogacy will be harmful to the resulting child, empirical evidence will have to play some role in the argument (whether directly or indirectly).

Why try and construct some principles to guide the "fair use" of empirical evidence in ethical arguments? The reason is that such principles can give us a set of criteria for judging the quality of the empirical evidence that is invoked: we will then be in a position better to evaluate the evidence-dependent ethical arguments themselves. The principles are necessary because while in some cases the evidence is clear and supports a particular and uncontroversial conclusion, it is far more common to find that the interpretation of empirical evidence is contested, and may involve an assessment of complicated, unclear, and contradictory results. Even so the use of empirical evidence in ethical arguments is important. The aim of this chapter is not to suggest that the use of ethical arguments employing empirical evidence is illegitimate but that we need to take care that the evidence used is of the best possible quality. It is suggested that the employment of principles of "fair use" (or something like them) will ensure that the empirical evidence used in ethical arguments meets this criterion. Any ethical argument that is then proposed that uses empirical evidence in its premises can be evaluated (to some extent) independently of its conclusion. It is important to see that the suggested "fair use" principles are only a minimum requirement applying to the empirical content of the argument. The principles will not, of course, guarantee that the argument employing the empirical evidence is valid or that the conclusion is true.

In the second section of this chapter I outline and defend some principles of "fair use." In the third section I illustrate the discussion by looking at the use of empirical evidence in ethical arguments about the Mumps, Measles, and Rubella (MMR) combined vaccine. In the fourth section I discuss a number of possible objections to this approach.

2. Some Possible Principles for the "Fair Use" of Evidence

The following suggested four principles are not supposed to be an exhaustive list of all the relevant criteria when judging empirical evidence. Instead, they are given to illustrate the types of things that ought to be taken into consideration when constructing or reviewing ethical arguments that employ empirical evidence. The suggested principles are as follows:

(1) Any argument appealing to empirical evidence on a topic should take into account all of the relevant published evidence.

(2) Where there is uncertainty in the evidence this should be acknowledged.

(3) Not all evidence is of equal value.

(4) Consideration of the evidence should lead on to the development of the ethical perspective on that issue.

Let us discuss each of these suggested principles in more detail.

A. Principle 1: Any Argument Appealing to Empirical Evidence on a Topic Should Take into Account All of the Relevant Published Evidence

This principle is hopefully uncontroversial. The idea is that we should not just use the evidence that supports our own preconceived ideas or the conclusion that we might tend to favor or are seeking to convince others is true. Anyone employing empirical evidence as part of their ethical argument, should attempt to conduct a systematic review of all of the published (or any known unpublished) evidence on the particular topic to ensure that they are not providing a misleading picture as to what evidence exists. Such a principle also has an important practical role as any ethical argument that uses a biased selection from the available evidence will be weaker than one that does not. One consequence of this proposal is that it follows that anyone interested in producing evidence-dependent arguments will need to become familiar with the empirical literatures most relevant to their topic. This may include evidence from medical, sociological, historical, psychological, and other sources depending upon what the argument is about. One of the things that endangers this principle is the way that certain pieces of evidence are given prominence in various ways. For example, the media might report a particular study without providing the relevant context of previous work performed in the field. This is just the most obvious case of a bias that tends to exist in favor of the most recently published work. Another source of danger is that there is a bias in favor of the "iconoclastic" work that is seeking to attack an established view or suggests that some routine or common practice might be problematic for some reason. This first principle seeks to ensure a cautious evaluation of each piece of evidence within the framework of all of the relevant evidence available. In essence, this principle seeks to ensure the production of a fair assessment of the literature on a topic, before an argument is constructed or a conclusion is reached. The more thorough the review of the literature used as the basis of such evidence-dependent arguments, the stronger the ethical argument becomes.

B. Principle 2: Where There Is Uncertainty in the Evidence This Should Be Acknowledged

Evidence-dependent ethical arguments differ from *a priori* moral arguments because the strength of the argument is directly related to the strength of the relevant evidence itself. This is a problem because there will be a natural reluctance in the proponent of such an argument to acknowledge any uncertainty in the evidence used, as such an admission will weaken the ethical argument that is being presented. However, where the evidence is weak, ambiguous, or unavailable the person proposing the argument should acknowledge this. Where further studies would be helpful this should be pointed out and final judgment suspended until the evidence is available. Again this proposal is at least partly pragmatic, in that it endeavors to ensure that a proposed argument is not held to be so strong it can resist all challenges, only for someone to point out at a later stage a weakness in the relevant evidence used. Given the fact that many forms of research involving human subjects will be judged to be unethical, many of the arguments proposed within healthcare ethics are likely to remain only at the level of speculation: the evidence is not, and never will be, available. However, many other arguments can evolve as the evidence on a subject grows. This is, I think, an important feature of this type of argument. The strength of the argument will fluctuate depending upon the amount and quality of the evidence available at a particular time. It will, I am sure, be helpful to researchers in relevant empirical fields if such uncertainty is acknowledged and suggestions are made about what sort of evidence might be most useful in relation to reaching a reasonable conclusion to the ethical arguments. This second principle is essentially an appeal for an honest assessment of the quality of the empirical evidence available to the advocate of the ethical argument under consideration.

C. Principle 3: Not All Evidence is of Equal Value

Once again, this should be an uncontroversial statement as it is clearly apparent that different studies have different value: they use different methods, seek to address different research questions, and may have different "weight" in our deliberations about an issue. The alternative view would have to be that all studies are of equivalent value, which is absurd. I am not suggesting that we should see, say, quantitative studies as superior to qualitative studies, or that the only things that will really count as evidence are meta-analyses of randomized controlled trials. This can be left open. Evidence needs to be judged in terms of the research questions that have been set. The proposal behind this principle is much more modest. It is that if, say, one epidemiological study involves fewer participants than another, then all things being equal, that with more participants is methodologically superior. Likewise the qualitative study investigating patient perceptions of some aspect of medical care that is designed to elicit the participants' views clearly, is a better study than one that does not. However, issues to do with study design are complex and controversial. Different people may prefer different types of study. It might be that some decisions will have to be taken and defended about the relative merits of particular forms of research, or more modestly, that within the formulation of a particular type of study, agreement will be sought as to what factors may result in a better study than others. Despite the fact that we need to leave room for disagreement about the relative merits of different methodologies, we can also see the importance of weighing the available evidence fairly.

D. Principle 4: Consideration of the Evidence Should Lead on to the Development of the Ethical Perspective on That Issue

The reasoning behind this principle is that there is a strong temptation to select evidence to fit a pre-determined conclusion. By contrast, I suggest that the evidence should have "priority": the ethical argument should be formulated in the light of a detached assessment of all of the relevant evidence. Of course, we may all be guilty of a certain type of "selection bias" in such cases, but the idea would be that discussion of an ethical issue where empirical evidence is relevant should begin with a review and discussion of the empirical evidence; or if there is no evidence available then this should be noted, as well as the fact that the argument, as a result, is hypothetical. This principle is an appeal for "evidence-based" ethics, and it follows from and reinforces the other three suggested principles. Evidence-dependent ethical arguments are only as strong as the relevant evidence used in the argument. These principles are an attempt to suggest ways to strengthen the empirical claims used in support of the ethical arguments, and thereby strengthen the ethical arguments themselves. This point can be emphasized by considering an example.

3. The Use of Evidence: Vaccination Using MMR Vaccine

I have chosen to use the issue of evidence related to the mumps, measles, and rubella (MMR) vaccine and the way that such evidence might be used in ethical arguments as an example, because of the ongoing discussions, particularly within the United Kingdom, about whether parents should be offered the choice of single vaccines instead of the MMR combination vaccine.[4] There are, of course, many different ethical arguments that could be formulated about vaccination policies in general and MMR in particular.[5] For example, it is possible to construct an ethical argument focusing on the idea that it is for parents to choose whether or not to expose their children to actual or perceived harm based upon their own assessment of the relevant evidence.[6] In this chapter I will not consider such an argument in detail, but rather consider the prior question about how we should respond to the relevant evidence about the MMR vaccine, using the principles as outlined above.

A. Evidence-Dependent Ethical Argument Should Be Based upon All of the Relevant Evidence

One of the problems about the way that the MMR issue arose in the public consciousness in the UK was that it resulted from media reports of a single piece of research published in *The Lancet*.[7] Discussions of this study tended not to report that it was very tentative in nature, was based on a sample of twelve children, and that the paper explicitly noted that a causal link between MMR and autism and bowel disease had not been established. In fact, the media focused not on the rather cautious claims in the paper itself but upon the oral comments of Andrew Wakefield at the press conference related to the publication of the paper.[8] The reported comments were not placed in the context of the extensive publications that already existed, the longstanding use of MMR with no reported problems in many parts of the world, nor the possible dangers of measles as a disease (even in developed countries such as the United Kingdom). Judgments about the evidence need to take into account all of this evidence, rather than being based on a single publication. If the *Lancet* study had been placed in such a context, it is unlikely that it would have had the same impact. Even at the time of publication there was strong evidence that the MMR vaccine was safe, and such evidence was based on extensive epidemiological analysis of hundreds of thousands of children.[9] This has been confirmed by subsequent studies.[10]

Of course, discussion of such empirical evidence is always difficult. It is always possible that new studies might produce results that overturn established beliefs. However, there is a need when weighing harms and benefits to ensure that all of the relevant evidence should be taken into account. The published evidence did not (and does not) support the conclusions that Wakefield sought to draw from the paper. While parents might, understandably, seek not to expose their child to what they perceive as the harm involved in MMR vaccination, we should note that such a judgment is not based on a fair and full evaluation of all the relevant evidence. Respecting parental judgments in such a case involves choosing to respect the parents' *perception* of the evidence. However, this does not, of course, change the evidence itself. If parents are truly basing their decision on best interests considerations then they should consider all of the relevant evidence. Scientists, healthcare professionals, and journalists are, in turn, under an obligation to report all of the relevant evidence fairly, even where strong views are held or disagreement exists.

B. Acknowledge Uncertainty

The *Lancet* paper was carefully phrased to suggest the need for further investigation of the reported results. However, the paper does not reference or report the published research suggesting that MMR is safe. As suggested above, empirical evidence on any issue is never definitive, as it might be overturned by further research in the future. For example, it is always possible that any intervention might cause harm and that this only comes to light at a later date. However, given the relative weight of the evidence on the two sides in this particular case, the onus of proof was on the opponents of MMR to formulate the need for further work carefully. At the press conference and in interviews this was not done.[11] Where there is uncertainty there is nothing wrong with suggesting the need for further research. However, there is also a need to consider the potential problems that might emerge from misunderstandings of the evidence and an obligation to be cautious in drawing conclusions from a single small-scale piece of research. This is especially important when, as in this case, such interventions affect young children. There have been previous scares about vaccines, with tragic results.[12]

C. Not All Evidence is of Equal Value

This is perhaps the vital consideration in the MMR story. The *Lancet* paper, as suggested above, was based on small numbers and explicitly said that no causal link had been established. On the other hand, large-scale epidemiological studies suggested that the vaccine was safe. This suggests that the dispute was not a disagreement with equal evidence on both sides. Clearly the better quality evidence counted in favor of MMR. At best, all that Wakefield *et al* had was a possible temporal correlation between MMR and the onset of autism as reported by some of the parents involved. A temporal association does not justify the inference to the existence of a causal link. It would take much more to demonstrate such a relationship between the two events. At best, the *Lancet* study suggested grounds for further investigation. Such investigation has been conducted and no credible evidence for any link between MMR and autism has been established.

D. Evidence Before Ethics

While it is right that parents decide whether to vaccinate their children (at least in most cases), it is vital that all of the relevant evidence is considered.[13] There is a real danger that the results of a single study are used to motivate all of the ethical arguments in relation to MMR. Such an approach does not fairly weigh the available evidence, nor does it consider the reality of measles as a disease, nor the reality of a more complicated vaccinations routine involving six vaccinations rather than two. Clearly, there is a potential danger that the evidence of a single study is selected to support a pre-existing view about vaccinations. An opponent of vaccinations, or someone uninformed about the benefits (as well as the potential harms) of vaccinations, might be influenced not to consider all the available evidence relating to judgments about what is in the best interests of a child. If judgments about harm and benefits are to be made, they must be made on the basis of all of the relevant evidence.

4. Possible Objections to the Principles Approach

The discussion in this section includes a consideration of a number of possible objections to the principles approach to evidence-dependent ethical arguments as outlined in this chapter. I have suggested that such arguments are, in themselves, quite legitimate as long as they conform to the principles as outlined above. Once we have such criteria in place for assessing the relevant empirical evidence, the discussion can then move on to an assessment of the ethical arguments that build upon such evidence. However, it might be possible to offer some objections to the approach adopted in this chapter. I will outline and discuss only four objections here.

A. The "Ontological Objection"

This objection focuses on the claim that the approach outlined above is naïvely committed to the idea that we are able to access information about a world independent of any observer; that is, that evidence tells us something about an objective world through the production of facts. Of course such a form of realism might be used to support such claims about evidence.[14] However, it is not clear that the supporter of the view outlined above needs to be committed to realism. She just needs to be committed to the weaker claim, that we can distinguish and grade different forms of evidence. For such an objection really to be a threat, it would have to go further and provide its own theoretical justification for doubting that we can justifiably distinguish between different forms of evidence and different pieces of research. This looks implausible but might be linked to some form of subjectivism or relativism.

B. The "Relativity Objection"

This objection focuses on the idea that there is a plurality of views about the nature of the world and how we might investigate it. From this premise is drawn the conclusion that we therefore have no good grounds to prioritize one such view over any other. This might then, in turn, be used to argue that the evidence-based approach outlined above is committed to an "imperialist" agenda in seeing science as the main (or only) possible framework for experiencing the world. However, once again, it is not really clear that the supporter of the principles above is forced to accept such a view (even if they wish to defend it) as a weaker claim will again suffice. In this case, the weaker claim only needs to be that not all perspectives are equal, and that one that is committed to the types of principles outlined above is superior to one that is not (at least when we are seeking to judge empirical questions).

C. The "Epistemic Objection"

This objection focuses on the idea that uncertainty is a constant in medicine in relation to interventions and outcomes, and therefore it is naïve to believe that we can agree what counts as relevant evidence and agree how we should weigh it in a situation of disagreement. On such a view, knowledge might be something which is unobtainable. All we have, at best, is something provisional. There is a degree of truth in such a view. It is rare that we can all agree what counts as relevant or decisive evidence. However, a commitment to the principles outlined here does not require that all uncertainty be removed. All the principles require is that we can judge that some evidence is better than others, and that where uncertainty does exist we acknowledge this.

D. The "Autonomy Objection"

This objection is different in nature to the other three, as it involves an ethical claim. The objection is that individuals should be able to decide what counts as relevant evidence for their discussion in the light of what they believe. On this view, even if "objective" evidence exists it might only be one issue to consider. In such a case, it is up to an individual to decide what to do, and if their own views clash with the "evidence," their autonomous decision takes precedence. However, this view confuses two things: the relevant evidence and our actions. Even if we accept that it should be up to individuals whether they accept the evidence or not in terms of their own actions, this is a different issue from what the evidence might be. The evidence continues to exist whatever the individual might decide. While in liberal democracies we might choose to give priority to autonomous individuals to decide what to do, it is important that we see that this does not change the evidence as such. If we are talking about public policy, rather than individual action, particularly where it concerns vulnerable and incompetent individuals such as young children, the requirement for evidence-based decision-making is much stronger. In other contexts, if an evidence-dependent argument is presented appealing to the idea of harm and this is then used as the basis for arguing that something should be restricted or banned, such as commercial surrogacy or preimplantation genetic diagnosis, then any evidence about harm needs to be clear and convincing.[15]

5. MMR and the Four Objections

The first three objections relate to general issues in the philosophy of science and are not specific to the MMR issue. The arguments will stand or fall independently of this particular case. If the discussion about the evidence in relation to MMR using the principles above is convincing, then there will be a *prima facie* case for dismissing these objections. However, the last objection is particularly relevant to the MMR issue as something like it can be seen to be at least implicit in many of the discussions about the vaccine. Such an argument can be based on the idea that it is for parents to make judgments about risk in relation to their children and there is no role for the intervention of the state (or other third parties). This view can be supported by an appeal to the idea of parental autonomy in relation to parents' decisions affecting their children. There may be general acceptance of such an ethical argument, unless the risk of harm is significant.[16] However, whatever weighting we give to parental decision-making in relation to their own children, the situation is different if you have responsibility for formulating public policy, as suggested above. In this latter case, it might be relevant to ignore options that increase parental autonomy if the evidence suggests that such an option is not justifiable for other reasons. Such a basis might be given for the Department of Health's policy of supporting MMR and refusing to fund single vaccines. This policy can not only be supported because it provides the best fit with the relevant available evidence, but also because two publicly-funded parallel policies will be more expensive than one, and in addition, a policy based on support for single vaccines is likely to result in a negative impact upon the public's health.

6. Conclusion

In this chapter I have outlined a set of principles to use in considering whether the evidence appealed to in support of ethical arguments fairly represents the relevant existing evidence on that topic. The principles are not supposed to be the last word on this issue, but will, I hope, prove to be useful in making judgments about the quality of the relevant empirical evidence used in the premises of evidence-dependent ethical arguments. I have also outlined and explored how the principles might be useful in the context of an example (the recent debate about MMR vaccination), and considered and rejected a set of objections to a principle-based approach to the evaluation of evidence in ethical arguments.

Acknowledgment

Thanks to the audience at the XVIIth ESPMH Conference on Philosophy of Medicine and Healthcare in Malta for comments on an earlier version of this chapter.

NOTES

1. Angus Dawson "Psychopharmacology," *Encyclopedia of Applied Ethics,* vol. 3, ed. Ruth Chadwick (San Diego: Academic Press, 1998), pp. 727–734; Susan Golombok, *Parenting: What Really Counts?* (London: Routledge, 2000).

2. R. M. Hare, *The Language of Morals* (Oxford: Oxford University Press, 1952).

3. Charles R. Pigden, "Naturalism," *A Companion to Ethics*, ed. Peter Singer (Oxford: Blackwell, 1991).

4. Tom Heller, Dick Heller, Stephen Pattison, and Tom Heller, "Ethical Debate: Vaccination Against Mumps, Measles, and Rubella: Is There a Case for Deepening the Debate?' *British Medical Journal*, 323:7317 (13 October 2001), pp. 838–840; Michael Jarmulowicz. "Single Measles Vaccine Should be Allowed"; *British Medical Journal* 324:7339 (23 March 2002), p. 733.

5. In general: Jeffrey B. Ulmer and Margaret A. Liu, "Ethical Issues for Vaccines and Immunization," *Nature Reviews: Immunology*, 2:4 (2002), pp. 291–296; Tim Dare, "Mass Immunisation Programmes: Some Philosophical Issues," *Bioethics*, 12:2 (April 1998), pp. 125–149; Marcel Verweij and Angus Dawson, "Ethical Principles for Collective Immunisation Programmes," *Vaccine*, 22 (13 August 2004), pp. 3122–3126; Angus Dawson, "Vaccination and the Prevention Problem," *Bioethics*, 18:6 (November 2004), pp. 515–530. In particular: Angus Dawson, "Risk Perceptions and Ethical Public Health Policy: MMR in the UK," *Poiesis and Praxis*, 3:4 (December 2005), pp. 229–241.

6. Angus Dawson, "The 'Best Interests' Argument and Childhood Immunisation," *Bioethics*, 19:1 (February 2005), pp. 72–89.

7. Andrew J. Wakefield, S. H. Murch, A. Anthony, J. Linnell, D. M. Casson, M. Malik, and M. Berelowitz, "Ileal-Lymphoid-Nodular Hyperplasia, Non-Specific Colitis

and Pervasive Developmental Disorder in Children," *Lancet*, 351:9103 (28 February 1998), pp. 637–641.

8. Michael Fitzpatrick, *MMR and Autism: What Parents Need to Know* (London: Routledge, 2004).

9. David Elliman and Helen Bedford, "MMR Vaccine: The Continuing Saga," *BMJ*, 322:7280 (27 January 2001), pp. 183–184; Annamari Patja, Irja Davidkin, Tapio Kurki, Markku Kallio, Martti Valle, and Heikki Peltola, "Serious Adverse Events after Measles-Mumps-Rubella Vaccination During a Fourteen-Year Prospective Follow-up," *The Pediatric Infectious Disease Journal*, 19: 12 (December 2000), pp. 1127–1134; Heikki Peltola, and Olli P. Heinonen, "Frequency of True Adverse Reactions in Measles-Mumps-Rubella Vaccine: A Double-Blind Placebo-Controlled Trial in Twins," *Lancet*, 1:8487 (26 April 1986), pp. 939–942.

10. Kreesten Meldgaard Madsen, Anders Hviid, Mogens Vestergaard, Diana Schendel, Jan Wohlfahrt , Poul Thorsen, Jørn Olsen, and Mads Melbye "A Population-Based Study of Measles, Mumps and Rubella Vaccination and Autism," *New England Journal of Medicine*, 347:19 (7 November 2002), pp. 1477–1482; Liam Smeeth, Claire Cook, Eric Fombonne, Lisa Heavey, Laura C. Rodrigues, Peter G. Smith, and Andrew J. Hall "MMR Vaccination and Pervasive Developmental Disorders: a Case-Control Study," *Lancet*, 364:9438 (11 September 2004), pp. 963–969.

11. Fitzpatrick, *MMR and Autism*.

12. E. J. Gangarosa, A. M. Galazka, C. R. Wolfe, L. M. Phillips, R. E. Gangarosa, E. Miller, and R. T. Chen, "Impact of Anti-Vaccine Movements on Pertussis Control: The Untold Story," *Lancet*, 351:9099 (31 January 1998), pp. 356–361.

13. Dawson, "The 'Best Interests' Argument and Childhood Immunisation."

14. Michael Devitt, *Realism and Truth* (Oxford: Blackwell, 2nd ed., 1991).

15. Angus Dawson, "The Human Fertilisation and Embryology Authority: Policy Making in a Contested Context," *Healthcare Analysis*, 12:1 (March 2004), pp. 1–8.

16. Dawson, "The 'Best Interests' Argument and Childhood Immunisation."

Eight

AN ASSESSMENT OF THE NORMAL FUNCTION MODEL AND IMPLICATIONS FOR ENHANCEMENT

Cathleen Schulte

1. Introduction

The ideal of maintaining and restoring human health through the provision of healthcare and medical research has become a moral and political imperative in many industrialized societies, and policies that aim to achieve this, in a just and cost-effective manner, are central to political manifestos. The concepts of health and disease also underpin many discussions in biomedical ethics. How we define disease will influence, for example, the way we think about disability, and as a result, affects arguments in areas such as preimplantation genetic diagnosis and gene therapy. More recently, the effects of disease have provided some of the moral justification for human embryonic stem cell research programs.

Embedded in these wider policy considerations are the implications that a concept of disease that is either too wide or too narrow will have for medical practice. First, the so-called "medicalization" of what are judged to be undesirable traits or behaviors (for example, depression, or developmental problems in young children) seems to shift social as well as personal responsibility to the medical domain. This is in spite of the fact that the influence of these different domains on the disease process cannot be separated easily. A wide conception of disease might therefore lead to an increase in medicalization, and a corresponding obligation to treat certain conditions within the medical rather than the social domain.

Second, the concepts of health and disease have been employed to identify the type of medical treatment that society, or the healthcare professional, has an obligation to provide. A distinction is often drawn between this and other forms of medical intervention that are seen as non-essential, primarily because they do not fit a definition of disease.

The concepts of health and disease are therefore used both in medical practice and as a policy tool, and we need to consider their content and where their boundaries might lie. The majority of definitions of these concepts carry at least some normative, or value, content. Some theorists, however, have proposed value-free accounts, and one of the most widely discussed is that of Christopher Boorse, in which he defines disease as an impairment of normal functional ability.[1] Because it seems to provide an objective standard for health and disease, this value-free definition has been used by Norman Daniels as one guiding principle in his wider theory of just healthcare. Daniels applies it not only to circumscribe the aims of healthcare but also to distinguish between what is and what is not medically necessary. In their recent book *From Chance to Choice*, Allen Buchanan and co-authors extend the principles of Daniels's original theory to consider the impact genetic technologies are likely to have on the goals of medicine and distribution of healthcare. This approach seems reasonable and promising. Nevertheless, it would seem that such a discussion should include at least some explication of different theories of function as encountered in the philosophy of biology. But Daniels, Buchanan, *et al.* offer no such analysis. In this essay I argue that without such analysis and in its current format, the normal function model, and its constituent concept of function, can be shown to have problematic implications for Daniels's theory.

2. Normative and Non-Normative Conceptions of Health and Disease

The social, political, medical, and scientific endorsement of the concept of health suggests that it possesses intrinsic value, and indeed, "the orthodox view is that all judgments of health include value judgments as part of their meaning."[2] The different normative positions can be further divided into strong and weak versions. The strong normativist position would claim that a condition should be classified as disease simply because it is judged by the individual (or a group of individuals) to be bad or undesirable. By contrast, the weak normativist position would claim that in order for something to be seen as healthy or diseased it must *also* be good or bad for the person concerned. This position does not rule out other non-evaluative criteria, for example the import of naturalistic concepts such as function.

To complicate matters further, in bioethical discussions normative and non-normative concepts of health and disease are frequently either mixed or viewed as incompatible. For example, in a discussion of disability, John Harris rejects Boorse's conception of "normal species functioning" as forming part of the definition of disability "because people might be normal and still disabled."[3] Instead, Harris defines disability as "a condition that someone has a strong rational preference not to be in and one that is in some sense a harmed condition."[4] However, rejecting the theoretical account and replacing it with a normative account obscures the fact that the two are not mutually exclusive, as one might fit the theoretical conception of disease *and* have a strong preference not to be in this state.

In his "biostatistical" theory Christopher Boorse argues for a departure from the prevalent idea that health and disease are defined with reference to the value-system of the patient, the doctor, or the normative community to which they belong.[5] Instead, he believes that health and disease can be described in theoretical terms based on the central assumption—one that he places within the classical tradition of the history of medical conceptions of disease[6]—that "an organism is theoretically healthy, that is, free of disease, insofar as its mode of functioning conforms to the natural design of that kind of organism."[7] His theory is based on the concepts of biological function and statistical normality where the normal function of any biological process can be said to fall within the statistical norm of that process occurring in a specified group of individuals (the reference class). Only those processes or traits that make a standard contribution to the survival and reproduction of a "sufficiently large sample of the population" and are therefore statistically significant will constitute a normal function.

Any notion of "the normal" and "the natural" may appear to be complex, possessing both empirical and normative content. However, Boorse rejects the need for any normative influence on these concepts and argues that "the nature of the species will be a functional design *empirically* shown typical of it."[8] For Boorse the functional design of a species, or species design, encompasses functional processes at every level of the physiological hierarchy "from organelle to cell to tissue to organ to gross behavior."[9] He defines disease as "a type of internal state which is either an impairment of normal functional ability—a reduction of one or more functional abilities below typical efficiency—or a limitation on functional ability caused by environmental agents."[10] So, health is, simply, the absence of disease.

Numerous challenges, both by normativists and non-normativists, have been made to this definition and it is neither possible nor the purpose of this piece to discuss the merits and deficiencies of Boorse's account.[11] Instead, I will consider one of the central concepts of his theory, the concept of function. I will then focus on the implications the function concept will have for the application of Boorse's definition to a wider theory of healthcare.

3. Function

The concept of function in the philosophy of biology remains controversial and it has been suggested that biology may need to incorporate different accounts of function in order to explain a trait's presence, its future changes, and how it contributes to the complex systems and abilities of the organism.[12] For reasons of space I cannot do justice to this ongoing and complex debate, but I hope to be able to demonstrate that all accounts of function are dependent on environmental context.[13]

A. The Etiological Account

In the philosophy of biology function claims are most often used to explain the *activity* of a structure or trait: for example, the function of the heart is to pump blood. It is, however, more difficult to explain the *existence* or presence of a trait by referring to its function. Without further qualification, it is not logically possible to argue that traits exist because they fulfill a function, and that therefore the function can explain the presence of a trait: that is, it does not make sense to say the heart is there because it pumps blood.[14] This is because functional equivalents, such as a mechanical heart, could also carry out that function. It cannot therefore be concluded that because an organism has a circulatory system, this organism has a (biological) heart.

There is one view of functions, the etiological theory of functions, which is able to explain the existence of a trait. Also referred to as the historical account, this theory is one of three major alternative accounts and is becoming the standard view among evolutionary biologists.[15] The theory bridges the logical gap that exists when we try to explain the presence of a trait from its activity by referring to the causal history of that trait, or its etiology. According to the etiological theory, the function of a trait is a consequence of the presence of that trait in a system, where the expression of this trait in the past played an essential role in the causal history of establishing the present trait.[16]

A generic definition of function on this view is:

"The function of X is Z" means:

(1) X has been naturally selected because it does Z;
(2) Z is a consequence (or result) of X's being there.[17]

In addition to its explanatory force, this definition ensures that other important criteria for a functional account are met. First, because traits are selected *for* a certain function the definition ensures that real functions are distinguished from accidental functions or mere dispositions. This is important since the function of a trait and its disposition can diverge. Second, it can accommodate the fact that functions may be displayed in only a minority of cases.[18]

This definition reflects the mainstream etiological view and there have been important critical developments. However, what is common to all these accounts is that a "*specified type of causal background*" is available (that is, a specified environment which interacts favorably with the functional trait).[19] The overall conclusion therefore that can be drawn from the etiological theory is also relevant to my argument: according to the etiological view functions arise in—and can only be defined in relation to—a specified environmental context.

B. The Goal-Directed Account

Boorse subscribes to a different view of functions, the class of goal-directed (or "current utility") theories.[20] These principally have in common a forward-looking account, which, unlike the etiological view, cannot explain *why* an organism currently has a particular trait.[21] Instead, the concept of goal-directedness focuses on why the trait *presently* contributes to a certain goal and why this trait may continue to persist. For Boorse, the "basic notion of a function is of a contribution to a goal."[22] In contrast to the etiological account therefore, Boorse's answer to the question "Why is trait X there?" is forward-looking: because it contributes to a certain goal. In addition, his view of functions also offers an answer to a different type of question: "How does S work?" where S is the goal-directed system in which the trait X appears.

For Boorse, organisms are objectively directed at *various* goals, for example, survival and reproduction. Consequently, his definition deliberately does not distinguish between "*a* function" and "*the* function" of a trait and what is required for a function X to be *the* function among possible other functions "is not any fixed general property but instead *varies from context to context.*"[23] This present contextual definition is in clear contrast to the etiological account where the function is explained from its causal history. What converts "*a* function of X" into "*the* function of X" is simply that one among all the functions performed by X which satisfies whatever relevant conditions are imposed by the "context of utterance."

This way Boorse arrives at the following definition of functions:

> "A function of X is Z" means that in some contextually definite goal-directed system S with contextually definite goal(s) G, during some contextually definite time interval t, the Z-ing of X falls within some *contextually circumscribed* class of functions being performed by X during t—that is, causal contribution to a goal of S.[24]

Putting this into the context of his theory of health and disease, Boorse concludes that the goal-directed system S is the individual organism, and the only functions that are relevant to health are the functions that support the individual organism's goals of survival and reproductive competence.[25]

C. The Capacity Account

This account was developed by Robert Cummins, who tackles the difficulty of trying to explain the presence of a trait by appealing to its function—the problem of possible functional equivalents—by suggesting an alternative functional explanation.[26] For him the function of a part is that of its effects that will contribute to the complexity of a containing system and where the system provides the appropriate background for that function. For example, because the usual background for a heart is within a circulatory system, it makes sense to say that the heart functions as a pump in this particular system.

According to this view, functional analysis can be conducted without having to refer to evolutionary mechanisms. It is therefore selection-neutral, but it still depends on the "background analysis of a containing system (the hive, the corporation, the eco-system)."[27] Importantly, functions can continue to be exercised even if (due to a change in the environment, for example) the function no longer contributes to the organism's ability or, to use Cummins's phrase, capacity to maintain the species. To ascribe a function to a trait is to ascribe a capacity to it; the singular capacities are then analyzed within the context of a containing system and emerge as functions. The pursuit of normal function in healthcare systems on this view would commit to the pursuit of the functional capacity of the organism regardless of wider environmental context and functional relevance.

4. The Normal Function Model Applied to a Theory of Just Healthcare

In his theory of just healthcare, Norman Daniels suggests that the aim of healthcare systems should be to meet "objectively ascribable" and "objectively important" healthcare needs.[28] These needs have to be fulfilled so that individuals can achieve or maintain species-typical normal functioning. Like Boorse, therefore, and with explicit reference to Boorse's account, Daniels defines disease as "deviations from the natural functional organization of a typical member of a species" and health as the absence of disease.[29] Normal species functioning allows individuals to operate within their normal opportunity range, that is their normal range of skills and talents, and thus construct their life plans and conceptions of the good.[30] Importantly, the range of talents is specific to the individual, thereby allowing for individual differences to be preserved. The requirement is therefore for the normal opportunity range to be fair but not equal. With this requirement, Daniels advocates the social structural view of the level playing field conception of equal opportunity. This conception demands leveling the effect of inequalities that are propagated by unjust social structures and institutions but does not go as far as the leveling of all social *and natural* differences. Daniels therefore believes that social institutions, such as a healthcare system, should be giving individuals equal opportunity to participate in society by keeping them functioning as close as possible to the species norm thereby making them normal, but not equal, competitors.[31]

Because of its role in defining the individual's "normal opportunity range," Daniels sees species-typical normal functioning as an appropriate and fundamentally just standard for societies and healthcare systems to pursue.

However, he does recognize some of the limitations of using a biological function concept and therefore aims to apply a weaker version that does not need to operate within the strict value-free constraints adopted by Boorse. In particular, he identifies two notions of environment, the natural and the social environment, and notes the difficulty in specifying "the range of environment taken as 'natural' for the purpose of revealing dysfunction."[32] For Daniels the difficulty arises when the specified environment is dominated by social criteria; for example, racially discriminatory environments might make being of a particular race a disease whereas dyslexia might not be regarded as a disability in non-literate environments. As I argue in more detail below, limiting the scope of environmental effects on function to such normative and transient influences is problematic. I have included Daniels's reservations here merely to illustrate that in his theory the normal functioning model does not *necessarily* exclude normative judgments, and indeed explicitly allows "normative judgements *about* disease."[33] Nevertheless, his definition of disease will mainly depend on Boorse's theoretical conception.

While there seem to be advantages to the application of a value-free concept of disease in a theory of healthcare, there are additional problems with this approach. The first of these concerns the unspecified and relatively uncritical import of the normal function concept. In the following I will refer to Daniels's theory interchangeably with that of Buchanan *et al.*, who incorporated the theory into *From Chance to Choice*. Daniels was a contributor to this project and the principle of the normal function model does not significantly differ from his original work.

A. Problem 1. Function

Daniels views his notion of disease as operating within weaker non-normative constraints than Boorse's strictly naturalistic version: "it will not matter if what counts as disease is relative to some features of social roles in a given society, and thus to some normative judgements, provided the core of the notion of species-normal functioning is left intact."[34] On functions he makes two further qualifications. He notes his awareness of the fact that Boorse's view of functions "fails to accommodate all cases that a successful account in the philosophy of biology would have to address" but does "not believe, however, that we must refrain from using a notion of normal functioning in ethics and political philosophy until a 'true' account of functions emerges in the philosophy of biology."[35] This view has several problematic implications. First, to expect that a single, "true" account of function will eventually emerge could be a dangerous assumption to make: several theorists have argued that the philosophy of biology may have to accept a pluralistic account of function in order to meet all the requirements this concept demands.[36] Also, the above qualifications have not significantly changed in content since they were made by Daniels in a much earlier paper, which raises the question of whether any serious attempt was made to investigate more recent thinking in the philosophy of biology.[37] This is significant since Daniels's theory seems unable to accommodate different notions of function and seems to depend on the application of a singular concept.

Daniels supports his method of including an undefined notion of function by arguing that "it is enough for [his] purposes if the line between disease and its absence is ... *uncontroversial* and ascertainable through publicly acceptable methods, such as those of the biomedical sciences."[38] However, it can be assumed that the same "biomedical sciences" will inevitably focus on the breakdown of biological function. Therefore, by failing to outline at least some of his understanding of function it is questionable whether throughout his analysis "the core of the notion of species-normal functioning *is* left intact."[39]

By acknowledging that his account fails to accommodate all cases that a successful account of function would have to address, but by nevertheless proceeding regardless of this insight, Daniels could be criticized for using a flawed heuristic. Jason Scott Robert has recently reminded us of the dangers of so-called "hedgeless hedging" strategies: "even though [such a] model may initiate the production of more adequate models, such models will themselves be so drastically different from the original model that its catalytic role may be overestimated."[40] Given that the restoration and maintenance of function is one of the cornerstones of Daniels's theory, using a simplified assumption as his premise may prove to be a dangerous strategy to pursue.

B. Problem 2. Environment

One of the problems with applying the normal functioning model to an ethical construct is that the model has its origin in explaining biological systems, and the existence and viability of such systems is determined partly by the environmental context in which they evolve. It has also been argued that it would be wrong to conceive of environmental context as a fixed and separate entity. Instead, the environment should be viewed as being causally constituted by the organism developing or operating within it.[41]

In Boorse's and Daniels's accounts there seems to be a considerable amount of cross talk concerning the impact of environmental considerations on normal species functioning, which in turn creates conceptual difficulties. For example, while Boorse's concern rests with naturalistic effects, such as the effect exercise or altitude might have on an individual's normal heart rate, Daniels seems to be concerned mainly about the normative effects an environment might have on functional ascriptions. He groups these effects under the term "socially created environment" but does not expand on its definition.[42] It seems that his understanding of a socially created environment would certainly include prevailing social values, such as attitudes towards race, gender roles, or homosexuality, but the actual extent to which the socially created environment determines functional context is not sufficiently acknowledged. However, if, as I have tried to demonstrate, function is dependent on context, then in order to make the normal functioning criteria morally relevant, we do need to be clear about the context in which it is placed.

It is therefore crucial to remember that, in addition to Daniels's notion, there is a second form of "socially created environment" which is devoid of any *overtly* normative content. It is socially created in the sense that it was created by human abilities such as spoken language and advanced tool making.[43] Civilizations are dependent on the expression of complex cognitive traits and these have enabled, among other things, the study and understanding of physical processes, and the development of sophisticated technologies and industries. More recently, the rapid advances in information technology have radically transformed traditional patterns of life and society. The environment is therefore socially created in a manner that is much more pervasive than Daniels implies. It does contain transient elements that are open to revision and social change, and which would fit his notion of "socially created." However, the underlying social, cultural, and economic fabric is indispensable to any Western societal framework we identify with, and is thus indispensable to a Western conception of healthcare ethics.

The socially created environment and biological functional traits are therefore far more interdependent than Daniels's account suggests. But there is one further important consideration. As long as they are able to provide for viable human life, social systems can change without biological constraint and therefore with a radicality not encountered in biological evolution. This has resulted in some biological functions being no longer synchronous with their environment and normal biological function even being purposely disrupted in favor of social change.

One well-documented example is female reproductive function.[44] The normal reproductive function of higher primate species females is marked by monthly ovulations and the concurrent ability to conceive. The corresponding reproductive pattern is still seen in contemporary hunter-gatherer tribes where women carry serial pregnancies and breastfeed for much longer than is usual in modern societies.[45] However, social change has meant that many women living in industrialized societies decide to overrule (at least for a time) their normal reproductive function in favor of pursuing their own value system. The pursuit of a normal species functioning standard can therefore operate in direct opposition to one of the fundamental concepts of Western bioethical (and increasingly medico-legal) thought, the concept of autonomy. Since human functions consist of both cognitive and physiological function, the two types of function cannot be studied in isolation, and depending on the development of one, it may be difficult to define the other.

C. Problem 3. Level of Application

Lastly, it is not clear at which level of system organization the restoration (or maintenance) of normal function should be directed. Should it be applied at the level of the organism, at organ level, or even at molecular level? Short-sightedness is normally "restored" to normal function with spectacles or contact lenses. However, what this restoration in fact involves is compensatory correction or simulation at the level of the whole organism: the *individual* can continue to function as though they had normal eyesight. But if we alter the level of application to a lower physiological level and still accept that *normal functioning* is the standard then there would be an obligation to provide for laser surgery (for example) on a general basis. But the follow-on question from this conclusion might be: to what extent do we have such obligations? Short-sightedness constitutes an impairment in our society and without correction would seriously restrict equal opportunity. But do we regard laser eye surgery as being as important as a hip replacement? Buchanan *et al.* argue that "judgments about the relative importance of treating different diseases and impairments will have some social variability" but if normal functioning at organ level is our main concern then there would be no difference between these conditions.[46] If we accept simulation of functioning at the level of the individual (for example, through the wearing of spectacles) then one further consideration arises. Because in Daniels's theory, normal functioning is ultimately aimed at protecting fair equality of opportunity, and following the above line of thought, there would be no reason why the simulation of function could not be applied to any disease or impairment. The consequence of this would be that even serious impairments, such as those affecting mobility, could be legitimately corrected at the level of the individual (with wheelchair use) and at the social level (better wheelchair access) and would not necessarily warrant, or demand, surgical or possibly genetic intervention. This conclusion need not even be as absurd as it might seem. Anita Silvers, for example, suggests that we are wrong to "normalize" function if normal is equated with most common, since the most common form of function can for some be disadvantageous and not very functional. Someone who walks with a feeble gait, although fulfilling the criteria of normal function at the individual level, might have more effective mobility when using a wheelchair. We should therefore not automatically endorse "any scale that illegitimately naturalizes such rankings by appeal to biological imperatives."[47]

The implementation of species-typical functioning as a guide to just health policy would require consistency in the selection of the appropriate target level of function. It may however be that in practice the acceptance of different functioning levels is more appropriate, which poses the question whether species-typical functioning can really fulfill the role of a universal standard and suggests that healthcare might have to appeal to a different criterion.

5. Framework Considerations

Descriptive premises play a prominent role in bioethics, from questions surrounding the moral status of the embryo to end of life decisions. However, they are frequently problematic mainly because they directly attribute moral worth to the natural order.[48] Therefore, if function, in the form of a descriptive concept, is to feature in a normative theory of health it must be able to demonstrate normative meaning.[49]

It could be argued that Daniels's theory contains an inherent normative component since the aim is to give individuals access to fair equality of opportunity. But because he does not analyze existing function accounts in the philosophy of biology, Daniels cannot uncover a logical problem specific to the restoration and maintenance of *biological* function.

In order to acquire normative meaning we need an inclusive and pluralistic view of biological function where neither the causal history nor the goal-directedness of functions can be separated from the relevant normative framework. Such a framework will be composed of three equal components which interact "horizontally." The three components for a functional account (function, natural environment, and social environment) form a triangular relationship with each component influencing the composition of the other (figure 8.1). In this schema the *abstract notion* of function can exist in isolation (and thus in a value-free form) but it cannot derive any content, whether descriptive or normative, without reference to an interdependent natural and normative environment.

Nevertheless, even this pluralistic conception of biological function creates concerns regarding the choice of the normal function standard for Daniels's wider theory of healthcare. Daniels has based his theory of healthcare on John Rawls's principles of justice.[50] These are principles which would be chosen by individuals in "the original position"—a hypothetical situation which places individuals behind a "veil of ignorance," that is, without knowledge of their own social and natural circumstances.[51] Rawls believes that in this position individuals would choose two principles which should govern the basic structure of society. First, each person should be granted equal rights to equal basic liberties. Second, social and economic inequalities are allowed only if they work as part of a scheme which improves the expectations of the least advantaged and are perpetuated by positions open to all under conditions of fair equality of opportunity.[52] The crucial extension of this idea in Daniels's theory of healthcare lies in the fact that Rawls does not include health in the list of social primary goods, since he assumes that everybody in the original position is "normal" and a fully cooperating member of society. Daniels argues that healthcare must be distributed in such a way as to achieve equality of opportunity and therefore healthcare institutions, as social institutions, will also be governed by the fair equality of opportunity principle.

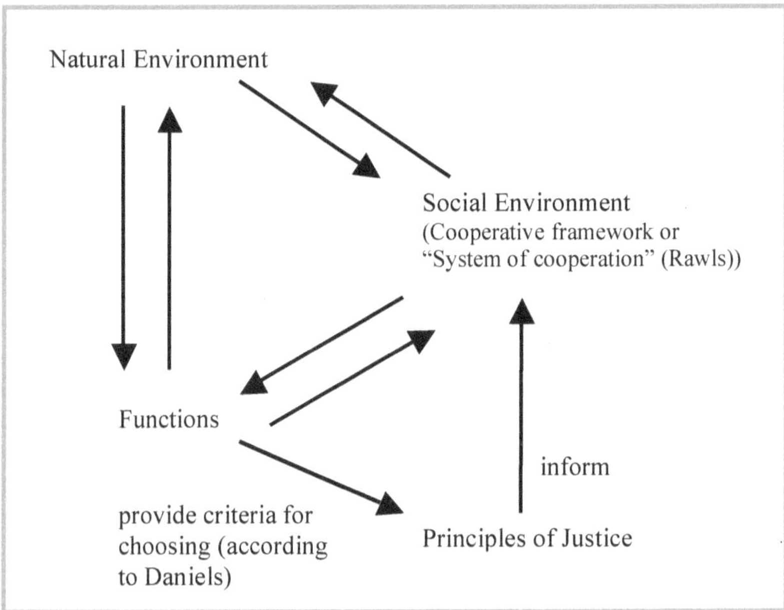

Figure 8.1 *The interdependency of function and environment, and their relationship to the principles of justice*

Since (for Daniels) equal opportunity can only be pursued if people are normal functioning competitors, from the original position it must be assumed that normal function *can* be obtained, otherwise the second principle of justice (containing the fair equality of opportunity standard) could not be achieved. Normal function is however dependent on the natural and socially created environment (or to use Rawls's term: system of cooperation), whereby the principles of justice inform the social institutions on how the system of cooperation is to be administered, thus creating a complex network around the concept of function (figure 8.1).

Therefore, while the principles of justice (containing the principle of equal opportunity) could not be determined or implemented without the concept of function, the cooperative framework, in relation to which function must be defined, cannot be justly operative without the principles of justice informing it. On the other hand, past systems of cooperation, although they at one time played a part in the selection of functions, will nowadays frequently be irrelevant to them. This situation is illogical and suggests that normal biological functioning cannot constitute a necessary aspect of access to equal opportunities. Species-typical functioning is too inflexible and too limited by evolutionary constraints to accommodate rapid social change. For these reasons it cannot provide an adequate criterion for a healthcare system based on the principles of justice, and does not generate the normative force that Daniels expects.

6. Implications for Enhancement

For Daniels (and for Buchanan *et al.*) the normal functioning model also provides a "qualified and limited defense" of what is known as the treatment-enhancement distinction. Eric Juengst has recently helped to clarify "enhancement" by arguing that the concept operates as a moral boundary concept in two types of conversations.[53] In the first conversation, it is used to define the proper limits of biomedicine and applies to any intervention that does not constitute treatment. The second conversation is concerned with the ethics of self-improvement and here the boundary is drawn to provide a moral distinction between enhancement and achievement. On this analysis, the normal functioning model finds its home in the "proper limits of biomedicine" conversation: restoring and maintaining someone's normal functional ability will constitute treatment. Any precise demarcation of the enhancement border, however, remains difficult since for the individual concerned all enhancements are inherently changes for the good. Equally, aligning normal function with justification for treatment can run into difficulties.

In biomedical ethics, the discussion surrounding the issue of how disease might affect equal opportunity most often revolves around genetic disorders. Until the development of genetic technologies such diseases were regarded as being the result of nature or chance; and beyond human control. Buchanan *et al.* take the view that it is precisely our newly acquired ability to test for some of these diseases that makes intervention, where possible, a requirement of justice. More often than not, the provision of treatment will meet this requirement. Nevertheless, for *some* individuals at the lower end of the normal functioning spectrum, justice may require enhancement of their functioning.[54]

However, it is worth remembering that the majority of diseases are not wholly and simply caused by natural inequalities. Most people suffer from chronic diseases, such as cancer, heart disease, and diabetes, for which the effects of the social structure are a contributory factor *in the widest sense.* Traditional ways of life have largely been abandoned and although we mostly perceive this as a positive change, there are trade-offs with regard to our health. This can be interpreted in two ways. If we follow Buchanan *et al.*

loosely and view normal function simply as a necessary requirement for equal opportunity, then the pursuit of equal opportunities might require the system of cooperation, which puts in place social structures and exercises its values through them, to change in such a way as to make diseases of this kind less likely. This could be achieved, for example, by returning our existing functions to their original context. However, considering that choice of lifestyle has become one of the hallmarks of modern societies and that large parts of the global economy are built on offering this choice, this type of approach might be considered unrealistic (bearing in mind that many people even in industrialized societies often do not have this choice).

The alternative, endorsed by Buchanan *et al.*, would be to view healthcare as a distributive resource which supports the pursuit of equal opportunity. This commits the cooperative framework to medical interventions that address (and prevent) such diseases and leads to the following conclusions about the nature of enhancements. If we continue to define normal function as the standard against which we measure the provision of healthcare, but if, at the same time, the environment has changed in such a way that normal (physiological) function has become sub-normal, then there will be a commitment to restore (individual) functioning by enhancing the original (physiological) function. This approach differs from treatment in one important respect and, moreover, demonstrates the significance of defining at which level of organization the normal functioning concept is to operate. The difference lies in the fact that treatment, both at the level of the physiological process and at the level of the individual, will only restore functioning to its original level. On the other hand, this type of enhancement at the physiological level will, at the level of the individual, only match the effect achieved by treatment, which means the *individual* is not enhanced. If, therefore, we view the treatment-enhancement distinction as drawing a moral boundary at the level of the individual then, in the context described, the distinction can be preserved.

There are other types of enhancement which at first glance are aimed at "correcting" malfunction and might therefore appear to constitute treatment. But rather than restore the original process to its functional level, this type of intervention will in effect only *simulate* functioning, thus returning the individual to their starting position where they *appear* to be functioning normally. One example of this kind involves the provision of fertility treatment for women. In many industrialized societies there has been a progressive rise in the average age at which women choose to have their first child. Increasingly women have to make use of medical interventions to support their ability to conceive at an older age. However, such "treatments" can never fully restore the natural fertility seen in younger women and arguably this simulation of fertility constitutes an enhancement of natural function.

We therefore need to consider whether it is in fact possible to retain the normal function criteria. The possibly irreversible changes to our environment are not an external, pathogenic threat to normal functioning but are integral to the function concept. As a result, normal species functioning in modern social structures will often mean the enhancement or simulation of a standard that has become a decontextualized and redundant concept. This will be true regardless of which theory of function we choose to consider. Any reference to such functioning becomes arbitrary and the distinction which underlies such cases collapses.

7. Conclusion

What this analysis has shown is that when applying unresolved biological premises to bioethical debate and in order for this debate to be meaningful, it is important to consider the philosophy of biology of such uncertainties adequately. I hope to have demonstrated that depending on the extent of such consideration and analysis, it is possible to arrive at very different conclusions. Normal species functioning is not a value-free concept and in its current format provides a confusing definition of health and disease on which to base a theory of healthcare.

Acknowledgment

This chapter is based on my dissertation for the MA in Healthcare Ethics and Law. It was written as the dissertation was completed in 2004.

NOTES

1. See Christopher Boorse, "A Rebuttal on Health," *Biomedical Ethics Reviews: What is Disease?* eds. James M. Humber and Robert F. Almeder (Totowa, NJ: Humana Press, 1997), pp. 3–134.

2. Christopher Boorse, "On the Distinction Between Disease and Illness," *Philosophy and Public Affairs*, 5:1 (Autumn 1975), pp. 49–68, at p. 50.

3. John Harris, "Equality and Disability Symposium: One Principle and Three Fallacies of Disability Studies," *Journal of Medical Ethics*, 27:6 (December 2001), pp. 383–387, at p. 384.

4. *Ibid.*.

5. Boorse, "A Rebuttal on Health."

6. Boorse, "Health as a Theoretical Concept," *Philosophy of Science*, 44:4 (December 1977), pp. 542–573, at p. 554.

7. Boorse, "On the Distinction Between Disease and Illness," p. 57.

8. Boorse, "Health as a Theoretical Concept," p. 555 (my emphasis).

9. Boorse, "A Rebuttal on Health," p. 7.

10. *Cf.* Boorse, "A Rebuttal on Health," p.7, 7n.

11. *Ibid.*; Larissa K. F. Temple, Robin S. McLeod, Steven Gallinger, and James G. Wright, "Defining Disease in the Genomic Era," *Science* 293:5531 (3 August 2001), pp, 807–808.

12. Marc Bekoff and Colin Allen, "Teleology, Function, Design, and the Evolution of Animal Behaviour," *Trends in Ecology and Evolution* 10:6 (June 1995), pp. 253–255.

13. *Nature's Purposes: Analysis of Function and Design in Biology*, eds. Colin Allen, Marc Bekoff, and George Lauder (Cambridge: MIT Press, 1998).

14. See Robert Wachbroit, "Normality as a Biological Concept," *Philosophy of Science*, 61:4 (December 1994), pp. 579–591, and Sandra D. Mitchell, "Dispositions or Etiologies? A Comment on Bigelow and Pargetter," *The Journal of Philosophy* 90:5 (May 1993), pp. 249–259.

15. Colin Allen and Marc Bekoff, "Biological Function, Adaptation, and Natural Design," Allen, Bekoff, and Lauder, *Nature's Purposes*, pp. 571–587.

16. Mitchell, "Dispositions or Etiologies?" p. 251.

17. Rachel Cooper, "Disease," *Studies in History and Philosophy of Biological and Biomedical Sciences*, 33:2 (July 2002), pp. 263–282.

18. Tim Thornton, "Mental Illness and Reductionism: Can Functions be Naturalized?" *Philosophy, Psychiatry, and Psychology*, 7:1 (March 2000), pp. 67–76, citing Ruth Millikan, *Language, Thought, and other Biological Categories* (Cambridge: MIT Press, 1984).

19. Mitchell, "Dispositions or Etiologies?" p. 252.

20. *Cf.* John Bigelow and Robert Pargetter, "Functions," *The Journal of Philosophy*, 84:4 (April 1987), pp. 181–196.

21. Bekoff and Allen, "Teleology, Function, Design and the Evolution of Animal Behaviour," p. 254.

22. Boorse, "Health as a Theoretical Concept," p. 555.

23. Boorse, "Wright on Functions," *The Philosophical Review*, 85:1 (January 1976), pp. 70–86, at p. 81 (my emphasis).

24. *Ibid.*, p. 82 (my emphasis).

25. *Ibid.*

26. Robert Cummins, "Functional Analysis," *The Journal of Philosophy*, 72:20 (20 November 1975), pp. 741–765, reprinted in Allen, Bekoff, and Lauder, *Nature's Purposes*, pp. 169–196.

27. *Ibid.*, p. 190.

28. Norman Daniels, "Health-Care Needs and Distributive Justice," *Philosophy and Public Affairs*, 10:2 (Spring, 1981), pp. 146–179, at p. 152; Norman Daniels, *Just Healthcare* (Cambridge: Cambridge University Press, 1985); also Allen Buchanan, Dan W. Brock, Norman Daniels, and Daniel Wikler, *From Chance to Choice: Genetics and Justice* (Cambridge: Cambridge University Press, 2000), esp. chs. 3 and 4.

29. Daniels, "Health-Care Needs and Distributive Justice," p. 155.

30. *Ibid.*, p. 154.

31. Buchanan *et al.*, *From Chance to Choice*, p. 109.

32. Daniels, "Health-Care Needs and Distributive Justice," p. 156n.

33. *Ibid.*, p. 156.

34. Buchanan *et al.*, *From Chance to Choice*, p. 122; *cf.* also Daniels, "Health-Care Needs and Distributive Justice," pp. 156–157.

35. Buchanan *et al.*, *From Chance to Choice*, p. 121.

36. See Allen and Bekoff, "Biological Function, Adaptation, and Natural Design."

37. Daniels, "Health-Care Needs and Distributive Justice," p. 156n.

38. Buchanan *et al.*, *From Chance to Choice*, p. 122n (my emphasis).

39. *Ibid.*, (my emphasis).

40. Jason Scott Robert, "Constant Factors and Hedgeless Hedges: On Heuristics and Biases in Biological Research," *Philosophy of Science*, 70:5 (December 2003), pp. 975–988.

41. Richard Lewontin, *Biology as Ideology* (New York: Harper, 1991), cited in Philip Kitcher, "Battling the Undead: How (and How Not) to Resist Genetic Determinism," *Thinking about Evolution: Historical, Philosophical, and Political Perspectives*, eds. Rama S. Singh, Costas B. Krimbas, Diane B. Paul, and John Beatty (Cambridge: Cambridge University Press), ch. 20, p. 400.

42. Buchanan *et al.*, *From Chance to Choice*, p. 122n.

43. Sean B. Carroll, "Genetics and the Making of *Homo Sapiens*," *Nature*, 422:6934 (24 April 2003), pp. 849–857.

44. Mel Greaves, "Cancer Causation: The Darwinian Downside of Past Success?" *Lancet Oncology* 3:4 (1 April 2002), pp. 244–251.

45. *Ibid.*

46. Buchanan *et al.*, *From Chance to Choice*, p. 123.

47. Anita Silvers, "A Fatal Attraction to Normalizing: Treating Disabilities as Deviations from 'Species-Typical' Functioning," *Enhancing Human Traits: Ethical and Social Implications*, ed. Erik Parens (Washington: Georgetown University Press, 1998), pp. 95–123.

48. Tuija Takala, "The (Im)Morality of (Un)Naturalness," *Cambridge Quarterly of Healthcare Ethics*, 13:2 (April 2004), pp. 131–134.

49. K. W. M. Fulford, "Teleology Without Tears: Naturalism, Neo-Naturalism, and Evaluationism in the Analysis of Function Statements in Biology (and a Bet on the Twenty-First Century)," *Philosophy, Psychiatry, and Psychology*, 7:1 (March 2000), pp. 77–94.

50. John Rawls, *A Theory of Justice* (Oxford: Oxford University Press, 1990 (revised)).

51. *Ibid.*, p. 118.

52. *Ibid.*, pp. 53, 72.

53. Eric T. Juengst, "What does *Enhancement* Mean?" *Enhancing Human Traits: Ethical and Social Implications*, ed. Erik Parens (Washington: Georgetown University Press, 1998), pp. 29–47.

54. Buchanan *et al.*, *From Chance to Choice*.

Nine

ON THE DISTINCTION BETWEEN POSITIVE AND NEGATIVE EUGENICS

Stephen Wilkinson

1. Positive and Negative Eugenics

Academic work on eugenics often utilizes a distinction between positive and negative eugenics. Much of this work assumes that the distinction is morally significant and that positive eugenics is worse than negative eugenics (other things being equal). Despite its pervasiveness and supposed importance however, the nature of the positive-negative distinction remains unclear and the terms "negative" and "positive" are used in several different ways in the literature. This chapter aims to provide clarification by analyzing and explaining some different accounts of the distinction and by showing how these relate to other key ideas such as the therapy-enhancement distinction and concepts of health and disease. The chapter also provides a short overview of the reasons for thinking that the positive-negative eugenics distinction is morally significant.

This chapter is exclusively concerned with a distinction *within* eugenics, not with how to differentiate eugenics from other categories. Nonetheless, something should be said first about the meaning of "eugenics." Francis Galton defines it as the study of "the conditions under which men of a high type are produced" and as "the science which deals with all influences that improve the inborn qualities of a race."[1] Eugenics however is not merely a field of study and, as Diane Paul notes, "it is less often identified as a science than as a social movement or policy, as in Bertrand Russell's definition: 'the attempt to improve the biological character of a breed by deliberate methods adopted to that end.'"[2] For the present purposes, Russell's definition will suffice. However, it should be noted that this is only a working definition and much more could be said about what eugenics is. Moreover, this working definition will almost certainly turn out to be too wide, since people might attempt to "improve the biological character" of humanity in lots of different ways, and I doubt that we want to classify all of these as eugenic.

Something should also be said about the different kinds of practices that are likely to fall under the general heading "eugenics." In contemporary bioethics, selective reproduction is the practice which appears most often to be called "eugenic." Eugenic selection of this kind aims to encourage the passing on of "good genes" or to prevent the passing on of "bad genes." Traditionally, eugenics strived to achieve this by selective breeding. Contemporary reproductive technologies, however, mean that selective breeding is not now the only possible method. Another is the *in vitro* selection of embryos (those with "good genes") using preimplantation genetic diagnosis (PGD), and similarly the preconception selection of ova and sperm (again, those with "good genes"). Based on the working definition of "eugenics," neither PGD nor gamete selection are *necessarily* eugenic (with much depending on the purposes to which they are put) but either *could* constitute eugenics if used deliberately to "improve the gene pool."

The following characterizations of the positive-negative distinction are fairly typical of those found in the ethics literature:[3]

> "positive eugenics" ... aims to increase desirable traits rather than reduce undesirable ones ...[4]

> positive eugenics attempts to increase the number of favorable or desirable genes in the human gene pool, while negative eugenics attempts to reduce the number of undesirable or harmful genes, e.g., genes that cause genetic diseases.[5]

> "Negative eugenics" refers to the elimination of diseases or defects, whereas "positive eugenics" refers to the enhancement of traits.[6]

> Negative eugenics is a systematic effort to minimize the transmission of genes that are considered deleterious, in contrast to positive eugenics, which aims to maximize the transmission of desirable genes.[7]

> The aim of negative eugenics is disease prevention and health promotion, not enhancement of normal capacities.[8]

On these definitions, most PGD presently practiced in the UK is *negative* eugenics (if it is eugenics at all) since its aim is to "screen out" conditions such as beta thalassaemia, cystic fibrosis, Duchenne muscular dystrophy, and Huntington's disease.[9] If however PGD could be used instead to select children with dispositions to be exceptionally athletic, or attractive, or intelligent, then this would be *positive* eugenics (on the assumption that these features are desirable).

Characterizing the positive-negative distinction may however be less straightforward than it at first appears. For in most, maybe even all, cases the same eugenic practice can be described as both "negative" and "positive." This arises most obviously in cases where the trait in question is a matter of degree, such as athleticism, attractiveness, or intelligence. For, in such cases, the negative feature is just the absence of the positive feature (and *vice versa*). So, for example, selecting *out* low(er) intelligence ("negative eugenics") might be the same practice as selecting *in* high(er) intelligence ("positive eugenics"). Moreover, this does not apply only to cases in which the desirable trait is a matter of degree. Take for example a single gene disorder such as cystic fibrosis, which is caused by a malfunctioning gene on chromosome 7.[10] Although the symptoms of cystic fibrosis can vary in their severity, whether someone has the condition or not is not itself a matter of degree. Nonetheless, the same problem applies. For while we would normally say that we were selecting *against* cystic fibrosis, and *against* this malfunctioning gene (both negative features), there appear to be no reasons for not also saying that we are selecting *in favor of* copies of chromosome 7 with fully functioning genes and *in favor of* future persons with fully functioning respiratory systems (both positive features). So if we tried to make sense of the positive-negative distinction solely in terms of "selecting out the bad" versus "selecting in the good," it would turn out to have little or no determinate meaning, for just about anything could count as positive or as negative if suitably described.

2. The Disease Account and the Normality Account

Two main responses to this are available. The first defines the positive-negative distinction in terms of disease avoidance and says that negative eugenics aims to reduce the incidence of disease, while positive eugenics aims to "improve the quality" of the population in other ways. We can call this the Disease Account. The second response is to distinguish between positive and negative eugenics by reference to their relationships with the normal. We can call this the Normality Account. On this account, what negative eugenics does is to select out subnormal (worse than normal) traits, while positive eugenics selects in supernormal (better than normal) traits. (For the present purposes, I shall leave to one side the difficult question of what counts as better or worse than normal.)

To see how these two construals of the positive-negative distinction differ from one another, consider the following embryo selection scenario. Embryo 1 is known to have a serious single gene disorder. Embryo 2 does not, as far as we know, have any genetic disorders. Nonetheless, testing reveals that 2 would be likely to have significantly below average intelligence (although not low enough to constitute an intellectual disability or disorder). Embryo 3 is generally normal but, testing reveals, would be likely to have a remarkably effective immune system and would be relatively unlikely to develop cancer. Embryo 4 is also generally normal, but testing reveals that 4 would be likely to have considerably higher than average intelligence.

We can see how the different accounts of the positive-negative distinction work by asking, for each embryo, whether selecting (or deselecting) it for implantation would constitute negative or positive eugenics (assuming, for the sake of argument, that it is eugenics of one sort or another).

Starting with Embryo 1 (which, for reasons that will emerge shortly, is the most complicated of the four) the Disease Account would classify deselecting 1 on the grounds that it has a serious disorder as *negative* eugenics; for it is an obvious case of disease avoidance. Proponents of the Normality Account would *probably* agree that this is negative eugenics because disorders, especially serious ones, generally do involve subnormal functioning of a bodily part or process. However, whether they would (or should) *necessarily* agree in such cases is a more difficult and open question. For one major question in the philosophy of health concerns whether diseases *necessarily* involve some form of subnormality (most likely, subnormal functioning). Indeed, some theorists, notably Christopher Boorse, have argued that health is to be understood as the absence of disease, with disease being understood as statistically subnormal function.[11] If Boorse is right, and this necessary connection between disease and subnormality exists, then the Disease Account and the Normality Account will be in total agreement on Embryo 1 type cases (both viewing it as negative eugenics). But if, as some of Boorse's critics argue, some cases of disease do not involve subnormal functioning then there will be some Embryo 1 type cases about which they disagree—that is, the cases which involve disease but not subnormality.

Turning now to the other embryos, deselecting Embryo 2 (which has no known disorders but probable low intelligence) would be positive eugenics on the Disease Account, since the reason for deselecting 2 is something other than disease avoidance, but it would be negative eugenics on the Normality Account, since the embryo is deselected for having a subnormal feature. Selecting Embryo 3 because it is likely to develop an exceptionally effective immune system would be negative eugenics on the Disease Account, because the goal is disease avoidance. On the Normality Account, though, this is positive eugenics because we are selecting 3 on the grounds that it has a supernormal feature. Finally, selecting Embryo 4 on the grounds that it is likely to develop a high level of intelligence would be positive eugenics on both accounts. For the selection does not aim to avoid disease and aims to bring about the creation of supernormal characteristics.

3. The Enhancement-Therapy Distinction

The positive-negative eugenics distinction is, as was suggested earlier, related to another central distinction in bioethics, that between enhancement and therapy. David Resnik outlines the importance of the therapy-enhancement distinction as follows:

> The therapy-enhancement distinction occupies a central place in contemporary discussions of human genetics and has been the subject of much debate. At a recent conference on gene therapy policy, scientists predicted that within a few years researchers will develop techniques that can be used to enhance human traits. In thinking about the morality of genetic interventions, many writers have defended somatic gene therapy, and some have defended germline gene therapy, but only a handful of others defend genetic enhancement, or even give it a fair hearing. The mere mention of genetic enhancement makes many people cringe and brings to mind the Nazi eugenics programs, Aldous Huxley's *Brave New World*, "The X-Files," or the recent movie "Gattaca."[12]

It is widely held then that, in controversial areas of practice and research, such as the application of new reproductive technologies, enhancement interventions are (other things being equal) more morally problematic and less acceptable than therapeutic interventions. This view will be examined briefly at the end of the chapter. For the present purposes, though, our main question concerns the relationship between the therapy-enhancement distinction and the positive-negative eugenics distinction.

The first point to make is that, if we are talking about eugenic selection, as opposed to modification, the term "therapy" is a misnomer. This is because "treatment" (like "therapy") implies that an individual's condition is cured or improved (if the treatment is successful). In eugenic selection cases however (such as that of Embryos 1–4 above) no one is cured of anything—but a (future) person who probably will not develop a given disease is chosen for creation instead of a different (future) person, who probably would have had that disease, had she been created.

In the case of "therapy" then I propose a distinction between "therapy" and "disease avoidance." The term "therapy" should be reserved for cases in which the disorders of determinate individuals are treated. Treatment can include both curative and palliative interventions, and can be applied to embryos and fetuses, as well as to existing persons. "Disease avoidance," on the other hand, is a wider category and covers any practice which aims to reduce the prevalence of disease. Thus curative therapy is just *one type of* disease-avoidance strategy. Others include selective reproduction, preventive medicine, and environmental health policies. One potentially significant difference between therapy and disease avoidance then is that therapy (when successful) necessarily benefits determinate individuals, whereas disease avoidance need not do so.

Slightly different considerations apply in the case of "enhancement." It could be argued that to "enhance" also implies that a determinate individual will be made better. However, our linguistic conventions and intuitions are rather weaker about this than they are in the case of "therapy" and it does appear (more) acceptable to talk about enhancement-selection, as well as enhancement-modification. A good illustration of this is the Human Genetics Commission's 2004 report, *Choosing the Future: Genetics and Reproductive Decision Making*, in which it says:

> **Embryo enhancement** refers to using techniques to enhance the genetic make-up of a child, and is prohibited. In theory, embryo enhancement might involve either the selection of an embryo with genetic characteristics indicative of desirable traits such as beauty or intelligence, or a process of genetic modification to enhance such traits.[13]

This looks like reason enough to allow "enhancement" to be used both for cases in which identifiable individuals are "improved," and for cases of selective reproduction in which "better" embryos are chosen for implantation rather than "worse" ones. Thus, we might say that the term "enhancement" is broader in its application than the term "therapy," the latter only applying to cases in which determinate individuals are affected.

4. Enhancement, Disease, and Normality

This still leaves us with the question of what enhancement is, a question which has much in common with the earlier attempt to distinguish positive from negative eugenics. The commonality is that, just as the positive-negative eugenics distinction can be understood either in terms of disease or in terms of normality, so can the concept of enhancement. Enhancement interventions can be understood either as measures which aim to "improve" people (or populations) in ways other than disease avoidance (like positive eugenics on the Disease Account) or as measures which aim to produce people with supernormal traits (like positive eugenics on the Normality Account). Thus, we can have a Disease Account and a Normality Account of enhancement.

As with the positive-negative eugenics distinction, both construals (the Disease Account and the Normality Account) are in the literature. In the three passages quoted below, for example, Elizabeth Cooke, William Gardner and Frances M. Kamm (respectively) contrast enhancement with the avoidance or prevention of disease:

> one may be inclined to redistribute as much as possible and be as "charitable" as possible, *going well beyond disease prevention, and into*

> *enhancement,* where height, good looks, physical strength, and intelligence, would be considered generous endowments of resources for one's future descendants.[14]

> Enhancement ... is the use of genetic engineering to supply a characteristic that a parent might want in a child that *does not involve the treatment or prevention of disease.*[15]

> enhancement itself may take two forms: (a) improving humans so that they fare better than any current human with respect to some characteristic, and (b) bringing people to have *good characteristics, whose absence in them would not be a disease*, that are now already common to many but not all humans (e.g., high intelligence).[16]

In contrast to this "disease account," Walter Glannon appeals to normal functioning, suggesting that enhancement "aims to raise cognitive and physical capacities *above the normal range of functioning* for persons."[17] And H. Tristram Engelhardt explicitly rejects the "disease account," stating that enhancements can be used to avoid disease: "One can engage genetic enhancement in order to avoid cancer. Increasing or enhancing resistance to cancer can be a contribution of love to those at risk of difficult deaths."[18]

5. Enhancement and Positive Eugenics

Both "enhancement" and "positive eugenics," then, are open to two different interpretations. Each can be taken to refer either to interventions which aim at "improvements" other than the avoidance of disease, or to interventions which aim to create supernormal traits. Does this mean that enhancement and positive eugenics are the same thing? The answer to this is a qualified "yes," the qualification being that this holds only if one adopts the same account for each (that is, either the Disease Account for both, or the Normality Account for both). Thus, it is theoretically possible for the two to differ, but only if we adopt a Disease Account of one and a Normality Account of the other. In principle, we could do this. However, in practice whatever rationale underlies preferring the Disease Account for one will most likely apply equally to the other (and similarly for the Normality Account).

More fundamental perhaps are the question of whether the difference between the two construals matters and the question of how we should deal with these ambiguities. The answer to the first is that it matters insofar as both "enhancement" and "positive eugenics" are seen by many as morally significant categories. Whether something is counted as "enhancement" or "positive eugenics" may therefore affect its (perceived) moral status. If it matters morally whether something is an enhancement or not, then it matters how "enhancement" (and similarly "positive eugenics") is defined, because practices may be less favorably treated if they are classified as enhancements. Moreover, the answer matters because it will determine what kinds of arguments are available in support of the view that "enhancement" and "positive eugenics" are morally worse than their opposites.

So clearly the definitions of "enhancement" and "positive eugenics" matter, but how are we to arrive at a single settled definition given the different interpretations outlined above? One possibility would be to decide in favor of one of the two accounts ("disease" and "normality"). However, there appear not to be any compelling reasons for favoring one over the other, since both usages appear coherent, are prevalent in the literature, and (as we will see shortly) can be allied with distinctive kinds of moral argument. My proposal then is that we permit both "enhancement" and "positive eugenics" to be used in either their "disease" senses or "normality" senses, but that we ask users of these terms to specify clearly which of the two senses is being invoked. In addition, for maximal clarity, I would suggest, where at all possible, using alternative terminology. For instance, rather than talking about enhancement and positive eugenics, one could talk of "supernormality selection" and the "production of supernormal traits" (if the "normality sense" is intended), or of non-health-related selection and the production of "non-health-related features" (if the "disease sense" is intended).

Perhaps some people will be left unsatisfied by this pragmatic answer and demand to know what enhancement (or positive eugenics) *really is*. However, asking such questions is not terribly helpful. For having said what the different meanings of the terms "enhancement" and "positive eugenics" are, and called for clarity in people's use of the terms, it is not obvious that asking which one is "really" enhancement (or positive eugenics) has much point.

In the remaining sections, I outline the main arguments for the view that enhancement (or positive eugenics) is morally worse than negative eugenics (other things being equal), noting at the outset that (for reasons of space) this can only be a superficial overview of what is a complex and fascinating topic. In the ethics literature, this view is widespread. As James Keenan puts it: "[For many] ethicists, enhancement stands as an activity that we should always avoid, a modern day bioethical intrinsic evil. They see enhancement as the point of no return on the slippery slope."[19]

As I suggested earlier, which arguments are available to support the view that positive eugenics (enhancement) is morally worse than negative eugenics depends on which understanding of these terms we are dealing with ("disease" or "normality"). Therefore, I will deal with each account in turn.

6. Moral Significance on the Disease Account

Why should disease avoidance be preferred to other kinds of "improvement"? One possible reason, as far as medical ethics and the regulation of healthcare are concerned, is that (arguably) disease avoidance is a core goal, if not *the* core goal of medicine. Thus, it has an importance and a legitimacy that many other goals lack. Resnik describes this view as follows: "A slightly different approach to these issues asserts that genetic therapy is on solid moral ground because it promotes the goals of medicine, while genetic enhancement promotes other, morally questionable goals."[20]

This "goals of medicine" argument is however flawed. One problem with it is that saying what the goals of medicine are is not easy, and it is far from obvious that disease avoidance is medicine's only goal, or even its main one. Other possible goals include promoting happiness and enabling people to exercise their autonomy, neither of which necessarily involve disease avoidance, and both of which may require doctors to go beyond mere disease avoidance. Another criticism of the "goals of medicine" argument is that it wrongly views as intrinsically valuable, something which is only instrumentally valuable (the avoidance of disease). What really matters (so the objection goes) is patient welfare (perhaps in conjunction with some other fundamental goods). Thus, doctors should not refrain from benefiting patients simply because what they require (or want) goes beyond the treatment of disease; and conversely, they should not treat (or strive to avoid) disease unless doing so benefits the patient.

A second argument for regarding disease avoidance as more legitimate and significant than other goals is that diseases are states that are necessarily bad for people, a feature which gives us a strong *prima facie* reason always to avoid them. This argument, though, is also flawed. First, and most obviously, many states, other than diseases, are bad for people. As Bernard Gert, Charles Culver, and K. Danner Clouser remind us, "many things can be wrong in an individual's life without her having a malady: for example, being in poverty, being neglected, or being in a runaway truck."[21]

Second, disorders vary considerably in the extent to which they impact on people's well-being. Clearly, whether harmless diseases exist depends on which theory of health is the correct one, not something that can be decided here. Nonetheless, it should be noted that, according to some major philosophies of health (such as the Boorsean one discussed earlier), (negative) welfare and disease are not necessarily or universally related to one another.[22] Thus, this argument is weak insofar as it rests on a contentious assumption about the nature of disease. Taken together these objections provide sufficient reason for rejecting this second argument.

The third and final argument for seeing disease avoidance as more legitimate than other (enhancement) goals is that the pursuit of enhancement goals is more likely to be vulnerable to charges of "playing God," "interfering with nature," or "changing human nature." Behind this is the idea that whereas disease avoidance, especially therapy, is restorative, reinstating natural functioning, other sorts of improvement do (or can) go beyond what nature provides. This argument however is also destined to fail. One major problem with it is that disease avoidance can, and often does, involve going beyond what nature normally provides. An obvious real life example of this is vaccination. Similarly, if we used the genetic testing and selection of embryos to reduce the incidence of cancer or heart disease in old age, this would clearly be "going beyond the natural" (if anything is) but equally clearly aimed at disease avoidance. Finally, and more fundamentally, the soundness of arguments in the "playing God" and "interfering with nature" categories has been rightly called into question by numerous philosophers. Hence, it is far from obvious that any arguments of this kind are valid.[23]

7. Moral Significance on the Normality Account

I want now to subject the Normality Account of enhancement (and positive eugenics) to the same scrutiny, asking why avoiding or removing subnormal traits should be generally preferable (other things being equal) to creating or selecting supernormal traits. I will briefly consider three arguments in turn: one broadly utilitarian, one broadly egalitarian, and a third based on what Derek Parfit terms the Priority View.[24]

First, the utilitarian argument. This states that avoiding subnormality is generally preferable to striving for supernormality because usually, and on average, avoiding subnormality will generate more net welfare per unit of resource. The premise on which this argument is based may well be true for, as Parfit reminds us, the "same increase in resources usually brings about greater benefits to those who are worse off."[25] However, this utilitarian argument to some extent bypasses our present concerns because our question is whether avoiding subnormality is preferable to promoting supernormality *all other things being equal.* But if avoiding subnormality will generate more utility than promoting supernormality then *other things are not equal*, and we have an obvious extrinsic reason for preferring subnormality-avoidance. Thus, the utilitarian argument, whilst expressing a significant practical truth, bypasses our main concern.

The second (egalitarian) argument says that (1) inequality is a bad thing and/or ought to be avoided or reduced, (2) subnormality avoidance is likely to reduce inequality, and (3) striving for supernormality is likely to increase inequality (except perhaps in societies where enhancement becomes almost universal, and where in effect "the norm" becomes a merely historical benchmark). So, it follows that avoiding subnormality is (nearly always) preferable to seeking supernormality, even where the different outcomes are the same in terms of total utility. This argument is structurally sound. It does however rely on two controversial (or otherwise problematic) premises which would need to be clarified and argued for in order to render the argument convincing.

The first premise is that subnormality avoidance is likely to reduce inequality. Expressed in such a general form the premise is hopelessly vague and we are left needing to know both what subnormalities are to be avoided and what things are to be equally distributed. In the first category, candidates include subnormal biological functioning, subnormal ability to support other people, and perhaps even subnormal aesthetic characteristics. In the second, candidates include health equality, equality of material resource, equal talents, and equal welfare.[26] Quite how the items in each of these categories relate to one another is difficult to fathom. For example, it appears fairly reasonable to suppose that if fewer people with genetic disorders (which, let us assume, involve subnormal biological functioning) existed, then this would help to equalize the levels of material resource, talent, and welfare. But even this is not obvious and is a complex empirical matter, since the material resource and welfare distributions will depend crucially on how society is organized, and examples of people with high levels of talent *and* high levels of disability are plentiful. So, in each case, it would have to be established empirically that subnormality contributes toward inequality. Perhaps this can be done but it would be a major undertaking.

The second premise is the commitment to egalitarianism itself. This is an enormous topic in political philosophy and this is not the place to rehearse the general arguments for and against different forms of egalitarianism. Nonetheless, the existence of fundamental objections to egalitarian theories of distribution should be noted.[27]

The third and final argument is, in many respects, the same as the egalitarian argument, but replaces the egalitarian premise with what Parfit calls the Priority View, the view that "benefiting people matters more the worse off these people are."[28] This view resembles egalitarianism in *some* respects and its supporters will often agree with egalitarians about what ought to be done. The main difference is that whereas egalitarians are concerned with something relational (equality), prioritarians are not. Parfit explains the point as follows:

> It may help to use this analogy. People at higher altitudes find it harder to breathe. Is this because they are higher up than other people? In one sense, yes. But they would find it just as hard to breathe even if there were no other people who were lower down. In the same way, on the Priority View, benefits to the worse off matter more, but that is only because these people are at a lower absolute level. It is irrelevant that these people are worse off than others. Benefits to them would matter just

> as much even if there were no others who were better off. The chief difference is, then, this. Egalitarians are concerned with *relativities*: with how each person's level compares with the level of other people. On the Priority View, we are concerned only with people's absolute levels.[29]

The Priority View argument then says that avoiding or removing subnormal traits is generally preferable (other things being equal) to creating or selecting supernormal traits because avoiding or removing subnormal traits is more likely to benefit those who are worse off. While it does seem to me that the Priority View is more plausible than many versions of egalitarianism, the Priority View *argument* faces the same problems that beset the egalitarian argument. First, the Priority View itself would have to be established. And second, for reasons given above, it is not obvious that subnormality avoidance will be coextensive with benefiting the least well-off (with much depending on the kinds of subnormality in question). The Priority View argument also faces a third objection which did not afflict the egalitarian argument. This is: can the Priority View be applied to possible future persons as well as to existing ones? Maybe it can, but some of its attractiveness depends on the intuition that benefiting those who are already worse off matters more morally. But in selection, as opposed to modification, benefit is not the issue. Instead, what is at issue is whether to create a possible future person. This is certainly not a decisive objection to the Priority View argument, but it is nonetheless another challenge that its proponents must face.

8. Conclusion

This chapter describes two accounts of the positive-negative eugenics distinction. The Disease Account says that negative eugenics aims to reduce the incidence of disease, while positive eugenics aims to "improve the quality" of the population in other ways. The Normality Account says that negative eugenics selects out subnormal (worse than normal) traits, while positive eugenics selects in supernormal (better than normal) traits. These accounts are also accounts of enhancement, with enhancement being the equivalent of positive eugenics in each case. It is suggested that we permit both "enhancement" and "positive eugenics" to be used in either their "disease" senses or "normality" senses, but that we ask users of these terms to specify clearly which of the two senses is being invoked. In addition, less ambiguous terminology should be used where possible. For instance, rather than talking about enhancement and positive eugenics, we could talk about "supernormality selection" and the "production of supernormal traits." Finally, the chapter has given an overview of the arguments for the view that the positive-negative eugenics distinction is morally significant. Most of these appear flawed. There may be some mileage in the Priority View argument but, as we have seen, it faces considerable obstacles.

NOTES

1. Francis Galton, *Essays in Eugenics* (Honolulu: University Press of the Pacific, 1909), p. 35.

2. Diane B. Paul, "Is Human Genetics Disguised Eugenics?" *Biology and Philosophy*, ed. Michael Ruse and David Hull (Oxford: Oxford University Press, 1998), pp. 536–549, at p. 537.

3. Richard Barnett, "Eugenics," *The Lancet*, 363:9422 (22 May 2004), p. 1742; Ruth Chadwick, "Genetics and Ethics" *Routledge Encyclopaedia of Philosophy*, ed. Edward Craig (London: Routledge, 1998); Ruth Chadwick, Henk ten Have, Jørgen Husted, Mairi Levitt, Tony McGleenan, Darren Shickle, and Urban Wiesing, "Genetic Screening and Ethics: European Perspectives," *Journal of Medicine and Philosophy*, 23:3 (July 1998), pp. 255–273, at p. 268; Rachel Iredale, "Eugenics and its Relevance to Contemporary Health Care," *Nursing Ethics*, 7:3 (1 May 2000), pp. 205–214, at p. 207; Tom Shakespeare, "Choices and Rights: Eugenics, Genetics, and Disability Equality," *Disability and Society*, 13:5 (1 November 1998), pp. 665–681, at p. 668.

4. Diane B. Paul, "Eugenic Anxieties, Social Realities, and Political Choices," *Social Research*, 59:3 (Fall 1992): p. 663–683, p. 663.

5. David B. Resnik, "The Moral Significance of the Therapy-Enhancement Distinction in Human Genetics," *Cambridge Quarterly of Healthcare Ethics*, 9:3 (July 2000), pp. 365–377, at p. 373.

6. Jean E. Chambers, "Women's Right to Choose Rationally," *Cambridge Quarterly of Healthcare Ethics* 12:4 (October 2003), pp. 418–428, at p. 418.

7. Bernice S. Elger and Timothy W. Harding, "Huntington's Disease: Do Future Physicians and Lawyers Think Eugenically?" *Clinical Genetics*, 64:44 (October 2003), pp. 327–338, at p. 335.

8. Walter Glannon, "Genes, Embryos, and Future People," *Bioethics*, 12:3 (July 1998), pp. 187–211, at p. 197.

9. HFEA (Human Fertilisation and Embryology Authority, UK), *HFEA Licenses PGD for Inherited Colon Cancer*, Press Release (1 November 2004), http://www.hfea.gov.uk.

10. Richard Twyman, "Cystic Fibrosis," Wellcome Trust Website, 30 July 2003, http://genome.wellcome.ac.uk/doc_wtd020856.html.

11. Christopher Boorse, "On the Distinction Between Disease and Illness," *Philosophy and Public Affairs*, 5:1 (Autumn 1975), pp. 49–68; Christopher Boorse, "Health as a Theoretical Concept," *Philosophy of Science*, 44:4 (December 1977), pp. 542 573; Christopher Boorse, "A Rebuttal on Health," *What is Disease?* eds. James M. Humber and Robert F. Almeder (Totowa, New Jersey: Humana Press, 1997), pp. 1–134.

12. Resnik, "The Moral Significance of the Therapy-Enhancement Distinction in Human Genetics," p. 365. See also W. Anderson, "Genetics and Human Malleability." *Hastings Center Report* 20.1 (1990), pp. 21-24.

13. Human Genetics Commission (UK), *Choosing the Future: Genetics and Reproductive Decision Making*, July 2004, p. 19

14. Elizabeth F. Cooke, "Germ-line Engineering, Freedom, and Future Generations," *Bioethics*, 17:1 (February 2003), pp. 32–58, at p. 37 (my emphasis).

15. William Gardner, "Can Human Genetic Enhancement be Prohibited?" *Journal of Medicine and Philosophy*, 20:1 (February 1995), pp. 65–84, at p. 65 (my emphasis).

16. Frances M. Kamm, "Genes, Justice, and Obligations to Future People," *Social Philosophy and Policy*, 19:2 (July 2002), pp. 360–388.

17. Glannon, "Genes, Embryos, and Future People," p. 197 (my emphasis).

18. H. Tristram Engelhardt, Jr., "Genetic Enhancement and Theosis: Two Models of Therapy," *Christian Bioethics*, 5:2 (August 1999), pp. 197–199, at p. 198.

19. James F. Keenan, "'Whose Perfection is it Anyway?': A Virtuous Consideration of Enhancement," *Christian Bioethics*, 5:2 (August 1999), pp. 104–120, at p. 113.

20. Resnik, "The Moral Significance of the Therapy-Enhancement Distinction in Human Genetics," p. 368.

21. Bernard Gert, Charles M. Culver, and K. Danner Clouser, *Bioethics: A Return to Fundamentals* (New York: Oxford University Press, 1997), p. 98.

22. *Ibid.*, p. 104.

23. Ruth Chadwick, "Playing God," *Bioethics News*, 9:4 (1990), pp. 38–46; William Grey, "Playing God," *Encyclopedia of Applied Ethics*, eds. Dan Callahan, Peter Singer, and Ruth Chadwick (San Diego: Academic Press, 1998); John Stuart Mill, "On Nature," *Nature, The Utility of Religion, and Theism* (Rationalist Press, 1874); Richard Norman, "Interfering with Nature," *Journal of Applied Philosophy*, 13:1 (1996), pp. 1–11.

24. Derek Parfit, "Equality or Priority?" *Bioethics*, ed. John Harris (Oxford: Oxford University Press, 2001), pp. 347–386.

25. *Ibid.*, p. 349.

26. Richard Arneson, "Egalitarianism," *Stanford Encyclopedia of Philosophy*, ed. Edward N. Zalta, http://plato.stanford.edu/entries/egalitarianism/.

27. Arneson, "Egalitarianism"; Brian Barry and Matt Matravers, "Justice," *Routledge Encyclopaedia of Philosophy*, ed. Edward Craig (London: Routledge, 1998); Parfit, "Equality or Priority?"

28. Parfit, "Equality or Priority?" p. 366.

29. *Ibid.*, pp. 369–370.

Ten

THE GENETIC FALLACY AND SOME OTHER CONCERNS IN BEHAVIORAL GENETICS

Niall W. R. Scott

1. Introduction

The issue of the genetic fallacy has been given recent attention in the fields of genetics, behavioral genetics, and the philosophy of biology. Concerns are raised about the political nature of debates in human biology regarding genetic explanation and causal accounts of human nature. What is at issue, as Lenny Moss puts it, involves questions such as "What should count as biology?" and "What should count as the nature of human nature?" as well as the concern that to divide "nature from nurture is to take sides in advance."[1]

Recent work by Neil Levy and Mianna Lotz that rejects the genetic argument for reproductive cloning, shows a problem in accepting a particular deterministic causal story of why cloned children may be preferred to adopted children.[2] It also introduces a broader issue about why we might want to raise concerns about accepting a material/efficient deterministic approach to behavioral genetics. Levy and Lotz hold that the presumed preference for cloned children depends on a belief in the importance of a genetic connection to our offspring, a causal relationship that makes false assumptions about the way one might care for biologically related children rather than adopted children. Although the title of their paper provides, in addition to empirical evidence, the philosophical reason why this assumption is false, the paper does not discuss the fallacy to which the title refers—the genetic fallacy.

In the essay "The Dream of the Human Genome," written in 1992 as a response to *The Code of Codes*, Richard Lewontin points out that the causal information that can be derived from DNA is difficult to interpret, in much the same way that it is difficult to pin down an exact meaning of a word, where that meaning is context-dependent.[3] In this paper I would like to challenge the causal approach to genetic behaviorism, and to argue that it is inadequate, since it does not consider the full possibilities available in a causal account. If an account is given solely in material terms, or in terms of what brings about physical change, then it is possible that what a behavioral trait is as a cultural, social, or moral norm will be read into the characterization of that trait's physical origin, without recognizing that it is not physically present. This, I hold, involves committing a genetic fallacy not just at the logical but also at the ontological level, following Nietzsche's version of the genetic fallacy in the *Genealogy of Morals*. If a full causal account is given that considers the Aristotelian idea of the four causes, including what a thing is for and what makes a thing what it is (its form), the mistake of thinking that somehow descriptions of behaviors emerge from a combination of genetic and environmental factors need not be made. In this chapter I will outline what a genetic fallacy is and present a slightly different reading from the logical definition to illustrate how the fallacy relates to the origin of a behavior and what that behavior is, with reference to behavioral research done on criminal and sexual behavior.

2. What a Genetic Fallacy is

The genetic fallacy concerns the relationship between a claim or thing and the origins of that claim or thing. The fallacy involves assuming that the nature of the source of the claim or thing is used to support or discredit that which comes after it. It is often referred to as a fallacy of irrelevancy regarding the origin or history of an idea.[4]

Usually the genetic fallacy is presented as a logical fallacy, belonging to that group of fallacies that involve *ad hominem* arguments. In this chapter I hold that it is possible to make a distinction between the genetic fallacy as it holds in the context of arguments, and as it holds in the context of things. As a form of *ad hominem* fallacy, the genetic fallacy describes the error in dismissing an argument as (1) invalid because of something that is wrong with, or mistaken in, its origins; or (2) invalid *because* of its origins (the fallacy of appealing to authority). In this sense the genetic fallacy is a logical fallacy and it is important to note that it considers the truth or falsity of a claim. There may well be good reasons for believing a claim or believing that one should dismiss a claim on the basis of its origins, but neither of these provides a logical criterion for accepting or rejecting an argument as valid or invalid. So the origins of an idea are to be distinguished from its justification.

This concerns the genetic fallacy as a logical fallacy. I would like to emphasize a spin on this. We can take the genetic fallacy as applicable to the relationship between things in general and their origins, thus moving from a fallacy concerning the structure of an argument to the relationship claimed concerning the content of what is argued about. This is to say that, in claiming that a thing is not the same as its origins, we can also make a claim in terms of the genetic fallacy about what can be said of a thing in relation to a causal account of how it came about. This can be maintained if we make a distinction between the cause of a thing and what that thing is.

3. The Fallacy in Terms of Causation

A causal story of how something came about does not give us an account of what it is. In the context of behavioral genetics, amongst other fields, it is important to bear this in mind. So we may well have an explanation of how a particular behavior came about—say, criminal behavior in a group or in an individual based on a combination of genetic, hereditary, and environmental explanations—but the origins of the mere behavior do not tell us what criminal behavior *is*. To uncover what criminal behavior is, we need to have an understanding of cultural, social, and moral values. We bring these understandings to bear on the group or individual in question in the assessment of their behavior on the basis of these values.

Nietzsche, in the second essay of the *Genealogy of Morals*, makes this clear in writing on the difference between the origin of law and the purpose of law:

> the cause and the origin of a thing and its eventual utility, its actual employment and place in a system of purposes lie worlds apart; whatever exists, having somehow come into being, is again and again reinterpreted to new ends, taken over, transformed and redirected by some power superior to it; all events in the organic world are a subduing, a becoming master, and all subduing and becoming master involves a fresh interpretation, an adaptation through which any previous "meaning" and "purpose" are necessarily obscured or even obliterated, however well one has understood the utility of any physiological organ (or of a legal institution, a social custom, a political usage, a form in art or in a religious cult), this means nothing regarding its origin.[5]

Moss argues that a genetic explanation of how a state of affairs came about, of the type where S1 leads to S2 leads to S3 leading to S*n*, allows that a gene can play a part in an explanation of how S*n* came to be, but that it is a contingent, not a necessary element of such an explanation. The presence of a gene in an explanation does not secure the soundness, adequacy, or completeness of the explanation. Avoiding a genetic fallacy, he holds, is a question of tidying up terminology, so that the nature of S*n* is in some disguised form present in the explanation of how S*n* came about. What is more, he maintains that whether or not a genetic fallacy is committed "must ultimately be seen as an empirical question."[6]

I maintain that there is more to consider, and that the genetic fallacy leads us beyond an empirical question. This difference between the origin of a thing and what it becomes or what it is, can be understood more clearly if we look at an Aristotelian account of causation, in which the aim is to investigate what a thing is. Aristotle distinguishes between four causes: the material which constitutes a thing, that is, the matter of which it is made; the efficient cause, that which brings about a change; the formal cause, that is, what a thing is, or its essence; and the teleological cause, the end or goal of a thing.[7]

Aristotle continues with an interesting point concerning the cause of a thing. He writes:

> People usually investigate the causes of coming to be thus: they see what comes after what, and what first acted or was acted on, and go on seeking what comes next. But there are two sources of natural change, of which one is not natural, since it has no source of change in itself."[8]

The thing that Aristotle considers not to be natural as a source of change is what a thing is; its end and what it is for.

4. Determinism in Behavioral Genetics

This issue is important in the role that biological determinism plays in accounts of human behavior, both in accounts that are grounded in a strong deterministic sense as well as in accounts that are weakly deterministic. From a strong determinist perspective, there is a direct causal relationship between genes and behavior, and although other factors such as environment are admitted to play a role, these are not important in the same way that genes are. Genes are sufficient to cause behavior, both in single and complex association.

A weak determinist perspective admits that genes are only a part of a broad, more complex set of conditions that bring about behavior, so genetics and the all encompassing term "environment" are both considered to be necessary for a full explanation of behavior. By and large in the realm of behavioral genetics, the strong version of genetic behaviorism is held to be false, not only on the grounds that we have insufficient knowledge of genetics but also, as Henry Tam claims, on ontological grounds.[9] He holds that over half the variance in the explanation of behavior is not genetic. We only have a measure of heritability provided by research into behavioral genetics, not an understanding of the mechanism through which genes act, and, according to Tam, there can be no full, strong genetic explanation to behavior.[10] Attempts to move away from a strict determinist view are not helped by perspectives promoted in the philosophy of biology by socio-biologists such as Michael Ruse and E. O. Wilson. Such positions hold that "the social behaviour of animals is firmly under the control of our genes, and has been shaped into forms that give reproductive advantages."[11]

However, Tam thinks that we may have good reason to accept a weak genetic determinism, which holds that genetics has a role to play in the cause of behavioral traits. This would have us accept that genetics is one of several relevant genetic causal factors that contribute to human behavior, but that we do have available the possibility of a full deterministic account of behavior. I still wish to challenge the way in which this is presented. The claim that I want to challenge is that what it means to provide a full deterministic account of human behavior, leads us to consider causation in material and efficient terms, but is not necessarily open to a broader, more Aristotelian account of causation.

When we apply only the notions of material and efficient cause to the case of behavioral genetics, all we have is mere behavior—action, but no warrant for bringing it under a description of a particular kind, for example criminal behavior, intelligent behavior, or heterosexual or homosexual behavior. In order to gain such a warrant, we need to import an additional account. An account of what makes a thing what it *is*, can be provided by, and come under the heading of, its formal and its teleological cause. In making this point, we bring in the two accounts that are, as Aristotle puts it, "not natural."

5. The Implications of the Genetic Fallacy for Behavioral Genetics

What does this mean in the context of behavioral genetics? At a basic level, even though there may be a genetic association in a causal account of say, criminal behavior, sexual orientation, or intelligence, this account is limited in that it does not recognize what the description of the behavior *does* in the causal account. More fundamentally, in attributing the description "criminal" to a certain kind of behavior, we are introducing a story about what we are holding these material causal explanations to be for.

There are statistical reasons for thinking that a behavior as a mere behavior belongs within a certain bracket, which excludes normative reasons. However, as accounts of the relationships between genetics and human behavior are presented, perhaps because of the emotive and political nature of what is at stake, the statistical meaning is quickly forgotten and the normative takes its place. So, the differences expressed genetically between those identified as exhibiting aggressive behavior related to a mutation in the gene producing monoamine oxidase, and those not, accounts for a certain proportion of the population.[12] The added normative description of the behavior as aggressive or antisocial behavior is not given by the mere statistical difference in the gene proportion: instead, it is a societal norm that is added to the genetic account. All too quickly it is assumed that we can in part account for a genetic origin of aggressive, antisocial, and criminal behavior without conceding that treating the behavior *as* criminal is an account that is imported into the causal story. In the case of monoamine oxidase deficiency, the work done by Brunner involving studies of aggressive male behavior in a Dutch family identified a pattern of inheritance to a sex-linked gene that coded for monoamine oxidase.

A mutation in this gene prevents the breaking down of serotonin and norepinephrine, and was linked by Brunner to lower levels of intelligence and a propensity to violent behavior. Upon publication of this work, the media declared the discovery of a "gene for crime," even though, as David Rowe notes, this abnormality has only been found in one family, and so can be presumed to be extremely rare.[13]

Yet Rowe, in his book *Biology and Crime*, goes on to show how "a single gene can influence a criminal disposition."[14] This suggests that, instead of crime's having a genetic origin, the criminal disposition is already present, and is something else that genetics has an influence *on*. This seems an acceptable way of expressing things. Genes may provide background conditions that bring about or can affect a certain behavior, but are not held to cause such behavior. So the mistaken claim that criminality or crime forms part of the causal explanation of behavior is not made. However, Rowe moves away from this position, and continues to give a causal account in material and efficient terms of the way in which genes determine behavioral characteristics. He holds that there is a causal asymmetry between genes and behavior, in that behavior can affect the expression of genes on the one hand, but environment cannot change a DNA sequence, except for the rarity of mutations. He holds this not only as a rejection of Lamarckianism, but also in support of the claim that there is a directional causal pathway of gene to environment:

> a gene's social environmental direction of causation is more plausible than the reverse. For instance if it were discovered that for a particular gene teenagers with a seven repeat allele hung out with delinquent friends more than those with a five repeat allele, it is more plausible that the allele created a tendency to choose delinquent friends than the reverse; hanging out with delinquent friends will not change a person's repeat number from five to seven.[15]

The problem with this hypothetical example moves on from the genetic fallacy of "locating" criminality in the causal account. It is not the explanation of causal direction, but rather the very idea that an allele can be held as a *cause* to create a tendency to hang out with delinquent friends. As is the case with MAOA deficiency, although such an allele may form part of the background conditions of the behavior, whether or not it is a cause of that behavior is going to be far from clear. There are too many other factors that deserve analysis—in this example, the nature, motivations, and reasons involved in friendship, the phenomenon of delinquency, and so on. And the social and cultural factors that pick out criminal behavior, many of which have little to do with aggression, do not have the features of a material cause. Consequently, a genetic causal account of behavior provides neither necessary nor sufficient conditions, provided these are still only background conditions for behavior.

A causal approach to behavior—even one in which terms such as "influence" and "predisposition" are used with caution—raises serious issues concerning ethical and social implications. So criticism can be leveled at the media and some scientists who promote the idea that a strict causal relationship between genes and behavior is common, as McGuffin, Riley, and Plomin do when they write: "Rarely is it mentioned that traits involving behaviour are more likely to have a complex genetic basis."[16] They continue by emphasizing the need to recognize the importance of the interplay between environmental factors and multiple genes. Much work has been done to move understanding toward this complexity in the case of research into genetic influence on sexual orientation, for example, dispelling the myth that the "gay gene" arose as a result of poor, inaccurate reporting of research by Dean Hamer on the possibility that a genetic *influence* on homosexuality could be linked to the Xq28 chromosome.[17]

They further emphasize the importance of recognizing the interplay between environmental factors and multiple genes. Yet they urge a move toward behavioral genomics, insisting that research demonstrates that "nearly all behaviours that have been studied show moderate to high heritability—usually to a somewhat higher degree than do many common physical diseases" and that "although environment plays a role, its contribution tends to be of the non-shared type, that is, environmental factors make people different from rather than similar to their relatives."[18] They insist however that these research findings need to be considered in probabilistic rather than deterministic terms. If this is borne in mind, some of the ethical concerns raised by behavioral genomics are seen to have little substance: for example stigmatization is less likely if the expression of a trait that leads to a condition is understood in probabilistic and not deterministic terms. It is unclear what argument lies behind this claim, especially regarding insurance, where the probabilistic likelihood of expressing a condition is all that would be required to alter a premium. A further issue concerning the understanding presented in media reporting of behavioral genetics, is that of the meaning of the term "heritability." The use of the term here differs from its colloquial sense. Here it is an expression concerning statistical variance, instead of the direct inheritance of certain characteristics.

The potential damage that can be done in research into the genetic origins of behavior is well illustrated by Schuklenk *et al.*'s excellent analysis of the ethical problems that are raised in framing such research in causal terms. Critical of Hamer's study, and the direct causal model, they point out that genes cannot specify any behaviors or psychological phenomena directly. The authors show, though without using the same terminology, that a genetic fallacy is committed in such research, underlining the specific meaning of heritability mentioned above:

> Importantly "gay genes" are not required for homosexuality to be heritable. This is because heritability has a precise technical meaning; it refers to the ratio of genetic variation to the total phenotypic variation. As such heritability merely reflects the degree to which a given outcome is linked to genetic factors; it says nothing about the nature of those factors nor about their mechanisms of action.[19]

For Schuklenk *et al*, research into sexual orientation can never be value-neutral, in that the motivation for uncovering the origin of homosexuality is rooted in social frameworks, which they claim are "pervasively homophobic."[20] Although this means that scientific research needs to recognize what elements from the social arena are read into causal accounts, but are not present in the material casual relationship between genes and phenotype, that is not to say that all genetic research into human behavior is to be dismissed. Instead, the importance that other accounts have on the material causal account need to be given a proper case in a full understanding of the relationship between a thing and its origins.

6. Considerations of the UK Nuffield Council's Report on Genetics and Behavior

The need to understand that behavioral genetics provides evidence in terms of statistics is emphasized in the Nuffield Report, where the importance of reading normal variation and behavior in the normal range as a statistical instead of a normative expression is emphasized and "no moral evaluation or judgement is implied."[21] However, the very identification of certain aspects of human behavior to be considered, such as looking into the genetic influences on aggressive behavior or intelligence, itself carries normative weight. This normative and political weight is well emphasized by Schuklenk as it relates to the issue of homosexuality.

An interesting example of ethical, legal, and social issues being added at the end of writings on research into behavioral genetics is found in the structure of the Nuffield Report *Genetics and Human Behaviour: The Ethical Context*. The scientific evidence is presented and evaluated first in the document, and the ethical, legal, and social issues are considered in the light of the report on scientific evidence. It is important to note however that the Nuffield report does outline well the limits of the empirical findings in relation to the causal relationship between genes and behavior, largely concluding that research is at different stages for different traits (the ones mentioned in the report are intelligence, personality, antisocial behavior, and sexual orientation). It also states that some areas of the human genome have been identified that may have an effect on human behavior, and "for most traits the route from such factors to a particular behaviour is unclear."[22]

In this approach, the science is being held to provide part of a causal account that will contribute to a better understanding of human behavior—ethical, legal, and social issues are considered in terms of responses to the research. In other words, given that this research is continuing and is being presumed to produce ever more accurate representations of the relationship between genes and behavior, what demands does it place upon, and what responses are required from, the ethical corner? What is asserted here is that the causal account—the foundation to the scientific approach—is one that needs to be properly understood. So, as Moss's position, set out earlier, states, whether or not the genetic fallacy is committed is an empirical question. This is most clearly expressed by the American Society for Human Genetics' (ASHG) 1997 statement on behavioral genetics, considering ethical and social issues. The role of the scientist in being able to communicate science clearly to the public is presented as crucial to ensuring that a sound understanding is gained in the context of genetic counseling and group differences. The result of this communication is: "Public knowledge, programme design, and policy developments should rest not on popular myths but on findings from the best available science."[23]

The Nuffield Report has as its aim to *consider* the ethics of undertaking research into behavioral genetics, and the implications of using, through genetic tests, the findings of such research to establish characteristics in practical contexts including education, employment, insurance, and legal proceedings. It also aims to determine the impact of the findings of behavioral genetic research on individual family members and social groups, and the "impact of genetic knowledge on the perception of those with relevant behavioural characteristics."[24] The report first considers the scientific evidence, then the ethical, social, and legal implications that (might) arise as a consequence of research. In each separate section on evidence produced through research, the validity of the evidence is questioned in terms of there not being enough empirical evidence to support a strong determinist view of genes as causing behavior, but that further research needs to be done.

The Nuffield report is careful to make sure that where research into behavioral genetics might lead to a diminishing of responsibility of the self in behavior, it opposes deterministic fatalism, which would be akin to the strong determinism mentioned above, and promotes the idea that human choice plays a causal role. However, an account that permits human choice is going to be an account of causation that needs not only much further investigation, but needs to be richer than empirical study can provide, as is suggested in the report.

Despite the Nuffield Council's rejection of a certain kind of determinism, behavioral genetics does depend on a methodological determinism, in that it depends on an assumption of a deterministic causal relationship between genes and behavior (no matter how minimal the contribution by genes may be) and environmental factors. In other words, it accepts a weak determinism concerning the role that genes play in human behavior.

So, the Nuffield report criticizes the misleading information given concerning the relationship between human sexual orientation and genetics in the label "the gay gene." Instead, it is underlined that genes play a role, have an influence, are involved amongst other aspects in the phenomenon named human behavior. These other aspects are usually cited as being environmental conditions, ranging from the cellular level to the extra-cellular level, as physical causes to the social.

In all this, it is implicit that the research into behavioral genetics will generate empirical evidence that demonstrates a relationship between genes and behavior to provide a better understanding of certain human behaviors that have been identified in the sphere of human social interaction. This relationship is expressed, then, through weak determinism, or, as Plomin suggests in his advocacy of a probabilistic approach, through a statistical likelihood that genes influence a particular behavior. Even though the relationship is expressed statistically, at the heart of it is an assumption of a causal relationship in terms of material and efficient causes—genetic, cellular, and environmental—that bring about human behavior in either a causal or a statistical account, where statistics are used to support the likelihood of the causal account being true. So there is always the chance that the features under investigation—the description of the behavior and what the nature of behavior is, be it criminal, sexual, or some other form—are likely to become part of the account of how the behavior came about. This leaves the way open for the genetic fallacy to be committed, not recognizing that nothing about the behavior is located in its origins. I hold that what the behavior in question *is* cannot be obtained through an explanatory account, nor can it be achieved through more empirical investigation.

NOTES

1. Lenny Moss, "Human Nature, the Genetic Fallacy, and the Philosophical Reconstruction of Anthropogenesis," *Kulturwissenschaftliches Institut: Jahrbuch 2004*, ed. Jörn Rüsen (Bielefeld: transcript Verlag, 2004).

2. Neil Levy and Mianna Lotz, "Reproductive Cloning and a (Kind of) Genetic Fallacy," *Bioethics*, 19:3 (2005), pp. 232–250.

3. Richard Lewontin, "The Dream of the Human Genome," *The Dream of the Human Genome and Other Stories* (London: Granta Books, 2000), p. 152; *The Code of Codes: Scientific and Social Issues in the Human Genome Project*, eds. Daniel J. Kevles and Leroy Hood (Cambridge, MA: Harvard University Press, 1992).

4. Julian Baggini, "Mental Manoeuvres: The Genetic Fallacy," *The New Humanist*, 117:2 (summer 2002), http://www.newhumanist.org.uk/volume117issue2.php.

5. Friedrich Nietzsche, *The Genealogy of Morals* (London: Penguin books, 1973)

6. Moss, "Human Nature, the Genetic Fallacy, and the Philosophical Reconstruction of Anthropogenesis."

7. Aristotle, *Physics*, *A New Aristotle Reader*, transl. J. L. Ackrill (Oxford: Oxford University Press, 1987), bk. II, ch. 3, 194a–195a.

8. *Ibid.*, bk. II, ch. 7, 198a.

9. Mark Philpott, "Not Guilty by Reason of Genetic Determinism," *Punishment Excuses and Moral Development*, ed. Henry Tam (Aldershot: Avebury, 1996).

10. *Ibid.*

11. Michael Ruse and E. O. Wilson, "The Evolution of Ethics," *New Scientist*, 108:1478 (17 October 1985), pp. 50–52.

12. H. G. Brunner, M. Nelen, X. O. Breakfield, H. H. Ropers, and B. A. Van Oost, "Abnormal Behaviour Associated With a Point Mutation in the Structural Genes for Monoamine Oxidase A," *Science*, 262:5133 (20 October 1993), p. 578–580.

13. David C. Rowe, *Biology and Crime* (Los Angeles: Roxbury, 2002), p. 89.

14. *Ibid.*, p. 90.

15. *Ibid.*, p. 97.

16. Peter McGuffin, Brien Riley, and Robert Plomin, "Genomics and Behaviour: Toward Behavioural Genomics," *Science*, 291:5507 (16 February 2001), pp. 1232–1249.

17. D. H. Hamer, S. Hu, V. L. Magnuson, N. Hu, and A. M. Pattatucci, "A Linkage between DNA Markers on the X Chromosome and Male Sexual Orientation," *Science*, 261:5126 (3 September 1993), pp. 321–327.

18. McGuffin, Riley, and Plomin, "Genomics and Behaviour: Toward Behavioural Genomics."

19. Udo Schuklenk, Edward Stein, Jacinta Kerin, and William Byne, "The Ethics of Genetic Research on Sexual Orientation," *The Hastings Center Report*, 27:4 (July–August 1997), pp. 6–13.

20. *Ibid.*

21. Nuffield Council on Bioethics, *Genetics and Human Behaviour: The Ethical Context* (Plymouth: Latimer Trend Company, Nuffield Council on Bioethics, 2002), sec. 1.8, p. 7.

22. *Ibid.*, sec 11.2, p. 111.

23. Stephanie L. Sherman, John C. DeFries, Irving I. Gottesman, John C. Loehlin, Joanne M. Meyer, Mary Z. Pelias, John Rice, and Irwin Waldman, "Behavioral Genetics '97: ASHG Statement. Recent Developments in Human Behavioral Genetics: Past Accomplishments and Future Directions," *American Journal of Human Genetics*, 60:6 (June 1997), pp. 1265–1275.

24. Nuffield Council on Bioethics, *Genetics and Human Behaviour, The Ethical Context.*

Eleven

EUGENICS: ENHANCING INDIVIDUALS OR POPULATIONS?

Niall W. R. Scott

1. Introduction

In this chapter I want to expand on some of the issues raised by Stephen Wilkinson in chapter nine, that arise from the definitions he has clarified and problems that emerge from those definitions. I also aim to discuss further moral issues concerning eugenics. In addition to Wilkinson's explanation of the distinction between positive and negative eugenics, there is the distinction that has been maintained for some time now in the literature between the new eugenics and the old or "historical" eugenics. This latter distinction aims to draw a line between questions concerning eugenics that have arisen in the light of developments and opportunities in modern biotechnology, and the eugenic social policies of the past. Such policies aimed to implement radical measures to curb the breeding behavior of those deemed to be contributing to the weakening of the human gene pool. I will first consider problems that arise in shifts from eugenics considered as individual reproductive decision making, to eugenics considered in terms of groups or populations. Here I will look at two cases, one of a couple opting to select a deaf child, the other of a "savior sibling" being born to help cure the disease of a family member. I then consider the context in which these choices are made and argue that it is not easy to treat them as discreet individual choices. Instead, they happen in a socio-political context and have group or population consequences. As a result, I hold that negative and positive eugenics share their goals. I discuss the goals of enhancement in recent work on liberal eugenics, and question whether the liberal approach to flourishing is acceptable when compared with an Aristotelian approach.

2. Questioning the Positive-Negative Distinction

One of the important differences between the new and the old eugenics is the shift in emphasis from enforcing or coercing human reproductive choices through policy, to the current situation in which individual choice is paramount. The main focus in this era of developing biotechnologies, with both its present and future possibilities, involves Prenatal Genetic Diagnosis (PGD), screening technologies and gene therapy, both somatic and germ line. Arguments that support new eugenics use the capacity for the exercise of autonomy to maintain that one can provide a moral defense for such practices.

Wilkinson's presentation of the distinctions between positive and negative eugenics demonstrates clearly why one may be motivated to oppose positive eugenics, especially where it involves enhancement. However, where negative eugenics involves therapeutic intervention it presents us with a challenge, since it would seem that we are morally obliged to intervene in someone's current condition, or in that of a future person, to prevent suffering and promote health. Wilkinson, in teasing out the complexities of definition, rightly demands clarity in the expression of the different senses of eugenics being used, mapped on to therapeutic and enhancement as well as disease normality accounts. I would like to introduce another request regarding definition, but one that challenges whether or not the positive-negative distinction can hold when eugenics is subjected to further scrutiny.

John Harris argues that where parents are in a position to make a choice about the health of their offspring, there is a moral obligation for them to make choices that reduce harm or suffering, be it through the promotion of therapeutic interventions, embryo selection, or somatic or germ line therapies.[1] He argues that, so far as this obligation is concerned, there is no significant moral difference between a range of interventions from embryo selection through to enhancement. That range includes gene therapy, which aims at the elimination of genetic disorder and the introduction of genetic material to enhance resistance to disease, but which may even aim at cosmetic enhancement: "There is in short no moral difference between attempts to cure dysfunction and attempts to enhance function where enhancement protects life or health."[2] It is clear then that with regard to the distinctions that Wilkinson has so carefully pointed out, Harris does not see the positive-negative distinction as morally significant. What is more, for Harris they are expressions of the same general move toward removing suffering, but simply stress different aspects. So the negative-eugenic act of deleting a deleterious gene for therapeutic reasons in an individual is going to provide enhancement for the human population more broadly, in so far as the potential harm caused by a malfunctioning gene has been removed.

3. Two Cases

I would like to suggest for a different reason that the positive-negative distinction holds in one sphere of argument, but not another. I wish to address this by considering it in a way that differentiates between eugenics at the individual level, and eugenics at the group or population level. This takes us back to the question of what eugenics is. I do not think it is especially easy to get away from the aspect of eugenics that aims at improving the human gene pool, as it features in some of the original definitions of the term, such as Francis Galton's: "Eugenics is the study of the agencies under social control that may improve or impair the racial qualities of future generations, either physically or mentally."[3] Diane Paul makes the point concerning attempts to invoke a different understanding of eugenics—one based on unintended effects brought about by individual reproductive choices rather than social policies—does not work. This is because it is not easy to demarcate between individual decisions and the political contexts in which they occur. She states: "A definition of 'eugenicist' that bars Francis Galton is, on the face of it, absurd."[4]

Let us look at two examples in recent history that involve couples making decisions about the nature of their offspring. First is the case involving the deaf couple Sharon Duchesneau and Candy McCullough, who in 2002 sought out a sperm donor with five generations of deafness in his family in order to give birth to a deaf child.[5] The couple's action drew criticism on account of its appearing to favor selection on the basis of a disability, but also defense on account of its upholding parental choice with regard to the nature of the parents' offspring. It also drew the request that attention be paid to the way in which deaf people are treated in current society, rather than to a fear of designing deaf babies.

The second case involves the birth of Jamie Whitaker to provide a suitable tissue match for his brother Charlie, who suffered from the blood disorder Diamond Blackfan Anemia.[6] This sparked controversy about parental selection of offspring for the therapeutic needs of another. Although the process was disallowed in the United Kingdom, Charlie's parents were able to travel to Chicago for the required services.

Both cases present highly complex issues when considered in terms of eugenics, and of the goals they were trying to achieve. We can look at both situations as involving individual choices. In doing this, a moral agreement or disagreement may well focus on the capacity for prospective parents to exercise their reproductive autonomy. We can also consider the consequences of the choices made. After all, they are choices *about* something; they are made with particular goals in mind. So, the moral debate concerning the acceptability of selecting a deaf child or selecting a child to provide therapeutic benefit to a sibling will engage with the question of whether it is acceptable to produce offspring solely with utility in mind. Is it right to produce a child in order to satisfy the need generated by a sick sibling? Is it acceptable to produce a child with a view to embodying the values of a couple and of the deaf community of which that couple is part? Of course, in both situations the parents will state that the reasons to have offspring are multiple and varied, but given the choice, children were born who could also fulfill a particular function. Yet still there remains the possibility of arguments against such selection for fear of the capacity to create a generation of humans valued primarily for the function they have been bred to serve.

Discussions on the acceptability of these two cases focus on the choices made available to the parents, given the available genetic technology. The Whitaker case presents us with an example that falls under the description of negative eugenics, since the aim of Jamie's selection and birth was that he should be of therapeutic benefit to his brother. Wilkinson, in chapter nine, has provided good reasons why on the one hand we would reject a disease argument based on the ambiguity of what the goals of medicine are and the nature of disease is in relation to health. On the other hand, we may well defend the parents' decision on egalitarian-priority-view grounds: that is, on the basis that it would benefit a person who is significantly worse off than others in not being able to generate red blood cells, and in being subjected to regular blood transfusions and a low life expectancy. John Harris would hold that this therapeutic intervention is morally obligatory for the parents, where the treatment and procedures are available.

Where the case of Duchesneau and McCullough can clearly be described as eugenic, it is not clear that the Whitaker case can. Duchesneau and McCullough made a choice about the nature of their offspring, preferring and selecting a sperm donor who was most likely to help them produce a deaf child. The child, having been born (deaf), holds genetic material that can be passed on to the next generation should he or she want to, maintaining the presence of the particular trait in the population. So here there is a direct relationship between a reproductive choice and a possible genetic future. For the Whitaker case, although it involves a reproductive choice, it is not immediately clear that it is an example of eugenic practice. If we go back to a definition of eugenics that stresses the importance of the effects of reproductive choices, then the Whitaker case will need to demonstrate a change in the genetic make-up of an individual that will not only enhance or improve the health or welfare of the individual, but also potentially improve or damage a future population. The therapeutic benefit to Charlie Whitaker is not similarly a benefit to his germ line. In this sense, he may still be a carrier of his condition and be able to pass it on. The rather difficult scenario that presents itself is that in his survival he is able to continue to pass on a deleterious trait, maintaining the form of anemia in the population, should he choose to reproduce. It is therefore not eugenic, in that no genetic benefit is being passed on and the trait is not being eliminated from the individual. However, it is eugenic in the sense that if this approach leads to the use of potential offspring in the treatment of certain conditions, a new kind of population will be generated.

The current definitional understanding of new eugenics *is* open to bringing about genetic health benefits to future offspring without the goal of improving the human species as a whole. In a far-fetched future scenario we could also imagine an individual being cured from a condition and then being discovered to carry a desirable trait dependent on the undesirable one. The natural responses that have been discovered concerning resistance to disease where traits are associated, indicate the lack of control and predictability we have over fighting disease. This is the case with sickle cell anemia resistance to malaria, or the recently discovered HIV-1 resistance associated with the chemokine receptor (CCR5) gene deletion, believed to be connected to exposure to bubonic plague.[7]

4. Health Goals and Social Goals

So, if we consider eugenics in terms of seeking out effects to improve certain features of the human population by either enhancing, reducing, or eliminating them as outlined above, the moral debate concerning these two examples changes significantly. In this case, what is of importance is not the parental choice *per se*, or the immediate consequence of the treatment or status of the child produced, but the societal effect and the population effect of such offspring in genetic terms. We can see then that the deaf child scenario is more likely to come out as a eugenic decision in so far as it clearly improves the chances of deafness being maintained in the population. It is interesting, though, that opposition to the birth of a deaf child comes from those who see deafness as a disability, and so as an undesirable trait. The two sides to this issue highlight the different ways in which certain features of humans can be promoted as desirable or not. These judgments arise in a social context. Wanting and valuing a deaf child affirms values held within a (the Deaf) community that does not experience deafness as a disability or impairment.

In the case of choosing to have a child who can provide therapeutic benefit to a sibling, the motivations of the parents are key to its moral assessment. However, if, as mentioned, the therapeutic benefit in tissue matching does not involve germ line intervention or a genetic intervention that has an influence on future generations, it may be that such a choice is not eugenic. If we hold to the idea that eugenics by definition has to involve a population and social element, this calls into question whether any therapeutic interventions can ever be truly eugenic when they do not affect groups or populations.

We could imagine a eugenic scenario in which whole populations of children were produced for therapeutic ends, creating a type of person that can affect the reproductive success of a group carrying a particular condition. It would be naïve to hold that we are only dealing here with individuals, or that we are speaking not of the betterment of humans in general, but of individuals. Just because the trait is maintained in the population but can be treated at a person-specific level, does not mean that eugenics can successfully be reduced to individual parental choice. These choices are going to have social consequences, but it is not clear to what extent they are going to have genetic and eugenic consequences. In the Whitaker case, the parents' choice could be fulfilled in one legally permissive location—the United States—but not in the United Kingdom. The capacity to go through with the decision to have a child needs to be recognized as occurring in a particular political and social context. If we stress this feature, the case cannot be treated as solely involving individual choice as new eugenics would want, but involves law, wealth, and policy, albeit as facilitators of choice, not in an enforcing or coercing role. There need be no mention then of historical eugenics.

Where negative eugenics aims at the laudable goal of eliminating disease, as with positive eugenics it is not easy to separate health purposes from social purposes. As has been presented above, even where negative eugenics is conceived of in terms of the health of the individual, the services that make interventions possible and available, the research that is developed to identify and target certain diseases, and conditions that present themselves to opt for elimination or enhancement will be socially motivated and arise in a socio-political context. It is from this corner that such interventions, negative or positive, will become possible and feed into individual reproductive choices. What is more, the emphasis solely on the individual's decision-making process regarding their genetic state or future in progeny can be argued to be more than just a concern for the individual. Although reproductive decisions and control are often seen as governed by individual autonomy, a person is given the right to make decisions regarding their reproductive choices, a right which arguably expands to the nature of their offspring. Ruth Chadwick has drawn attention to public health issues that arise in eugenics: gene therapy is a public concern, and draws on additional questions of resource allocation and collective identity.[8] As is clearly illustrated by the cases above, these cannot be separated from the context in which they happen. Other examples of eugenic choices that have population effects, or are guided by populations rather than individuals, are provided by genetic conditions that are more prevalent among certain groups. Although when it comes to defining eugenics Diane Paul insists too that "eugenics cannot be defined in terms of the social policies that account for its sordid reputation," it must be conceded that definitions of eugenics, though not derivative of policies, have contributed to the formulation of such policies.[9] This is largely due to eugenics' being open to implementation on a grand scale in the human population, even if it comes through individual choice motivated by the promotion of health and reduction of suffering.

My concern is that, despite the definitional distinctions maintained between positive and negative eugenics, it is not easy to present the broad goals aimed at as so distinct that someone might provide moral support for or condone negative eugenics, but have reasons to reject positive eugenics. I think that there are not only good reasons for rejecting both, but that positive and negative eugenics merge when populations are considered. Diane Paul points out that "most geneticists employ a narrow definition that identifies eugenics with a social aim and often coercive means."[10]

The main issue that develops from this concerns the way in which eugenics conceives of its aims. The health goals of the new eugenics genetic technologies are perfection or the betterment of the human being and the human race to alleviate current and future sufferings. Let us move on to look at this with regard to human flourishing and Nicholas Agar's liberal eugenics.

5. Flourishing: "Never Call a Man Successful Until His Life is Over. Only the Grave is Security Against Misfortune."[11]

At the heart of new approaches to eugenics there is still, I hold, a flaw in the way that goals are conceived—the general goal of enhancement or improvement is based either on a mistaken view of the good and/or on a picture of human development in terms of improvement that is fundamentally unhealthy to human flourishing. Nicholas Agar presents a particular view of human flourishing in his approach to eugenics. [12] His presentation of flourishing is in terms of genetic enhancement. It does not consider the possible accounts of human flourishing that present a different view of happiness or even success. Aristotle's account of flourishing sees it as pursuing optimal human *being* given the circumstances one finds oneself in despite the odds, instead of having an ideal goal of health or human perfection at which to aim.[13] Agar does reject a monistic view of flourishing in favor of a pluralistic one, characterizing the monistic view as, for example, the Nazi approach embodied in a particular racially biased conception of the optimal human. Another monistic view he considers is the hedonistic utilitarian conception of flourishing, condemning its pursuit of happiness and reduction of suffering as "leaving no room for meaningful choice about enhancement."[14]

The pluralistic view of flourishing he presents incorporates a careful approach to enhancement technologies, and recognizes that there are many ways in which humans can excel. Agar rejects flourishing as aiming at an ideal. He is also clear about the damage that some kinds of enhancement technologies can do, and equally clear that they should be opposed: "While there is no uniquely best way to use enhancement technologies, some uses of them are just plain wrong."[15] He goes on to reject enhancement technologies that can do harm (in what sense are they then truly enhancement technologies I wonder?), and enhancements that have a serious negative impact on a child's choice of life plan. This seems to be a reasonable approach, but if there are many ways in which humans can excel, why focus so strongly on genetic enhancement? Is this the *best* way in which humans can excel? Perhaps not. It may be the best way that biotechnologists, molecular biologists, or bioethicists can try to excel, but this is quite different from flourishing in terms of humanity as a whole. Where eugenics is directly involved in altering the human gene pool, it is not just individual flourishing that needs to be considered. It is hard to think of flourishing in genetic enhancement or therapeutic health goals without an idea of what one is aiming toward.

It seems at first that Agar's view has much in common with Aristotle's. Aristotle asks what might be required for human flourishing, where flourishing is synonymous with happiness and the virtuous life. However, Aristotle's position would differentiate between things that can be used as a means to the achievement of flourishing, and human flourishing itself, which he holds is worth pursuing for its own sake. For Aristotle, it is only happiness that is worth pursuing for its own sake; all other things are worth pursuing only in so far as they promote or are conducive to human flourishing. Human genetic enhancement is a means to a presumed good of health, and health is worth pursuing as a means to support a flourishing life. Health may well be necessary to flourish, but it is not sufficient. However, a person can be healthy to a reasonable measure, still suffering some ailments, and yet still lead a flourishing life. It all depends on what we take health to be. A plant that is growing incredibly well in arid, malnourished conditions can be said to be flourishing if its context is taken into account. As Aristotle puts it:

> A good shoemaker makes the neatest shoe out of the leather supplied to him and the same with all other kinds of craftsmen. And if this is so the happy man can never become miserable—although he cannot be entirely happy if he falls in with fortunes like those of Priam.[16]

The comedian Dylan Moran, talking about potential and happiness in his recent stand up show *Monster*, catches an image of true happiness in the sense that Aristotle might have meant:

> Look at the people who use their potential; the great athletes of the world, the Beckhams and the Roy Keanes of this world. People, charging, running up and down the field swearing and shouting at each other. Are they happy? No. They're destroying themselves. Who's happy? You. The fat fucks watching them, with the beer cans balanced on your ninth belly, roaring advice at the best athletes in the world.[17]

Returning to flourishing within a certain place, one may well argue here that we now find ourselves in a biotechnological context, a context that affords us current and prospective approaches to treating human conditions and thereby reducing suffering. The liberal eugenics position is fairly balanced in that it recognizes that great caution must be taken because of the potential dangers attendant on the use of new technologies. These dangers, though, are not just genetic. They also concern what is valued in different measure by different people.

To borrow an illustration from a colleague, it depends on what one's goals are.[18] An athlete, in running the 100 meter sprint, can have the goal of being the fastest runner possible and faster than anyone else. Any means used to achieve this goal can be thought to be legitimate, if we accept the goal being aimed at. It could be, though, that the athlete's goal is to run the 100 meters to the best of his or her ability. It might happen that this ends up in the runner being the fastest in the world, but it will not necessarily. This latter goal is not contained in the idea of running to the best of one's ability.

Agar *does* recognize that there are different ways in which humans can excel. This does not mean however that all ways in which humans can excel are commendable, morally acceptable, or worth pursuing. The reference to the possibility of enhancement technologies that, if applied, will cause harm and suffering to individuals, goes deep and makes me question the value of the effort being put into genetic technologies and their eugenics potential compared to other ways that can be given more attention that lead to a successful, flourishing life. A problem here lies with predictability—it is not known what the results of applying gene therapies may be regarding exposure to other conditions and disease. The warning scenario presented in Margaret Atwood's Science Fiction dystopia *Oryx and Crake* illustrates how the development of a drug to provide temporary sterility and enhance sexual pleasure leads to the lowering of resistance to an Ebola type virus.[19] I think it is irresponsible to dismiss this and other stories as scaremongering science fiction—note the example of HIV1 above.

If we apply this to human health we can scrutinize the goals of health. It would seem fairly uncontentious that the pursuit of health is a good thing for the individual who aims at a happy, flourishing life, but this becomes rather challenging where what counts as healthy varies from one individual to another, and where the notion of health is not restricted to a medical understanding. It becomes an even more complex issue when we consider it in terms of eugenics. The goals of eugenics aim at improving human health conceived in genetic terms. This involves not just the individual as outlined above, but populations. It is a difficult but serious question that needs to be answered in the application of genetic technologies to human flourishing. Are we conceiving of flourishing in too narrow and too limited a sense when we give so much attention to medical health?

6. Closing Remarks

The attractive nature of the term "enhancement" and recent work on liberal eugenics both serve to resurrect the concept of eugenics. The aim is to place the use of new genetic technologies to eliminate diseases and conditions that cause immense suffering in a different field from the eugenics of the past.

It is important to bear in mind that eugenics is concerned with betterment of the human population, be that under the negative or positive definition. There is a marked shift in emphasis through these definitions from the level of interventions articulated in social aims to the level of interventions articulated in terms of biotechnology. The latter looks to alterations in traits, the former alterations in populations. But changes in traits have population effects. So reducing the attention of what eugenics aims to do to the molecular/individual level does not alter the general effects that are brought about in populations. The challenge presented by liberal eugenics regarding human flourishing opens up space for genuinely interesting engagement with the question of what it is we take flourishing and happiness to be. I think more effort needs to be devoted to the development of a richer view of enhancement that is not focused on the genetic betterment of humans, even if this means living with suffering as part of the human condition.

NOTES

1. John Harris, "Is Gene Therapy a Form of Eugenics?" *Bioethics* 7:2–3 (April 1993), pp. 178–187.

2. *Ibid.*

3. Francis Galton, *Inquiries into the Human Faculty* (London: Macmillan, 1883), p. 44.

4. Diane Paul, "Is Human Genetics Disguised Eugenics?" *Biology and Philosophy*, eds. Michael Ruse and David Hull (Oxford: Oxford University Press, 1998), pp. 536–549, at p. 540.

5. "Couple 'Choose' to Have Deaf Baby," BBC News (8 April 2002), http://news.bbc.co.uk/1/hi/health/1916462.stm.

6. "Brother's Tissue 'Cures' Sick Boy," BBC News (20 October 2004), http://news.bbc.co.uk/1/hi/health/3756556.stm.

7. Enrique Gonzalez, Rahul Dhanda, Mike Bamshad, Srinivas Mummidi, Reni Geevarghese, Gabriel Catano, Stephanie A. Anderson, *et al.*, "Global Survey of Genetic Variation in CCR5, RANTES, and MIP-1α: Impact on the Epidemiology of the HIV-1 Pandemic," *PNAS*, 98:9 (24 April 2001), pp. 5199–5204.

8. Ruth Chadwick, "Gene Therapy," *A Companion to Bioethics*, eds. Helga Kuhse and Peter Singer (Oxford: Blackwell, 1998), pp. 189–197, at p. 195.

9. Diane Paul, "Is Human Genetics Disguised Eugenics?" p. 537.

10. *Ibid.*

11. Douglas S. Hutchinson, "Ethics," *The Cambridge Companion to Aristotle*, ed. Jonathan Barnes (Cambridge: Cambridge University Press, 1995), pp. 195–232, at p. 203.

12. Nicholas Agar, *Liberal Eugenics: In Defence of Human Enhancement* (Oxford: Blackwell, 2004); Nicholas Agar, "Liberal Eugenics," *Bioethics: An Anthology*, eds. Helga Kuhse and Peter Singer (Oxford: Blackwell, 1999), pp. 171–186.

13. Aristotle, *Nicomachean Ethics*, transl. J. A. K. Thomson (London: Penguin, 1955), 1100a10–1101b31, p. 82–86.

14. Nicholas Agar, *Liberal Eugenics*, p. 101.

15. *Ibid*, p. 103.

16. Aristotle, *Ethics*, 1100b27–1101a20, p. 84.

17. Dylan Moran, "Monster, Live," Dublin (Universal Pictures, April, 2004) DVD, ch. 3.

18. This example comes from Dr Peter Lucas (personal communication).

19. Margaret Atwood, *Oryx and Crake* (London: Virago, 2004).

Twelve

HARM, LAW, AND REPRODUCTIVE CLONING

Anna Smajdor

1. Introduction

> If there is to be a total prohibition of any form of reproductive cloning, it is important that it is supported by principled arguments why such a technique should be banned even if it were shown to be safe, effective, and reliable. Without such arguments, an indefinite absolute ban could not be considered rational.[1]

In 2005 the United Kingdom House of Commons Select Committee on Science and Technology published a report on reproductive technologies and the law.[2] Among a number of controversial suggestions, it mooted the idea that the legislation passed to criminalize reproductive cloning was hasty and irrational. Much of the rest of the Select Committee's report focused on the presumptive freedom of individuals to pursue their own ends, and the need for restrictions on this freedom to be based on sound evidence of harm.

The following statement from Mill is included in the report:

> The only purpose for which power can be rightfully exercised over any member of a civilised community, against his will, is to prevent harm to others. The only part of the conduct of any one, of which he is amenable to society, is that which concerns others. In the part which merely concerns himself, his independence is, of right, absolute. Over himself, over his own body and mind, the individual is sovereign.[3]

The committee's attitude is further exemplified by the following statements:

> The state should not prevent someone having a child—by assisted reproduction or other means.[4]

and

> The state should intervene only in carefully defined and justified circumstances, where there are specific harms in reproductive decisions.[5]

In this discussion I want to explore the kinds of harm which might be thought to justify a ban on reproductive cloning. It is commonly assumed that the harms which would be suffered by cloned children themselves are probably sufficient to warrant a complete ban. However, I suggest that (a) many of the supposed harms which would afflict clones have been overstated, and (b) children born as a result of cloning cannot be said to be harmed by being brought into existence. I argue that, while the Select Committee's Millian stance may be the correct one to take with respect to the law and assisted reproductive technologies (ARTs), it is misguided in so far as it is applied to the *children* born of ARTs. If compelling grounds for a legal prohibition of cloning are to be found, they must be based on other concerns: harm to society, for example, or threat to public resources.

2. What is the Harm of Reproductive Cloning?

John Stuart Mill claimed that the only just reason for interfering with someone's liberty is the prospect of their infringing someone else's liberty, for example by harming them.[6] This injunction leaves scope for whole swathes of immoral action that are not preventable by law. However, this is not unreasonable. Some actions are unamenable to proscriptive legislation. It might be possible to pass a law against lying, but it would be impracticable to try to enforce it. Law and morality play different roles in society, and this is why we can ask of an action *both* "Is it legal?" and "Is it right?"

In societies whose values are informed by a variety of different cultural, moral, and religious influences, it is hard to see how the state *could* undertake to enforce the moral views of all its citizens, in all their nuances and subtleties. This being the case, while there may be acts that are considered morally reprehensible by some or even all members of society, it does not follow that they should be illegal. In this discussion, I want to separate the legal from the moral question, in the context of human reproductive cloning, to establish that, while cloning might be morally wrong, it should not necessarily be prohibited by law.

While we cannot necessarily agree about all aspects of morality, harming others or restricting their liberty might be regarded universally as something to be avoided (I recognize that this is a contentious claim in itself: harm is not an easily defined concept, and even if it were, it still leaves the question of who, or what, we should avoid harming; I will address these problems later in my discussion). So, while we need a general agreement not to interfere with one another in order for society to function, we also need to agree that, should the exercise of one individual's freedom cause harm or loss of liberty to another, the *prima facie* rule of non-interference may be overridden in the interests of preventing this harm. Following on from this point, it seems reasonable to assert that legislation which restricts people's actions should, as Mill says, be employed only where there is reason to think that an individual's actions *will* cause harm to someone else. This is not to say that harm to others is the only morally relevant consideration, but that it is the only morally relevant consideration *to the state and to legislators.*

Suppose then that a would-be "parent" has found scientists—and surrogates where necessary—who are willing to assist in cloning him or her (that is, the third parties are not being coerced in any way). If unchecked by the state, the free exercise of these individuals' liberty will result in a cloned child. Can we justify impeding this liberty on the grounds that the clone will be harmed?

3. Risks to Cloned Children

> The use of this technique to create a child would be a premature experiment that exposes the developing child to unacceptable risks.[7]

Cloning is an intricate and highly uncertain procedure. It is widely known that Dolly the sheep was the sole successful result of 277 attempts. This in itself might seem to argue for caution where cloning human beings is concerned. John Harris has said that the safety consideration is "the one decent argument against cloning."[8] However, biologist Lee Silver has suggested that in fact cloning would be *safer* than natural conception because it bypasses the most common birth defect: having the wrong number of chromosomes.[9] Other common genetic birth defects come about through recessive genetic diseases, for example cystic fibrosis or Tay-Sachs. Again, this danger is circumvented if the cloned cell comes from a healthy adult. (There is a question here of course, as to what would happen if the cell did *not* come from a healthy adult. Silver does not address this possibility; I will explore this issue later on.)

Silver also observes that despite the apparently unpromising fact that 277 eggs were used in order to obtain only one live clone, it is important to remember that only 13 of the eggs actually started to develop into embryos, and of these, 12 were miscarried early in pregnancy. The implication is that only the "fittest" cloned embryos would survive to be born anyway; a kind of natural filter mechanism would weed out the worst results. Therefore, Silver seems to imply, cloning would not necessarily result in children with grotesque birth defects or genetic abnormalities, since such abnormal embryos would be unlikely to reach the stage of birth.

One can compare this with what we know about the apparent precariousness of natural conception: very few fertilized eggs result in live births, as frequently there are genetic or other anomalies which result in failure of the embryo to develop. In many cases, the woman will never know she has been "pregnant," since the embryo is not miscarried as such, but merely re-absorbed into the woman's body.[10]

In the light of this, the fact that only one out of thirteen fertilized eggs resulted in a live clone, does not look so shocking. And as Daniel Brock has suggested, if it is possible to bring the risk of failure or early miscarriage within the range of "normal" pregnancy, or of widely-accepted ARTs such as *in vitro* fertilization (IVF), it would seem that there are no grounds for a permanent ban on cloning based on these early harms.[11]

Brock assumes that the moral issue is for us not to exceed the degree of "natural" danger involved in conception. One could argue against this on the grounds that what we do deliberately is morally different from what occurs naturally. However, this type of argument focuses on the character and motives of the agent, rather than the harms involved, and is therefore not central to my discussion. For now, I will accept Brock's contention that a similar or lower risk level to that involved in "natural" pregnancy would be acceptable at least in the eyes of the law.

Silver's comments do not address the harm which repeated failed cloning attempts and miscarriages might cause to the woman who gestates the embryo. The effects of ARTs in general upon women may be regarded as a cause for concern.[12] However, this is a separate argument. For the moment, I assume that harms suffered by women in the process of cloning would be voluntarily risked by autonomous adults, and therefore do not necessarily constitute grounds for a ban.

4. Unknown Unknowns

> It is theoretically possible, although unlikely, that something totally unknown could go wrong.[13]

Any experimental procedure is likely to carry unforeseen consequences, since it is simply not possible to cover every eventuality in advance. Gregory Pence's remark, above, seems very optimistic. Reports have suggested that children conceived using IVF techniques are at increased risk of certain harmful conditions.[14] Similarly unpredictable consequences could result from attempts at cloning. Such a view was certainly shared by The National Bioethics Advisory Commission, which cited "unknown risk" in its assessment of safety issues, as part of the justification for recommending a ban on human cloning.[15]

One of the problems inherent in evaluating what have been termed the "unknown unknowns" of new technologies is that by definition, such risks are impossible to foresee. Perhaps because of this fact, it is difficult to articulate an argument for legislating against a procedure on these grounds. It may be that the best we can do is to attempt a reasonable guess at what results *might* ensue from particular technologies, adopting a worst-case scenario, and weighing this up against the supposed benefits of the technology.

5. Experiments on Human Beings

Is it unethical to perform any procedure that might be regarded as an experiment on a human being, or on what will eventually become a human being? Some people think so: Leon Kass cites this as a conclusive reason not to clone, claiming that in the absence of any consent-obtaining mechanism, such experimental procedures are intrinsically unethical.[16] But if we rule out experimental procedures in cases where we cannot obtain consent, the first caesarean sections would not have been permissible, nor the first IVF pregnancies.

It is also relevant here to consider the issue of prescribing drugs for babies (and children to a lesser degree). 65% of drugs prescribed for newborn babies have never been tested on this age group, because of obvious consent issues.[17] To some extent this means that the prescription of such drugs to babies is in itself experimental. This may not be an ideal situation, but it is by no means clear that it would be better for these babies if these drugs were simply refused them.

Cloning would certainly be an experimental procedure, initially, at any rate. However, this does not answer the question of whether cloned children would be harmed. They might be in some cases, but not necessarily in all. Kass's concern, of course, is not solely that cloning as an experimental procedure would harm the child. His claim implies that to experiment on human beings in this way is *in itself* morally wrong, whether or not anyone is actually harmed by it. However, I do not have room in my discussion to address these issues, and as I have argued, even though such concerns may be morally valid, it is not necessarily the case that they should therefore be enforced by law.

6. Identity Problems

> The idea that one could make through somatic cell nuclear transfer a team of Michael Jordans, a physics department of Albert Einsteins, or an opera chorus of Pavarottis, is simply false.[18]

Many of the arguments against cloning have focused on the idea that clones would be harmed because they would lack the unique identity possessed by naturally begotten human beings. But, assuming that the "parent" of a cloned child would be an adult, the clone would necessarily grow up in a different temporal (and possibly geographical) environment. Therefore, even if they were *absolutely* identical genetically, there would still be some significant differences in terms of environmental influence. It has been argued that much of the formation of neural networks in the brain is not governed by genetic factors at all. As George Johnson describes:

> In the reigning metaphor, the genome, the coils of DNA that carry the genetic information, can be thought of as a computer directing the assembly of the embryo. Back-of-the-envelope calculations show how much information a human genome contains and how much information is required to specify the trillions of connections in a single brain. The conclusion is inescapable: the problem of wiring up a brain is so complex that it is beyond the power of the genomic computer.[19]

This makes us wonder how the brain *does* get wired up. Johnson's description is of a more or less random arrangement of neural tangles, which are acted upon by experience and learning, so that gradually pathways and connections are formed. Whatever the genetic make-up of the individual, the formation of these pathways and connections is neither predictable nor controllable by any technological means currently available to us.

Another point to be made with reference to the possible lack of unique identity in clones is that, as various commentators have pointed out, clones would be *less* similar to their genetic "parent" than identical twins are to each other.[20] Identical twins share both the temporal and uterine environment, and mitochondrial DNA from the mother's egg. A clone, on the other hand, would not be derived from the same egg as its "parent," and would therefore receive an entirely different dose of mitochondrial DNA (I have focused here on the idea of adults cloning themselves; it might also be possible to clone embryos, in which case, the arguments would be slightly different in that the genome in question would not already have lived). Yet, as Richard Dawkins says: "Hell's foundations don't quiver every time a pair of identical twins is born."[21] One might question how Dawkins knows this, perhaps! However, if we do not think that identical twins suffer from the lack of some kind of essential uniqueness of identity, it seems illogical to suppose that clones would do so, especially since they would be less similar in genetic and environmental terms to their "parent" than identical twins to each other (again it is necessary to observe here that the decision to clone yourself incorporates a degree of responsibility which is not present in identical twins; this is a morally relevant point, made by Habermas among others, but it concerns the agent's motives rather than necessary harm to the clone, and therefore while I recognize its validity, it does not detract from my argument).

But if a clone's life were not in fact predetermined by her genetic similarity to her "parent," she might still suffer as a result of a misguided conviction that she was living a life that had already been lived. This line has been argued by a number of philosophers, and has been disputed by others.[22] However, while this misapprehension might indeed affect some clones, it seems plausible that not all would necessarily feel this way. Much would depend on the knowledge and assumptions of particular parents.

Therefore, again, it does not seem to be cloning itself which is intrinsically the cause of any harm. Moreover, many other misapprehensions might cause psychological suffering to children (for example, the belief that certain races or sexes are inferior, or of less moral worth than others), yet we do not as a rule assume that children who might suffer from such beliefs should therefore not be born.

So sharing a similar or identical genome with another person may not *necessarily* impinge upon anyone's personal uniqueness, largely because personal identity is not reducible to genetic components. Perhaps here, though, it is relevant to consider another comment by Leon Kass:

> One is shortchanging the truth by emphasizing the additional importance of the intrauterine environment, rearing, and social setting: genotype obviously matters plenty. That, after all, is the only reason to clone, whether human beings or sheep.[23]

Kass has a good point here: it seems peculiar to argue in favor of cloning if part of your argument is that there is nothing particularly special or important about reproducing another individual's genome. However, it is not necessarily the case that all would-be cloners simply want to see themselves duplicated exactly: for some people it might be that they have no other means of producing genetically related children. Even in the case of people who *do* want to duplicate themselves, it is not clear that this constitutes harm to the child.

7. Psychological Burdens to the Child

Perhaps cloned children would suffer through confusion over family relationships.[24] Hitherto, two genetic parents have been the *sine qua non* of human reproduction. Anyone created by cloning would be treading new ground in terms of family relationships. Would the original cell donor be thought of as the child's father/mother? Or—more correctly, perhaps—as its sibling?

A cloned child might feel totally alone in the world, an artefact, a product of science and machinery rather than the offshoot of a family tree. Or she might feel prefigured, pre-empted in all respects. Perhaps clones would feel a hideous sense of being observed by a society watching with bated breath for evidence of abnormalities, or by the donors/parents, seeking signs of themselves in the children.

Any exploration of how clones might feel is necessarily speculative. Yet surely if a clone knew of its origins it could not help but feel profoundly affected by the utter difference of its beginnings from those of other human beings. Such feelings might become less intense if cloning became widely accepted in the way that IVF, for example, has. It is worth noting that while there were dire predictions about the psychological repercussions of ARTs in general, evidence of serious psychological suffering has not been forthcoming. Partly, of course, this is due to the complexity of performing studies on such subject groups, as well as the fact that in many cases, ARTs move ahead so quickly that children are not old enough to contribute effectively to studies of their psychological welfare. However, studies that have been carried out seem to indicate that children born into "non-traditional" family structures as a result of ARTs are not psychologically damaged; nor do family relationships involving such children appear dysfunctional, or abnormal.[25]

One of the problems in evaluating psychological suffering is that it is necessarily a subjective phenomenon. Events are dealt with in diverse ways depending on individual outlook and circumstances. While the knowledge of being a clone might well constitute some degree of psychological pressure, the degree of psychological *harm* involved would surely depend on a multitude of factors.

8. How Much Harm?

A discussion of the harms involved in cloning must eventually turn to the question of how *much* harm a child would have to suffer in order to justify legal prohibitions on the procedures which would engender them. Perhaps we should attempt to answer this question by ascertaining what degree of suffering would entail that it would be better for a child never to be born. As Ruth Macklin has claimed:

> Evidence, not mere surmise, is required to conclude that the psychological burdens of knowing that one was cloned would be of such magnitude that they would outweigh the benefits of life itself.[26]

Many people have taken issue with this approach, finding it to be morally dubious. John Arras, for example, claims that

> The fact that unconceived or unborn children could end up having lives that were on balance worthwhile cannot function as an all-purpose excuse for imposing grievous pain, suffering, and deprivation on them.[27]

However, this complaint seems to beg the question. It suggests that it is immoral to inflict pain and suffering on unconceived children. Yet, clearly, it is impossible to do so: unconceived children do not exist and thus cannot be harmed. To argue otherwise seems to lead into a logical trap whereby we are forced to posit the existence of an unconceived child in order to claim that it is immoral to harm it.

Derek Parfit articulated the idea that, if a child's existence is contingent upon a particular action (for example, its parents' having had sex on a particular date), then that child cannot be said to have been *harmed* by the performance of that action if its life will be on balance worth living.[28] For example, suppose a woman is being treated for syphilis. She could wait before becoming pregnant for her cure to be complete, but she does not. Her child is therefore born with congenital syphilis.

Parfit suggests that the child has not been harmed by its mother's choice, since if she had waited, a *different* child would have been born (free from syphilis). Applying Parfit's ideas to reproductive cloning, it seems evident that, since the child would owe its very existence to cloning, it could not have been said to have been harmed by the technique, provided it had a minimally acceptable quality of life.

On Parfit's view, we could still say that a parent who clones herself acts immorally even though the child has not been harmed *per se*. This is because the parent could have chosen to conceive in better circumstances: in other words, a (different) child would have been born and would have had a better chance of leading a worthwhile life. The parent has chosen from two sets of circumstances, and has made the sub-optimal choice; it is here that the moral condemnation can be applied.

On this view, although the cloned child itself is not harmed (assuming it has a marginally worthwhile life), we might—perhaps—be able to argue that harms *do* ensue, which could make it justifiable to place a legal ban on cloning. However, the nature of these putative harms is difficult to articulate, and still more difficult to quantify. The implication is that there might have been a "better world outcome" had the woman made a different choice. But should the law really enforce that people choose the "best world option" in reproductive decisions? It might be that the "best world option" would be for *everyone* to refrain from having children, since it is often claimed that there are probably too many people in the world.

While reproduction is certainly a moral issue, we do not usually require of people that they forego the fulfillment of their reproductive desires for the sake of avoiding some kind of sub-optimal outcome. Moreover, the idea that there may be a simple binary choice between two options may be unrealistic in many situations. For some people who want to clone, it may be their only chance of having genetically related offspring. It is not necessarily a choice between a "natural" child or a clone. Even if a person is *not* infertile, she may still regard cloning as the only circumstance in which she would contemplate having a child, and again this seems to negate the validity of the "better option" argument.

9. Comparing Existence with Non-Existence

Finally, and perhaps most importantly, it seems to me that too much moral weight has been placed on the idea that there is a threshold which distinguishes between lives which are and are not worth living. If we suppose that such a threshold could prove useful, it is not enough just to assume its existence given the moral work that it is supposed to do: namely, to tell us what kind of conceptions are permissible and which reproductive technologies ought to be illegal.[29] Even if there were accurate measures for suffering, it is not clear how this could satisfactorily be used to show us whether some lives should not be lived. The question can be stated as follows: is it better for a potential entity (a) not to exist, or (b) to exist and suffer horribly?

Suppose I give birth to a child who suffers horribly from a disease that causes constant pain. There is no hope for a cure; moreover, the child will never gain any of the faculties that we think valuable in human beings. Would it be better *for that child* that it should never have existed? Many people might think that the answer for this is obviously "yes." However, while I do not dispute that this *might* be the case, I cannot see how it can be proved, or even how one might argue the position. Is it better never to be born than to live in pain? Is it somehow better for the world that there should be less suffering in it …?

To my mind, these questions are simply unanswerable. It is not clear that we can speak of existence as being a harm or a benefit in any kind of meaningful way at all. To do so seems to result in some bizarre logical anomalies. Suppose a congenital condition causes 50% of those affected to suffer so badly that they wish they had never been born. Would we wrong such individuals by conceiving them? If we could answer this in the affirmative, we should then be able to ask whether we would then benefit the 50% who would find value in their lives by conceiving them? This seems to follow from the previous point.

But this is absurd: we cannot benefit people by causing them to exist. If we *could*, we might find that *not* to conceive the 50% described above might be construed as a harm to them. If not to conceive the preconceived can harm them, then we are all guilty of harming infinite hordes of potential people who might reasonably be expected to benefit from life. This seems clearly nonsensical.

This leaves us in a difficult position with regard to the morality and legality of conceiving children. According to what I have just suggested, one could conceive a child with appalling genetic disorders specifically to obtain a sadistic enjoyment from its suffering, yet it would still not be true to say that the child had been harmed by being brought into being. Intuitively, however, people do think that to conceive a child in such circumstances *must* be wrong. I whole-heartedly agree with this. However, its wrongness does not lie in the fact that it *harms the child*. I should add here that, while my argument may seem shocking in terms of suggesting that one cannot be harmed (or benefited) by being born, I am not suggesting that one cannot be harmed after birth (or even before, for example during gestation). If a child were born to gratify the whims of a sadist, it might well be necessary for the state to intervene to prevent harms being perpetrated on that child.

In fact, although many arguments against cloning rest on claims relating to the harm suffered by clones, it seems likely that for many people, their objections would not necessarily evaporate if cloning were shown to be safe. In effect, moral objections to cloning are properly centered around deontological concepts of human dignity or rights. My argument in this discussion is not that deontological or non-utilitarian concerns are irrelevant, but that they are not in themselves sufficient to warrant prohibitive legislation, at least in a legislative context which purports to be based on Mill's harm principle.

The Select Committee report that I cited earlier in my discussion was controversial in rooting its arguments in harm-based considerations at the expense of deontological reasoning. As I have suggested, this approach has some challenging implications in terms of legislation. The committee believed that safety issues are currently a sufficient justification for legislation against cloning, but that once these are resolved further arguments would be necessary to justify a continuing ban. Since I have suggested that harm to clones themselves is not a compelling argument, we may question whether cloning could be banned on grounds of harm to others?

We might argue with Patrick Devlin that there are social harms that would ensue from a failure to legislate against cloning. To allow cloning might erode social cohesion and lead to public outrage. Alternatively, there might be serious resource-based considerations which might justify a ban. However, these possibilities need careful evaluation, which cannot be undertaken here.

10. Conclusion

To conclude, then, I suggest that if

> (1) we accept the Select Committee's claim that: "the state has no right to intervene in the choices of people to procreate unless evidence of harm can be shown";[30]

and we agree that

> (2) we cannot harm (or benefit) an entity by bringing it into being;

then it follows that there are no *prima facie* grounds for the State to ban cloning *unless* there is evidence of harm to entities other than the cloned child; perhaps to society at large. I think it possible that an argument could be made based on such harms, but as yet little effort seems to have been made to identify these harms or to incorporate them into legislation.

NOTES

1. House of Commons Science and Technology Committee, *Human Reproductive Technologies and the Law*, Fifth Report of Session 2004-05, Vol. 1 (2005), p. 35–36.
2. *Ibid.*
3. John Stuart Mill, *Utilitarianism and On Liberty*, ed. Mary Warnock (London: Fontana Press, 1962). Cited in *ibid.*, p. 17.
4. House of Commons Science and Technology Committee, *Human Reproductive Technologies and the Law*, p. 49.
5. *Ibid.*, p. 177.
6. John Stuart Mill, *Utilitarianism* (Indianapolis: Bobbs-Merrill Co., 1957).
7. National Bioethics Advisory Commission, *Report on Human Cloning* (1997), ch. 6.
8. John Harris, *On Cloning* (London: Routledge, 2004), p. 109.
9. Lee Silver's comments are discussed by Gina Kolata in her book *Clone: the Road to Dolly and the Path Ahead* (London: Penguin, 2002).
10. Allen J. Wilcox, Clarice R. Weinberg, John F. O'Connor, Donna Day Baird, John P. Schlatterer, Robert E. Canfield, E. Glenn Armstrong, and Bruce C. Nisula, "Incidence of Early Loss of Pregnancy," *The New England Journal of Medicine*, 319:4 (28 July 1988), pp. 189–194, at p. 191.
11. Daniel Brock, "Cloning Human Beings: An Assessment of the Ethical Issues Pro and Con," *Clones and Clones: Facts and Fantasies About Human Cloning*, eds. Martha Nussbaum and Cass Sunstein (New York: Norton, 1998), p. 158.
12. Christine Overall, Rayna Rapp, Laura Purdy, Andrea Dworkin and many others have argued that ARTs are not necessarily a boon to women.
13. Gregory Pence, *Who's Afraid of Human Cloning?* (Lanham, MD: Rowman and Littlefield Publishers Inc., 1998), p. 131.

14. Bengt Källén, Orvar Finnström, Karl Gösta Nygren, and Petra Otterblad Olausson, "In Vitro Fertilization (IVF) in Sweden: Risk for Congenital Malformations After Different IVF Methods," *Birth Defects Research. Part A, Clinical and Molecular Teratology*, 73:3 (March 2005), pp. 162–169.

15. National Bioethics Advisory Commission, *Report on Human Cloning*, ch. 6.

16. Leon Kass, *The Wisdom of Repugnance: The Ethics of Human Cloning* (Washington, DC: The AEI Press, 1998).

17. Simon Crompton, "Testing Times," *The Times* 21 August 2004.

18. National Bioethics Advisory Commission, *Report on Human Cloning*, ch. 2.

19. George Johnson, "Soul Searching," The Week in Review, *New York Times* 2 March 1997.

20. E.g., Richard Dawkins, Gregory Pence, Stephen Jay Gould.

21. Richard Dawkins, "What's Wrong with Cloning?" Nussbaum and Sunstein, *Clones and Clones*.

22. For the former see, for example, Søren Holm, "A Life in the Shadow: One Reason Why We Should not Clone Humans," *Cambridge Quarterly of Healthcare Ethics* 7:2 (Spring 1998), pp. 160–162; and Jürgen Habermas, *The Future of Human Nature* (Cambridge: Polity, 2003). For the latter see Matteo Mameli, "Reproductive Cloning, Genetic Engineering, and the Autonomy of the Child: The Moral Agent and the Open Future," *Journal of Medical Ethics*, 33:2 (February 2007), pp. 87–93.

23. Kass, *The Wisdom of Repugnance*.

24. See, for example para 4.7 of the report of the Human Genetics Advisory Commission, *Cloning Issues in Reproduction, Science and Medicine*, December 1998. Available at http://www.advisorybodies.doh.gov.uk/hgac/papers/papers_d.htm (accessed 19 April 2007).

25. Emma Lycett, Ken Daniels, Ruth Curson, and Susan Golombok, "Offspring Created as a Result of Donor Insemination," *Fertility and Sterility*, 82:1 (July 2004), pp. 172–179. See also Emma Goodman, Fiona MacCallum, and Susan Golombok, "Follow-Up Studies on the Psychological Consequences of Successful IVF Treatment," *Biomedical Ethics*, 3:2 (1998), pp. 40–43.

26. Ruth Macklin, "Human Cloning: Don't Just Say No," *U.S. News & World Report*, 122:9 (10 March 1997), p. 64.

27. John Arras, "AIDS and Reproductive Decisions: Having Children in Fear and Trembling," *Milbank Quarterly*, 68:3 (1990), pp. 353–382.

28. Derek Parfit, *Reasons and Persons* (Oxford: Clarendon, 1984).

29. See, for example, Harris, *On Cloning*, p. 109.

30. See note 1, House of Commons Science and Technology Committee, *Human Reproductive Technologies and the Law*, p. 21.

Thirteen

AN ANALYSIS OF SOME ARGUMENTS FOR AND AGAINST HUMAN REPRODUCTION

Matti Häyry

1. Background

I recently published in the *Journal of Medical Ethics* an article entitled "A Rational Cure for Prereproductive Stress Syndrome,"[1] and three colleagues, Rebecca Bennett,[2] Søren Holm,[3] and Sahin Aksoy,[4] presented in a later issue some critical comments on my arguments. Since limitations of space did not allow me to address all the concerns that they raised in the "official" response,[5] I will in this chapter revisit the topic, and clarify some of the arguments I put forward in the original article.

2. The Irrationality of Having Children

In the article, I made two main claims, one concerning the rationality and the other the morality of human reproduction. I will start from the rationality thesis, and the points and arguments that Bennett, Holm, and Aksoy present against it.

A. My Rational Case

I claimed in the article that *having children is irrational*,

- *if* (1) deliberately allowing the worst outcome of our actions is irrational;
- *and if* (2) having children allows the worst outcome.

The first if-clause defines a notion called the "maximin" rule, and many people, including me, believe that it gives a good account of one type of rationality. This type of rationality is particularly applicable in this context, where we can create out of nothing the very possibility of the worst outcome. The second if-clause makes an assertion that we can interpret either empirically or conceptually. Both I and my three critics chose the conceptual route.

I argued that having children allows the worst outcome of our reproductive choices (the creation of a possibly bad life, where the alternative is no life),

- *if* (3) the restriction of the analysis to the comparative value of life versus non-existence of possible future individuals, as experienced by themselves, makes good sense;
- *and if* (4) some individuals would genuinely prefer non-existence to their own life.

In defense of the first clause, I implied that the restriction makes good sense to me. In defense of the second, I referred to accounts of wrongful life cases, where individuals have themselves made the claim that they would rather not have been born at all.

My practical conclusion in the article was modest: (5) "Possible parents could be told that, according to at least one philosopher, it would be all right for them not to reproduce at all."[6] This was my suggested "rational cure for prereproductive stress syndrome"—the state in which people want to have children and see it as a goal so important that almost everything in our collective power has to be done to grant their wish.

B. "Not Strongly Irrational"

Holm argues against (1) that deliberately allowing a *low probability* of the worst outcome is *not* irrational. He starts from the premise that to make my argument work I would need to regard the maximin rule as the only criterion of rationality. But if I do so, I should never, for fear of micro-organisms, eat food which has not been fully sterilized in an autoclave—something that Holm seems to think would be ludicrous. On the other hand, if I do not regard the maximin rule as the only criterion of rationality, I cannot defend directive counseling against having children.

I have a very simple counter-comment to this. I do *not* regard the maximin rule as the only definition of rationality. Nor do I need to do so, because I do *not* advocate directive counseling—a choice I tried to make clear by the cautious formulation of conclusion (5). So this point does not dent my view, although it would have been accurate against someone who actually claims that maximin is the only measure for rationality.[7]

C. "Life Cannot Be the Worst Outcome"

Aksoy argues against (2) that having children cannot bring about the worst outcome, because the worst possible outcome of reproductive choices is always non-existence. He refers to his own previously formulated view,[8] according to which existence "is essential and prerequisite to everything good or bad, and deserves to be protected and respected."[9] He also quotes Spinoza, who in his work published in 1677 wrote: "No one can desire to be happy, to act well and live well, who does not at the same time desire to be, to act, and to live, that is to say, actually to exist."[10]

My primary reason for not being impressed by these statements in the present context is that they do not address choices before a being is or is not brought into existence. I can fully agree with Aksoy that human existence, once it is "here," so to speak, is the basis of all experiences. I can also agree with Spinoza that being alive precedes desires concerning the content of one's life (if this is what he meant). But I fail to see the relevance of these statements to the choice to reproduce or not to reproduce. All they demonstrate is that as the foundation of our experiences, life can have positive instrumental value to us, if our experiences are good. By the same token, it can have negative instrumental value to us, if our experiences are bad. It does not, however, have any value, good or bad, when it is not present.

D. "The Role of Others Is Misrepresented"

Holm has two main lines of argument against my claim (3). He sets off by stating that restricting our attention to the lives of possible future individuals does *not* make good sense. This is because the choice to reproduce or not to reproduce can also have an impact on the lives of others. The choice can affect the existing children of the potential parents. And if everyone decides to abstain, this can, among other things, decrease my future pension.

Holm is obviously right in saying that the decision will affect the other children of the potential parents. But my restriction is based on the idea that the changes in their lives are of a different order from the impact of the choice on new individuals. Whatever the personal and social significance of having new siblings is, it does not create, out of nothing, the possibility of a life that the one living it would prefer not to have. The process of being born, on the contrary, does allow this possibility. This is why I think that giving priority to the interests of siblings, or indeed the interests of parents, in reproductive choices would in most circumstances be frivolous.

Holm is also right in saying that my future pension could be smaller, if everybody abided by my rules, since this would eventually lead to a diminishing population. Then again, this is speculation, as we do not know how other institutions would be arranged to adjust to the situation. Perhaps the salaries of midwives, pediatricians, and school teachers could be transferred gradually to the pensions pot. In any case, I would be ready, if necessary, to bear my share of the economic burden caused by this development.

Holm also argues, taking the opposite angle and focusing on my remarks about John Rawls, that since rationality—as opposed to morality—centers on the well-being of the decision maker, its scope cannot be extended to the plight of others. Rational agents *as rational agents* are not, he says, moved by the fate of others—so not, in reproductive choices, by the fate of the possible future individuals.

This remark is brought on by my apparently ill-considered inclusion of Rawls's theory of justice in the discussion. Although I tried to use his ideas merely as an illustration of the maximin rule in action, not as a part of my own argument, I seem to have misled at least one of my readers. Holm is absolutely right in saying that in the Rawlsian model rational individuals only think about their own good, not about the good of others. But there are other instances of maximin decision making in which other-regarding factors can enter the picture. The New York health authorities, for instance, arguably made a rational choice, when in 1947 they vaccinated five million people against smallpox, thereby guaranteeing the safety of the population of eight million, although forty-five people became seriously ill and four died as a consequence.[11] We can, I believe, talk about decisions like this in terms of maximin rationality without directly involving the interests of those making the choice.

E. "Having Savior Siblings Is Rational"

Bennett notes against my claim (3) that ignoring the interests of a potential child's existing siblings does in certain circumstances seem irrational. A case in point is when these siblings suffer horribly from conditions that tissue transplants from the new individuals could cure or substantially alleviate. Producing these "savior siblings" would, according to my adopted account, seem rational. We could remove certain suffering by allowing only a slight possibility of suffering—surely an acceptable trade-off?

Well, no. While I congratulate Bennett on her perceptiveness, I must also point out that such trade-offs are *not* in line with the maximin rule. The remark is good from the viewpoint of maximizing expected utility, which is another feasible way of construing what rationality means.[12] But since the worst possible outcome of creating "savior siblings" is that there will be, in the end, *two* lives that those living them would prefer not to have (instead of just the already existing one), maximin rationality does not support this choice.

I should perhaps add, though, that creating a "savior embryo" or "savior fetus" would escape this objection. If no one is, in the end, born, the worst outcome could, in my original sense, be averted. But we have to face some thorny questions if this route is taken—for instance, the question of instrumentalization, that is, using the unborn individual as a mere means to the ends of others.

3. The Immorality of Having Children

What about my thesis concerning the morality of human reproduction, and the objections presented to it by my critics?

A. My Moral Case

I also claimed in my article that *having children is immoral,*

- *if* (6) bringing about avoidable suffering is immoral;
- *and if* (7) having children has this effect.

I took the first statement to be self-evidently true, and supported the second by specifying two senses in which it is, I believe, true. Having children brings about avoidable suffering

- *in the sense that* (8) all human beings suffer at some point in their lives;
- *and in the sense that* (9) potential parents cannot guarantee that their child's life would not become at some point in time (physically, mentally, or socially) overwhelmingly miserable.

My critics did not challenge the truth of these statements, but they did contest their ethical implications.

Since I know that we can bring about suffering in many other ways besides human reproduction, and since I understand that people's views on having children differ considerably, my practical conclusion from premises (8) and (9) was even more modest than my inference from the analysis of rationality: (10) "In principle, and in an equal discussion between competent participants, my moral views may entitle me to reproach individuals who decide, or have decided, to have children. There is, however, seldom much point in my doing so."[13]

B. "(Nearly) Everybody Has an Interest to Exist"

Aksoy and Bennett both dispute my claim (6)—that bringing about avoidable suffering is immoral—by arguing that it would be good for all, or at least most, potential individuals, to exist, and that to help them to come into being is always morally acceptable, despite the suffering produced as a side effect.

According to Aksoy, allowing *any* suffering that our potential children can experience is right, because existence is in and of itself valuable, and non-existence is the paragon of evil. In his view, it is "immoral to 'sentence' someone to non-existence while you have the chance to bring them into life."[14]

Bennett, in her turn, argues that bringing about *some* suffering is permissible, if good things in life depend on this. In her words, it "is in the interest of any child whose life will be likely worth living overall, that he or she is brought to birth."[15]

My main conceptual difficulty with these critiques is that I do not know *who* Aksoy and Bennett are talking about. Who exactly is the absent someone who is sentenced to non-existence; and who precisely is the unborn child whose interests would be served by bringing her to birth? How can we attribute experiences and interests to beings who have not existed in the past, do not exist now, and will possibly never exist in the future?

Apart from this metaphysical problem, I have a couple of normative issues to raise. Aksoy seems to say that even individuals whose lives would be utterly miserable—filled with suffering and nothing else—*must* be brought into existence, when we have that chance. If this is his message, I disagree, and so do many others.[16] I think that to force suffering human beings to live would be inhumane. Aksoy's view also implies that we should spend our entire lives trying to make babies. Women should aim to be with child all the time, and men should probably focus on perfecting the techniques of ectogenesis and male pregnancy. This is not an impossible idea, of course, but it is not one that is likely to have wide popularity, either.

Bennett, on the other hand, resorts to the language of "worthwhile lives" (an expression, by the way, that I did not use in my original article). This is undoubtedly a good move in that it helps her to avoid the criticism leveled at Aksoy's more stringent view. But drawing the line between "worthwhile" and "unworthwhile" lives in a universally acknowledged, or even widely accepted, way is not easy. So while Aksoy can be accused of committing himself to an absurdly stern view, Bennett defends a position which seems to require further specifications.

C. "The Good of a Good Life Outweighs the Bad"

Some tentative specifications are given in Bennett's critique of my claims (7) and (8)—which state that since all lives contain some pain and anguish, reproduction allows suffering in the relevant moral sense. She argues, level-headedly, that habitually banning otherwise good and useful activities just because some transient suffering ensues from them would be odd. Unless the suffering that reproduction causes is "great and overwhelming" or "so great as to outweigh the good of life," we should enable and encourage "the experience of being alive." As Bennett continues, we can take the "view that as long as life can be considered generally beneficial rather than generally harmful, creating this life is not immoral," and "as long as the suffering a life contains is likely to be outweighed by positive experiences, choosing to bring such a life into being is morally acceptable."[17]

The same logic applies, I suppose, to my claims (7) and (9). According to these, any human life can become, in Bennett's terms, a "life not worth living." The world is an insecure place, and many people suffer inordinately. This suffering can be due to physical, psychological, or social conditions, or it can be deliberately inflicted by other people. Parents cannot guarantee that their children will not fall victim to this kind of irreversible suffering at some point in the future, however healthy and happy they are when they are born. But Bennett's objection to this could be that if the probability of suffering is very small, reproduction should, nevertheless, be allowed in the name of the good it produces in the majority of cases. She does not say this in so many words, but she could feasibly take this line.

D. To Avoid Suffering or to Maximize Expected Net Good?

Bennett's remarks on various outcomes and probabilities introduce, as she acknowledges, an alternative account of morality to the one summarized in my claim (6). Instead of trying to check avoidable suffering we should, according to her, attempt to maximize the balance of good experiences over bad. In terms of ethical theory, hers is, of course, a viable option. But why should it be adopted in the current context?

Bennett's argument appears to be that my view, if taken to its conclusion, would lead to absurd recommendations. She writes: "If Häyry really believes that the morally preferable course of action is one which avoids suffering where this is possible it seems that he should be encouraging not only the avoidance of human reproduction but also the ending of existing human lives including his own."[18]

I agree that *if* the same rules applied to all possible and all actual human beings, Bennett's corollary would be inescapable. I do not, however, believe that this is the case. We should allow individuals who already exist, and who are capable of assessing the value of their own lives, to decide for themselves whether they would like to continue their lives or not. This applies to all autonomous human beings. In addition, we should, as a general rule, allow other individuals who exist and who are in some sense aware of their existence to continue their existence. This applies to all beings who fulfill the "awareness" criterion of moral personhood.[19] And even beyond this, we should probably make a distinction between all individuals that exist and the elusive, fictional entities that do not and will not ever exist.[20]

If these divisions are made, my outlook regarding the immorality of reproduction does *not* commit me to the view that existing people should kill themselves *en masse*. And this means that I do not need to extend the morality of maximizing expected net good, whatever its appeal in other areas, to reproductive decision making.

4. Summary and Conclusions

I have argued in this chapter that if to allow the worst outcome of our actions is irrational, and if to cause suffering is immoral, then to have children is irrational and immoral. I have also spelled out the premises of my argument, and claimed that they remain intact in the face of the objections presented by Bennett, Holm, and Aksoy.

I have not argued—either here or in my original article in the *Journal of Medical Ethics*—that the accounts of rationality and morality I have evoked are the only ones. All I have said is that to apply the maximin rule to reproductive choices makes good sense, because in these choices we can actually refrain from creating beings whom we can harm merely by creating them. Nor have I argued—here or originally—that anyone should give would-be parents directive anti-natal counseling. All I have implied, by arguing that abstinence is a rational and moral choice, is that no one should probably give them directive pro-natal counseling, either.

In the light of these observations, I still believe that it would be all right for people not to reproduce. And I still think that people would not be horribly manipulated if someone told them this.

Acknowledgment

This article was produced as a part of the project *Ethical and Social Aspects of Bioinformatics* (ESABI), financed between 2004-2007 by the Academy of Finland (SA 105139). My thanks are due to the Academy for the support, to Dr Tuija Takala for her helpful comments, and to Peter Herissone-Kelly for checking my English.

NOTES

1. Matti Häyry, "A Rational Cure for Prereproductive Stress Syndrome," *Journal of Medical Ethics*, 30:4 (August 2004), pp. 377–378.
2. Rebecca Bennett, "Human Reproduction: Irrational But In Most Cases Morally Defensible," *Journal of Medical Ethics*, 30:4 (August 2004), pp. 379–380.
3. Søren Holm, "Why It Is Not Strongly Irrational to Have Children," *Journal of Medical Ethics* 30:4 (August 2004), p. 381.
4. Sahin Aksoy, "Response to: A Rational Cure for Pre-Reproductive Stress Syndrome," *Journal of Medical Ethics* 30:4 (August 2004), pp. 382–383.
5. Matti Häyry, "The Rational Cure for Prereproductive Stress Syndrome Revisited," *Journal of Medical Ethics* 31:10 (October 2005), pp. 606–607.
6. Häyry, "A Rational Cure for Prereproductive Stress Syndrome".
7. John Rawls, *A Theory of Justice* (Oxford: Oxford University Press, 1972), pp. 152–157, at p. 175.

8. Sahin Aksoy, "To Value Life and Existence," *Eubios Journal of Asian and International Bioethics* 7:4 (July 1997), pp. 102–104.

9. Aksoy, "Response to: A Rational Cure."

10. *Ibid.*

11. John M. Last, *Public Health and Human Ecology* (Ottawa: Appleton and Lange, 1987), p. 354.

12. Julian Savulescu, "Procreative Beneficence: Why We Should Select the Best Children," *Bioethics* 15:5–6 (October 2001), pp. 413–426; Matti Häyry, "If You Must Make Babies, Then At Least Make the Best Babies You Can?" *Human Fertility* 7:2 (2004), pp. 105–112.

13. Häyry, "A Rational Cure for Prereproductive Stress Syndrome."

14. Aksoy, "Response to: A Rational Cure."

15. Bennett, "Human Reproduction."

16. *Ibid.*, Rebecca Bennett and John Harris, "Are There Lives Not Worth Living? When Is It Morally Wrong to Reproduce?" *Ethical Issues in Maternal-Fetal Medicine*, ed. Donna Dickenson (Cambridge: Cambridge University Press, 2002), pp. 321–334; David Archard, "Wrongful life," *Philosophy* 79:309 (July 2004), pp. 403–420.

17. Bennett, "Human Reproduction."

18. *Ibid.*

19. Matti Häyry, *Liberal Utilitarianism and Applied Ethics* (London and New York: Routledge, 1994), pp. 104–112.

20. Matti Häyry, "There Is a Difference Between Selecting a Deaf Embryo and Deafening a Hearing Child," *Journal of Medical Ethics* 30:5 (October 2004), pp. 510–512.

Fourteen

DOES THE BABY-SELLING OBJECTION TO COMMERCIAL SURROGACY MISUSE IMMANUEL KANT?

Stuart Oultram

1. Introduction

Does the baby-selling objection to commercial surrogacy misuse Kant? In this chapter I suggest that there are strong reasons for suspecting that it does. The chapter is split into two sections. In the first section, I briefly explain both how the baby-selling objection to commercial surrogacy is generated, and how that objection is founded upon Kantian moral philosophy. In the second section I move on to examine whether or not this appeal to Kant constitutes a misuse of his ideas.

2. What is the Baby-Selling Objection to Commercial Surrogacy?

The baby-selling objection to commercial surrogacy originates from the fact that upon completion of the arrangement the commercial surrogate mother, unlike her non-commercial counterpart, receives payment beyond that required to cover her expenses: she financially profits from her role in the arrangement. Yet to its critics this feature of commercial surrogacy arrangements represents more than just a procedural one, it represents a moral one. In short, this is the very reason commercial surrogacy is held to be morally unacceptable.

The reason why critics claim this is based upon the belief that the extra profit-creating payment which the commercial surrogate enjoys constitutes a payment *for the child itself.* As a consequence because commercial surrogacy, according to its critics, results in the sale of babies, commercial surrogacy is, like any other practice that involves the sale of human beings, morally objectionable.[1] As Sara Ann Ketchum notes, "The most straightforward argument for prohibiting baby-selling is that it is selling a human being and that any selling of a human being should be prohibited because it devalues human life and human individuality."[2]

In this respect commercial surrogacy, to its critics, is no different from a practice like slavery, in so much as those participating in commercial surrogacy—the commissioning couple (the eventual parents of the child), the commercial surrogate (the woman who carries the fetus and gives birth to the child), and the commercial surrogate agency (which administers the arrangement)—are conceiving of, or treating, the commercial surrogate child as a thing rather than as a person.

Given the above, it should come as no surprise that the Kantian underpinnings of the baby-selling objection lie within Kant's second formulation of the categorical imperative, *the formula of the end in itself*, which commands us to "act in such a way that you always treat humanity, whether in your own person or in the person of any other, never simply as a means, but always at the same time as an end."[3]

It is the distinction between persons and things which the formula of the end in itself encapsulates, and the reason why we should avoid treating persons in the same way we treat things, that resonate within the baby-selling objection. According to Kant, things are objects of inclination whose value is dependent entirely upon external factors. For example, an automobile is a thing, or object of inclination, the value of which is entirely dependent upon its ability to fulfill the function for which it has been designed: namely, getting people from point A to point B. As a consequence if it is unable to fulfill this function, due to a damaged engine for example, its value is substantially reduced to the point where it may become necessary to dispose of it. In such a situation it becomes valueless. This is what it means to be a means to an end. By contrast an end in itself is something the worth of which is an intrinsic part of it. That is to say that simply by existing, an end in itself is valuable. As Allen Wood nicely illustrates,

> when people bow their heads or doff their hats to their country's flag or to a religious object, they may have no end to be effected, except perhaps the successful performance of the gesture .... But they certainly do act for an end, namely, the value of the revered object. It is for the sake of this value that they perform the act of respect.[4]

For Kant, persons are ends in themselves and so should be treated as intrinsically valuable. As he states,

> Rational beings ... are called *persons* because their nature already marks them out as ends in themselves—that is, as something which ought not be used merely as a means—and consequently imposes to that extent a limit on all arbitrary treatment of them (and is an object of reverence).[5]

Briefly, the reason for this is that while a thing's value depends entirely upon the value exterior agents, typically human beings, invest in it, human beings, or persons, are capable of self-motivation. That is to say, we posses our own goals, motivations, and aspirations, and we regard persons as being intrinsically valuable, and so regard ourselves as being intrinsically valuable. Consequently Kant notes:

> This is the way in which a man necessarily conceives his own existence [as an intrinsically worthwhile end in itself rather than a value-dependent means to an end]: it is therefore so far a *subjective* principle of human actions. But it is also the way in which every other rational being conceives his existence on the same rational ground which is also valid for me; hence it is at the same time an *objective* principle.[6]

That is to say that if we think that we are, and should be regarded as being, intrinsically valuable ends in ourselves, we should regard everyone else in the same way.

So if we take, for purposes of illustration, the practice of slavery, we can clearly see what Kant means. What makes the practice of slavery wrong is the fact that human beings are bought and sold by others who then treat them as property. In addition, as a slave your will, freedom to act, and freedom to follow your aspirations are subsumed by the will of another being. In Kantian terms a slave is treated as a means to an end or an object of inclination whose value is dependent upon being able to fulfill the task for which he or she has been bought. However, the slave is a human being and as such constitutes a person in so much as she possesses all the qualities which mark her out as an intrinsically valuable end in itself. Consequently, because it is wrong to treat an end in itself as a means to an end, it is wrong to treat a human being as a slave.

3. How does the Baby-Selling Objection to Commercial Surrogacy Misuse Kant?

As we have seen, the baby-selling objection to commercial surrogacy, through its invocation of Kant, creates a powerful, and deeply negative, image of commercial surrogacy. As a result, it also lays a definite moral charge against those who participate in such arrangements: namely that they are treating babies not as intrinsically valuable human beings, but as a commodity to be made and sold to order. Commercial surrogate babies are, to use Kant's terminology, treated as objects of inclination or as a means to an end whose value is dependent only upon fulfilling that end.

Yet the problem is that it remains unclear whether this characterization of commercial surrogacy is an entirely accurate or fair one. Consequently, it also remains unclear whether the linked moral charge that commercial surrogacy contravenes the formula of the end in itself is an entirely accurate or fair one either.

To contravene the formula of the end in itself, those participants within the commercial surrogacy arrangement must conceive of the eventual commercial surrogate child in a certain way. However, despite the limitations of current empirical data, I would argue that it remains unclear whether the participants do in fact conceive of the surrogate child in the way in which advocates of the baby-selling objection claim that they do. The reason for this will become apparent if we take a look at each participant in turn—the commissioning couple, the commercial surrogate mother, and the commercial surrogate agency.

Beginning with the intentions of the commissioning couple, they are, I think it is fair to say, likely to be just like those of any other couple, irrespective of their chosen method of reproduction: namely, to have a child, to found a family, and to be parents. In this respect the commercial surrogate child, indeed any child, will be a means to an end in so much as it represents the means by which its parents fulfill their desire to be parents. Yet typically parents do not disrespect the humanity of their children, because the most fundamental part of being a parent is to allow and encourage your child to reach its full potential. In this respect, to their parents, children are never merely a means to an end. As John Robertson notes:

> The mere presence of selfish motives does not render reproduction immoral, as long as it is carried out in a way that respects the child's interests. Otherwise most pregnancies and births would be immoral, for people have children to serve individual ends as well as the good of the child. In terms of instrumentalism, surrogate motherhood cannot be distinguished from most other forms of reproductive situations.[7]

Therefore, unless there is some peculiar facet within the psychological make up of the commissioning couple which makes them prone to disrespect the humanity of their child, I think it would be reasonable to conclude that the commissioning couple does not break Kant's rule any more than any other parent does.

With regard to the commercial surrogate mother, I think it would be fair to say that her motives for having the child will be different to those of most other pregnant women, in so much as she becomes pregnant with a child that is not her own. So what are these other motives? In his study of commercial surrogates Philip Parker highlighted the following motivational factors in a woman's decision to become a commercial surrogate:

> Several factors appear to have a complementary relationship in determining each applicant's decision to be a surrogate mother, including 1) the perceived desire and need for money, 2) the perceived degree of enjoyment and desire to be pregnant, and 3) the perception that the advantages

> of relinquishment out-weighed the disadvantages. This last factor consisted of two motivational components. First, the women often expressed a strong wish to give the gift of a baby to a parent who needed a child. Second, the women felt (often unconsciously) that surrogate motherhood would help them master unresolved feelings they had regarding a loss of a foetus or baby through abortion or relinquishment. I should note that in 89% of the women who said a fee was a necessary condition, it was never a totally sufficient reason for being a surrogate.[8]

However, in her study of commercial surrogate mothers, Elizabeth Roberts highlights the fact that many commercial surrogates felt that in being asked to carry and care for the commissioning couple's child they were undertaking a sacred duty and that the child they were carrying was very special indeed. As Roberts notes:

> Still another surrogate spoke of the "sacred trust" that a surrogate mother was given in being commissioned to carry a baby .... "You get what you pay for. You can't enter into it in the spur of the moment. Making a baby is a beautiful and sacred thing .... If someone says 'I'm going to carry this baby for you,' it's as sacred of a trust as you can make."[9]

Given this, I do not think it would be unreasonable to say that some commercial surrogate mothers are guilty of thinking of the child they carry purely as a means to some other end, such as the means to relieve guilt, and not as an end in itself. However, at the same time, it would also be reasonable to conclude that there are going to be some commercial surrogate mothers who do not conceive of the child in this way, or whose motivations occupy the middle ground in so much as they acknowledge they have a responsibility toward the child they carry, while at the same time also acknowledging that the child will help them go on holiday this year. Therefore, I think it would be fair to say that there is a question mark over the commercial surrogate as to whether or not she is guilty of breaking Kant's imperative.

Assessing whether or not the commercial surrogate agency contravenes Kant's imperative is problematic because I have yet to find any empirical data on the motivations of those who work for commercial surrogate agencies. However, I would speculate that when it comes to the motivations of agencies, we are going to get a very similar sort of result to the motivations of commercial surrogates. We can reasonably expect that some agencies are going to be motivated by profit margins (assuming of course they are not charitable or not-for-profit organizations), while some will believe that what they are engaged in is special work and will care deeply about all the participants, including the commercial surrogate child, while some will have a mixture of motives some of which may well contravene the formula of the end in itself. As such I think it reasonable to conclude that there is a similar sort of question mark hanging over commercial surrogate agencies to the one which hangs over commercial surrogate mothers. However, as I noted earlier, it may not necessarily matter if these motivational question marks remain.

So if we were to assume that commercial surrogate mothers, and agencies, have a mixture of motives, this in and of itself would not be sufficient to justify the assertions of the baby-selling objection: namely, that it constitutes an infringement of the second formulation of the categorical imperative. This is because there are instances in which people can be treated as a means to an end without triggering an infringement of the formula of the end in itself, as Maxwell Charlesworth illustrates:

> It is not easy to formulate the principle [the formula of the end in itself] appropriately since there are clearly occasions where it is quite moral to employ another person to perform some services for reward. For example I can employ someone to carry bricks for me or dig trenches ... without necessarily using or exploiting that person as a means to an end or using him or her as a thing or instrument.[10]

So in cases where commercial surrogate mothers, and agencies, have mixed motives, this may be acceptable so long as neither is guilty of treating the child solely as a mere means to an end. In this respect, commercial surrogate mothers might, from a motivational point of view, be like nannies who love their charges but who nevertheless will not do the job for that love alone. Commercial surrogacy agencies might be like dating agencies that help bring people together, but that still have overheads to cover.

Although, if it were the case that in fact the motives of commercial surrogates, and agencies, were wholly selfish, and therefore involved conceiving of the child as being *merely* a means to an end, then it might be reasonable to conclude that there has been a breach of Kant's imperative. Yet, to my mind, this would still leave a question mark over whether or not the fact that *some* commercial surrogate arrangements might be guilty of contravening Kant's imperative is enough to justify the baby selling objection in its typical form, that is, that *the practice* of commercial surrogacy is wrong because it contravenes Kant's imperative.

However, at this point I would argue that, to my mind, any infringement on behalf of the surrogate or agency could be thought of as not in fact mattering enough morally to sustain the baby-selling objection in its typical form. The reason for this is that of the three participants within the arrangement, the relationship which would seem to count the most morally, and where no infringement of Kant's imperative can occur, is in relation to the motives of the commissioning couple, who as we have already seen are unlikely to be guilty of disrespecting the child's humanity.

After all, it will be with the commissioning couple that the child will spend the rest of its life, and it will be the commissioning couple, as the child's parents, who will subsequently have the most influence over that child's life. By contrast, the involvement of the agency and the surrogate with the child, and so the time they spend treating the child's humanity as a means only (assuming they do) is relatively short. As long as they fulfill their side of the arrangement and ensure that the child is conveyed safely to the commissioning couple, which of course is in their interests, it would not, I think, be unreasonable to argue that it does not matter whether they conceive of the child as a means only, or at the same time as an end in itself. In this respect, we could argue that we should only apply the formula of the end in itself to the commissioning couple, because the commercial surrogate agency and mother do not matter enough morally to warrant the application of the formula of the end in itself (although I acknowledge the fact that Kantians are unlikely to find this argument entirely satisfactory).

4. Conclusion

As we saw in section one, in claiming that commercial surrogacy contravenes the formula of the end in itself, the baby-selling objection to commercial surrogacy lays a powerful moral charge at the feet of the commissioning couple, the commercial surrogate mother, and the commercial surrogate agency. Yet, as we saw in section two, this charge may first of all be false in so much as it involves false assumptions, especially with regard to the commissioning couple, about the motives of those involved. Second, even when it is correct about the motives of those involved it is unlikely to be correct in every instance.

In this respect although the baby-selling objection to commercial surrogacy, *in its typical form*, may not misuse Kant I would argue that its invocation of him does not obviously yield the kind of blanket moral condemnation of commercial surrogacy that advocates of the baby-selling objection, in its typical form at least, want.

NOTES

1. See Elizabeth Anderson, "Is Woman's Labour a Commodity?" *Philosophy and Public Affairs*, 19:1 (Winter 1990), pp. 70–92.

2. Sara Ann Ketchum, "Selling Babies Selling Bodies," *Feminist Perspectives in Medical Ethics*, eds. Helen Bequaert Holmes and Laura Martha Purdy (Bloomington: Indiana University Press, 1992), pp. 284–294, at p. 286.

3. Immanuel Kant, *The Moral Law: Groundwork of the Metaphysic of Morals*, transl. H. J. Paton (London: Routledge, 1948), p. 91.

4. Allen Wood, "Humanity as End in Itself," *Kant's Groundwork of the Metaphysics of Morals: Critical Essays*, ed. Paul Guyer (New York: Bowman and Littlefield, 1998), pp. 165–188, at p. 171.

5. Immanuel Kant, *The Moral Law*, p. 90, Kant's emphasis.

6. *Ibid.*, p. 91, Kant's emphasis.

7. John A. Robertson, "Surrogate Motherhood: Not So Novel After All," *The Ethics of Reproductive Technology*, ed. Kenneth D. Alpern (Oxford: Oxford University Press, 1992), pp. 45–56, at p. 51.

8. Philip Parker, "Motivation of Surrogate Mothers: Initial Findings," *American Journal of Psychiatry*, 140:1 (January 1983), pp. 117–118, at p. 118.

9. Elizabeth Roberts, "'Native' Narratives of Connectedness: Surrogate Motherhood and Technology," *Cyborg Babies: From Techno-Sex to Techno-Tots*, eds. Robbie Davies-Floyd and Joseph Dumit (London: Routledge, 1998), pp. 193–211, at p. 198.

10. Maxwell Charlesworth, *Bioethics in a Liberal Society* (Hong Kong: Cambridge University Press, 1993), p. 79.

Fifteen

PROZAC, AUTHENTICITY, AND THE ARISTOTELIAN MEAN

John McMillan

1. Introduction

There is a tendency to think that the main way in which philosophy can contribute to bioethics is by encouraging people to formulate arguments for moral positions. This is an important aim: by thinking more critically about the reasons for moral beliefs, inconsistencies and inadequate justifications can be revealed.

One other way in which philosophy can contribute to bioethics is by explicating aspects of our moral psychology. For example, philosophical theories of moral responsibility can be used to unpack the assumptions implicit within the compulsory treatment of those with mental illness. Another important contribution of philosophy is to explicate what is behind our preferences about what makes our lives worth living. An important application of these ideas is to the impact that psychotropic medications might have upon how people assess their well-being. This chapter will demonstrate how philosophical explications of well-being can be applied so as to help interpret psychological change that is causally related to medication.

In *Listening to Prozac*, Peter Kramer[1] raises questions that should concern all those who are interested in what new psychiatric medications might mean for how we understand ourselves. Some of these questions concern the personality changes that he observed in some of the patients that he treated with Prozac. Kramer also expresses some frustration at the fact that ethicists have written so little that can be of help when thinking through such changes.

While he is right that ethicists have been of little help, there are some useful threads of moral theory that can help to unpack these questions. In particular, there has been a renewed interest in the philosophy of "well-being," and some of the points made in this debate are useful for thinking through personality change and Prozac.

One of the features of recent welfare theories has been an acknowledgment of the importance of life and its experiences being real or veridical. Most of these theories illustrate this importance with thought experiments about clearly unreal or non-veridical experience that suggest that there is something important missing from a life that consists of only these experiences. There is also an obvious connection here between some of Peter Kramer's worries about Prozac and worries shared by thinkers such as Carl Elliott and Walker Percy.[2]

Although welfare theories stress the importance of authenticity, they often do not give us much guidance about what happens when experiences fail to be real, veridical, or authentic. It is at this point that I think we might borrow some ideas from Aristotle. He believed that the virtuous person is one whose emotional reactions to the world are in harmony with their doing the right thing and thinking the right thing. What I want to propose is that one way that experiences can become inauthentic is when our passions or emotional reactions cease to be in harmony with our conception of the kind of person that we are.

I think this is an important issue, both for accounts of well-being and also for those people who are worried about the implications for authenticity of some psychiatric medications. To explore this further, I will begin by outlining Peter Kramer's description of one woman's response to Prozac. Then I will consider what implications the changes Kramer observes might have for our understanding of personal identity. The third section will draw upon points that have been made about the importance of authenticity for well-being. It is in this section that I will outline an Aristotelian account of inauthenticity. In the fourth section I will consider what I think are some of the stronger objections to this line of thought. While I will not be arguing for a moral conclusion, I will be showing how explicating concepts gives us a better understanding of important questions.

2. Tess

Tess contacted Peter Kramer for treatment of her clinical depression. Her childhood had been particularly harsh in that she had taken primary responsibility for looking after her nine siblings. Her need to provide a family environment for her siblings continued after her marriage at the age of seventeen, with the effect that pressure was exerted upon this relationship. Kramer creates an image of a person whose upbringing was lacking in many important ways and who still managed to respond with responsibility beyond her years. Her ability to manage in the face of huge challenges is one of the keys to understanding the changes that occurred when she took Prozac. Although Tess had not been given a great start in life she pursued a successful career as an administrator in a large corporation, as well as continuing to care for her mother. She presented to Kramer with depression that had lasted for several months. Although she was a very successful person in many aspects of her life, she did not consider herself so successful in her personal life.

A colleague referred her to Kramer after an unsuccessful course of psychotherapy. Kramer originally prescribed imipramine, but symptoms of her depression persisted, and there were some side effects from the medication. When Prozac was released by the US Food and Drug Administration, Kramer asked Tess whether she would like to try it. After two weeks of her taking Prozac, Kramer observed marked changes in Tess's behavior.

> In retrospect, she said, she had been depleted of energy for as long as she could remember, had almost not known what it was to feel rested and hopeful. She had been depressed, it now seemed to her, her whole life. She was astonished at the sensation of being free of depression.[3]

Tess's improved mental state resulted in many other changes in her lifestyle: she started dating men, she found that people approached her much more readily, the nature of her relationships changed. Her work also became more satisfying. She was able to handle the stress of tough negotiations better and not take conflict within her work environment personally. Kramer was amazed at the degree to which Tess's life improved.

> I had never seen a patient's social life reshaped so rapidly and dramatically: low self-worth, competitiveness, jealousy, poor interpersonal skills, shyness, fear of intimacy—the usual causes of social awkwardness—are so deeply ingrained and so difficult to influence that ordinarily change comes gradually if at all. But Tess blossomed all at once.[4]

The main reason why Kramer is impressed by the efficacy of Prozac is its ability to help with these deeply held habits and skills, all of which are important parts of an individual's personality. This sort of change is not typical for those taking antidepressants and seems to have surprised Kramer. Initially he prescribed Prozac for the usual reason, to help terminate depression and to return Tess to her premorbid self. However, the change that occurred was a transformation rather than a restoration.

So the aim of Kramer's treatment was to return Tess to her "normal" state of mind. Yet for her, Prozac had much wider effects. It had many positive effects over many areas of her life. It influenced the management style in her work, her relationships with men, and the way in which she handled difficult aspects of her past.

When an anti-depressant has the effect of lifting strong depressive affect, this can be a release from a burden that the person has been carrying. Tess described the "astonishing" feeling of being free from depression. It is also plausible to think that it would be difficult for her to imagine a time when she was not burdened in this way. Kramer does not confine his claims about Tess to this modest thesis. He also makes claims about Prozac's ability, for a significant minority of patients, to transform their sense of self.

> I believe that Tess's story contains an unchronicled reason for Prozac's enormous popularity: its ability to alter personality. Here was a patient whose usual method of functioning changed dramatically. She became socially capable, no longer a wallflower but a social butterfly.[5]

If a person has been depressed for a long period of time it would be usual to expect that this would result in their being perceived as having and experiencing a different sort of personality. Still, this does not amount to an ability to transform an individual's sense of self. In the following passage Kramer makes explicit his thesis about the self.

> When one pill at breakfast makes you a new person, or makes our patient, or relative, or neighbor a new person, it is difficult to resist the suggestion, the visceral certainty, that who we are is largely biologically determined.[6]

Gradually Kramer took Tess off Prozac. She had been off Prozac for a period of about eight weeks when she contacted Kramer to see if she could resume taking the medication. Tess had started to believe that some feelings characteristic of her ailment had begun to return: she had less confidence, and increased feelings of vulnerability. These feelings were not sufficient for considering Tess to be getting unwell again; they were feelings that she associated with her "old personality." In fact, her attitude toward the person that she is when on Prozac raises profound questions about the nature of personal identity and notions of the self.

3. Prozac and Personal Identity

Tess said

> "I am not myself." I found this statement remarkable. After all, Tess had existed in one mental state for twenty or thirty years; she then briefly felt different on medication. Now that the old mental state was threatening to re-emerge—the one that she had experienced almost all her adult life—her response was "I am not myself." But who had she been all those years if not herself?[7]

If it is possible for a medication radically to transform who it is that somebody thinks they are, this raises deep questions about the nature of identity and its relationship to the brain. However, it is difficult to know how to take this claim about a change in identity. On one of the standard theories of personal identity, Kramer's claim is hard to understand. In his paper "Personal Identity," Derek Parfit gives the following analysis: "X and Y are the same person if they are psychologically continuous and there is no person who is contemporary with either and not psychologically continuous with the other."[8]

In one way Tess has not been psychologically continuous. The kind of personality that others attribute to her and that she attributes to herself changed when she started taking Prozac. The complicated part of Parfit's analysis is how he describes psychological continuity. He identifies a number of factors involved in ascriptions of identity, the most important of which is memory. The original question that Parfit seeks to address is, how do we know that a person is the same person at another time? So if a person had the same memories, believed that these events happened to them and that they really happened, we would count this as evidence of them being the same person. Before she took Prozac, Tess had some of the same memories that Tess after taking Prozac does. Thus if we accept that memories play an important role in psychological continuity, then we have good grounds for believing that after Tess took Prozac she was still the same person.

The confusion here lies between the issue of "What sort of person do I want to be?" and "Who am I?" When Tess says that she is not feeling herself, she is saying that she is not the person that she can be when she is helped along with Prozac. The person that she was before taking Prozac is undoubtedly the same person. Perhaps even at that time Tess was not happy with the person that she was. She may have been irritated with things about her life, so when she has the ability to get on top of her depressive affect through Prozac, and to do something about these habits, she is becoming the person that she would prefer to be. When she does this her personality has changed in some way. Furthermore, her personality changes because it is something that she desires and has striven towards. Thus she could quite plausibly change who she is in this way, without negating who she was before.

It is quite possible that prior to taking Prozac Tess was not aware of any other way that she would like to be. The fact that she ended up in relationships that were not fulfilling may have been something about herself that she simply accepted. So she may never have thought that at another time she could be someone else. If this is the case then at that time she is who Tess is. The fact that at an earlier time she identified with a different sort of personality does not negate the fact that at an earlier time she was the same Tess. In fact Kramer describes how the new Tess came to describe the old Tess as mildly ill. So presumably if the old Tess accepted who she was at that time then she was making some sort of mistake.

Kramer talks about his discomfort with the apparent ability of Prozac to transform his patients' personalities. He notes that for some patients it can be an alienating (he uses "dislocating") experience suddenly to find themselves transformed.[9] He does make a comment that suggests he would agree with my reading of personality change: "Tess used her change in mood as a springboard for psychological change, converting pain into perspective and forgiveness."[10]

Here it sounds as if Kramer attributes Tess's change in personality to her ambition and motivation. The depression (which Prozac lifted) was limiting the degree to which Tess could be the sort of person that she wanted to be. That is, the absence of depression enabled Tess to work through the pain associated with her past and to forgive those who had caused her that pain.

While I do not think that the changes in personality that Tess and others have experienced on Prozac raise concerns about anyone's becoming, literally, a different person, I do think that there are other interesting questions that such changes raise. Although the new Tess may be psychologically continuous with the old Tess, there is still the vexed question of whether we should help people be better than well. Tess is not clinically depressed, hence to prescribe medication cannot be considered an attempt to return her to her premorbid self.

A satisfactory answer as to whether or not Kramer should give Tess more Prozac should consider a number of factors. If Kramer gives Tess Prozac when she is not unwell so that she can become better than well, is he acting any differently from the person who sells amphetamines on the street corner? What would this kind of role mean for the medical specialty of psychiatry? If we decided that it is acceptable to prescribe people Prozac when they are not, strictly speaking, unwell, and if other people respond to Prozac in the same way that Tess has, does this mean that we should make Prozac much more readily available, perhaps to the extent that we can buy it off the supermarket shelves? If we did this, could America and Britain become nations filled with Dale Carnegies and Richard Bransons? How long does Tess want to take Prozac for and is she aware of the risks?

All these questions are important, but I need to put them to one side for the time being. The central question that I want to consider is: might prescribing Prozac to Tess make her happier but inauthentic?

4. Authenticity and the Aristotelian Mean

I mentioned at the start of this chapter that I wanted to draw upon observations from the philosophy of well-being. One plausible theory of well-being is hedonism. It states that what it is that produces value in our lives is happiness. Those elements of our lives that produce happiness for us can thereby be considered constituents of our well-being.

Hedonism does imply that psychiatric treatments that make us happier do make our lives go better. It does appear that on a hedonistic account Prozac makes Tess's life go better for her. However, this is not the main point that I want to raise here. Rather it is one of the objections to hedonism that will be useful for unpacking the question of authenticity and Tess's well-being.

There are different versions of hedonism, and while I do not want to go into too much detail here, there is one important feature of some versions that I need to mention. In its simpler versions, happiness is understood as consisting simply of pleasurable mental states. A number of philosophers think that this version of hedonism fails to capture the importance for well-being of our experiences being real. In other words it is not sufficient that our lives involve pleasurable mental states; we also want to be a certain kind of person and do things that we think are valuable.

In *Anarchy, State, and Utopia*, Robert Nozick developed this objection with his example of the "Pleasure Machine."[11] This device attempts to show that we not only desire experiences to be good, but that we also require that they be real:

> Superduper neuropsychologists could stimulate your brain so that you would think and feel you were writing a great novel, or making a friend, or reading an interesting book. All the time you would be floating in a tank with electrodes attached to your brain. Should you plug into this machine for life, preprogramming your life's experiences?

Note that Nozick asks us whether we would choose to live our lives in the experience machine, and not merely whether we would choose to spend an hour or two in it after dinner. If we changed the scenario so that bars housed experience machines and patrons could plug into the machine for a couple of hours and then hop into taxis to go home (presumably it would be disorienting for a while after being plugged in) then we would have quite different intuitions about it. In fact being able to know what it would be like to do things which I will never actually be able to do, such as racing for Ferrari in the Italian Grand Prix, may be something which makes my life go better.

The point of the experience machine example is that we not only desire certain experiences, but that it is also important that we *really* are a certain type of person and that these experiences happen to us. Nozick's conclusion is "what we desire is to live (an active verb) ourselves, in contact with reality." Since the experience machine provides us with the best of experiences, what seems to be missing is the importance of the causes of our experiences.

The experience machine produces good experiences in such an artificial way that we can have little doubt that its experiences are unreal. How, if at all, can we know when the experiences that we have while taking a drug such as Prozac fail to be authentic?

One line of thought would be to suggest that experience is inauthentic when it is inconsistent with an individual's sense of who they are. By an individual's sense of who they are, I mean something different from the philosophical notion of personal identity. By an individual's sense of self I mean an individual's conception of who they are or of what sort of person they are.

Typically, if you were to ask a person what sort of person she is, she would tell you about some of the things that she likes doing, where she is from, what is important to her, and what she has done in the past. Describing yourself as a kind of person, then, seems to involve creating a set of descriptions each of which captures an aspect of your identity. We can describe this set of descriptions as an individual's narrative about the person that she is. So, experience can become inauthentic when it is inconsistent with an individual's narrative about the person that she is. In *Welfare, Happiness, and Ethics*, Wayne Sumner offers an example that helps to illustrate the point nicely:

> Asta keeps a diary. She has received a letter informing her that her son has been killed in the war and reassuring her that he died quickly, without pain. She records the comfort she has derived from this reassurance: "You can bear your children dying. What is unbearable is to think of them suffering, to think of that particular person, the child you carried, bleeding and in agony." Later she is visited by the sergeant who found her son on the battlefield and carried him back to the lines, and who knows the true circumstances of his death. She writes of that encounter: 'I would have given ten years of my life to have been able not to ask. But bargains like that can't be made. Either you're the sort of person who can hide from things or else you're not. I'd rather be so unhappy I want to die, and see the facts and look them in the face, than delude myself.' She asks the sergeant to tell her the truth.[12]

For Asta, to live more happily but in an ignorant way fails to comply with her narrative about the kind of person that she is. There are related although distinct ways in which her experience may fail to be authentic. If Asta decided against asking the sergeant about her son's death and lived more happily, she would be in a situation in which her reactions to the way in which her son died would be reasonable given what she (falsely) believes to be the circumstances surrounding his death. Falsely believing that her son died painlessly was unsustainable for Asta. Of course, this is something that other people may be able to deal with, and for them it may be possible not to ask the sergeant the truth. It is also possible for experience to fail to be authentic because our reactions to certain events are reactions that fail to conform to our conception of the sort of person that we are. If Asta had taken a drug before asking the sergeant about how her son had died and found, upon hearing the awful truth, that she was not upset or did not care, then she might think that the drug had caused her normal reactions to lived events to become inauthentic.

So, there are normative constraints involved in the assessment of our reactions to things that happen to us. In order for experiences to be authentic our reactions must fit within normative constraints for the person involved, and an important determinant of these constraints is the kind of person that this person thinks she is.

The idea that there is something important about the reactions that we have to lived events is one that can be traced back at least as far as Aristotle. In the *Nicomachean Ethics*, Aristotle is concerned with important questions about how we ought to live. He thinks that, instead of focusing upon abstract rules or aiming to maximize the good produced by our actions, we ought to aim at developing excellent characters and doing what the virtuous person would do. While I am not saying that we ought to follow Aristotle's moral advice, his ideas about what makes for an excellent character can shed some light on authenticity.

Aristotle's doctrine of the mean in respect of the passions is the idea that for every emotional reaction there is an intermediate state that is neither excessive nor deficient that is the mean state for that emotional reaction. Let us take the example he gives for anger. The "mean" that Aristotle thinks applies to anger he calls "mildness":

> The person who is angry at the right things and towards the right people, and also in the right way, at the right time, and for the right length of time, is praised. This, then, will be the mild person, since it is his mildness that is praised; for being a mild person means being undisturbed, not led by feeling, but irritated at whatever reason prescribes and for the length of time it prescribes. And he seems to err more in the direction of deficiency, since the mild person is ready to pardon, not eager to exact a penalty.[13]

Thus mildness is the criterion for anger, as it does provide that anger can be justified in some situations, as well as tending to minimize angry reactions. To have one's emotions in a mean, says Aristotle, is to feel and manifest each emotion at such times, on such matters, toward such people, for such reasons, and in such ways as are proper.

I am not concerned here with Aristotle's claims about what makes for an excellent character. Neither I am concerned with whether certain reactions are virtues or vices. But what does seem relevant is Aristotle's highlighting of the ways in which we evaluate our reactions to lived events. If after taking a drug we notice that the way we react to events no longer falls within our mean of reaction, then we may question the cause of this excess or deficiency of reaction. Realizing that a drug has brought about a new reaction may or may not be a worrying experience. In many instances the absence or deficiency of reactions such as anger or sadness is a liberating experience. However, if a very significant number of our passions became deficient or excessive then this might become more troublesome. I mentioned earlier that part of the reason that Nozick's experience machine looks unattractive is that it artificially causes all of our life's experiences, and that if we had the option of plugging into the machine for a few hours it would start to look much more attractive. Perhaps when passions become generally excessive or deficient as compared to previous settled means, worries about the causation of these reactions will become more significant.

What is so striking about Tess is that she has experienced exactly this kind of profound and widespread change in her reactions, yet does not find the fact that they are related to her taking of Prozac worrying. What seems to be an important part of Tess's endorsement of the changes that she experiences is that she has a coherent and consistent personal narrative about the person that she is when taking Prozac. The initial stages when she felt "dislocated" may have been partly due to her reactions and feelings failing to conform to the "mean" for her reactions.

5. Problems with Authenticity

It is not hard to think of examples of experiences being authentic but bad. Most of us would believe that when a person is having a leg amputated it is a good idea to provide them with anesthetic. Arguably the pain that a person would experience upon having a leg amputated is authentic. In other words the pain caused by having a leg removed is a reasonable reaction given what is happening to that person. A doctrine that believed experiencing pain of this sort contributed to a good life would be Calvinist in the extreme. Experiential authenticity is the view that in order for the reactions and activities of a life to constitute a good life they must be authentic. Therefore, the fact that the pain of a leg amputation is authentic does not mean that it will contribute to a life's going well. We can think of authenticity as being necessary but not sufficient for well-being.

Pharmacological Calvinism is a general mistrust of drugs used for non-therapeutic purposes and a conviction that if a drug "makes you feel good, it must be morally bad."[14] The Muslim and Mormon prohibitions on alcohol seem to be a form of pharmacological Calvinism. An important component of religious worries about alcohol (in addition to the behaviors that it may lead to) is that it may make experience inauthentic. It is likely that these groups are worried that even the occasional use of a small amount of alcohol may produce inauthentic experiences.

Many would disagree that the occasional use of alcohol invalidates experience. Many view the use of small amounts of alcohol as being a useful social lubricant for making conversation easier. Recall that when I discussed the experience machine I suggested that it makes a big difference whether we are being asked to plug in for a few hours or for the rest of our lives. Even if alcohol does make our reactions to lived events inauthentic, the occasional use of alcohol would seem to be analogous to spending a few hours in the experience machine.

It does not follow from what I have said about authenticity that religious worries about alcohol are irrational. If the occasional use of alcohol really does alter a person's reactions to lived events, to the extent that it clashes with her self-conception, then it may be that it really does violate her authenticity. In any case psychiatry ought to determine experiential authenticity on the basis of what is authentic for the patient being treated. Hence if a patient does have stronger beliefs about the violating of her authenticity through pharmacological means, then she may be the best judge of this.

A number of Kramer's patients felt discomfort with the changes they experienced on Prozac. He describes a young patient "Phillip" who did not like its effect upon him. He was mildly depressed and his problems stemmed from the way his peers treated him. Phillip responded well to Prozac and became "better than well." He hated feeling fine and missed his old bitterness. Kramer was worried about the severity of Phillip's depression and got him to agree to stay on Prozac for six months. Kramer describes Phillip's feelings about the effect of Prozac: "On Prozac, Phillip felt better than well and he hated it. He had been prematurely robbed of his disdain, his hatred, his alienation."[15]

Phillip's preferences make good sense if we take into account experiential authenticity. If Phillip could really change the way that his peers responded to him it would be understandable if he did. After all, it is hard to see what would be desirable about being on the receiving end of humiliating treatment. Phillip's dislike of Prozac is due to the unreality of the feelings that it produced in him. Phillip's peers continued to hassle him when he was on medication, but the degree to which these episodes upset Phillip decreased. Phillip must have been aware that his reactions to events happening around him were not "normal" for him. In other words, when subjected to humiliation at the hands of your peers it is reasonable to become angry and bitter at your treatment. As feeling quite happy when getting a hard time would not have conformed to what Phillip considered a reasonable reaction to lived events, Phillip's experiences while on Prozac would have failed to be experientially authentic.

I have suggested that people who judge that their responses or experiences are inauthentic would feel that their response was not within what they think of as being the range of reasonable reactions for them. In other words, if they found themselves in a social setting and responding with much more social bravado than they take to be within the mean for themselves, then they might start to see their reactions as pathological in some way, as reactions that are not authentic for them.

I have suggested that in order for experience to be authentic it must fit within normative constraints for the person involved, and that an important determinant of these constraints is the kind of person that a patient sees herself as. It is important to bear in mind that there are worse things than being in an inauthentic state. Phillip feels bitter, isolated, and resentful, but does not find these feelings so bad that the unreal feeling of Prozac is better. If his depression becomes more severe it seems likely that the better but not real feeling of Prozac will be what is best for Phillip.

If Kramer is satisfied that Tess can integrate the experiences that she has on Prozac into a coherent personal narrative, then he should not be concerned at her becoming better than well. Given that her experiences on Prozac are given meaning and integrated into her sense of who she is, it is not as if her experiences are caused by Prozac. So for people like Tess, Prozac is not like Nozick's experience machine, since she is an important cause and the ultimate judge of her experiences.

NOTES

1. Peter Kramer, *Listening to Prozac* (London: Fourth Estate, 1994).

2. Carl Elliott, *A Philosophical Disease: Bioethics, Culture, and Identity* (New York, London: Routledge, 1999); Walker Percy, *The Thanatos Syndrome* (London: Deutsch, 1987); Walker Percy, *Love in the Ruins* (London: Paladin, 1989).

3. Kramer, *Listening to Prozac*, p. 7.

4. *Ibid.*, p. 8.

5. *Ibid.*, p. 11.

6. *Ibid.*, p. 18.

7. *Ibid.*, p. 18.

8. Derek Parfit, "Personal Identity," *Philosophy as It Is*, eds. Myles Burnyeat and Ted Honderich (London: Allen Lane, 1979), p. 195.

9. Kramer, *Listening to Prozac*, p. 14.

10. *Ibid.*, p. 10.

11. Robert Nozick, *Anarchy, State, and Utopia* (Oxford: Basil Blackwell, 1974), pp. 104–108.

12. Wayne Sumner, *Welfare, Happiness, and Ethics* (Oxford: Clarendon Press, 1996).

13. Aristotle, *Nicomachean Ethics*, transl. Terence Irwin (Indianapolis: Hackett Pub. Co, 1985), p. 105.

14. Kramer, *Listening to Prozac*, p. 274.

15. *Ibid.*, p. 291.

Sixteen

THE CASE OF SELF-DEMAND AMPUTEES: A DILEMMA FOR PROFESSIONAL BIOETHICS?

Floris Tomasini

1. Introduction

> All men by nature desire to know.
> Aristotle, *Metaphysics*

> A hospital in Scotland acknowledged this morning that it had carried out limb amputations on two patients who had nothing *physically* wrong with them. Falkirk and District Royal Infirmary said that they were both suffering body dysmorphic disorders.
> BBC transcript of "Complete Obsession," a *Horizon* documentary.

Self-demand amputees are persons who need to have one or more healthy limbs or digits amputated to fit the way they see themselves. They want to rid themselves of a limb that they believe does not belong to their body identity. For this reason they have been classified as having an amputee identity disorder, rather than body dysmorphic disorder or apotemnophilia.[1] In fact, sometimes this desire to rid themselves of one or more limbs or digits is so obsessive and strong that, if refused treatment, they will self-harm in order to rid themselves of the offending appendage. This poses some challenging questions at the margins of professional bioethics.

My purpose in this chapter is to provide a number of normative and professional ethical perspectives on whether or not it is possible to justify the treatment of self-demand amputees. In doing so I proceed dialogically, moving between empirical context and normative theory revealing the taken for granted normative assumptions (what I call the natural attitude—a technical term borrowed from phenomenology) that provide ethical limits to justifying the treatment of self-demand amputees.[2] While I critically examine both Kantian responses against, as well as utilitarian responses for, amputation on demand, I conclude that neither normative tradition can fully incorporate an understanding of *what it is like to be* a self-demand amputee. Ethical justification, I argue, falls short of the recognition that there may be a problem, since neither theory can justify the apparent non-rational desire of amputation on demand. To end, I briefly introduce a metaethical idea, "the struggle for recognition," opening up the theoretical possibility of a hermeneutics of recognition before ethics that may be more sensitive to the problem of radical embodied difference exemplified by self-demand amputees.[3]

2. A Strong Kantian Justification against Amputation on Demand and its Partial Refutation

> Amputation of an organically healthy limb is anathema to me as a surgeon. The very thought of it disgusts me, when the limb(s) poses no imminent threat to life. I cannot see how it can be justified when it undermines the intrinsic worth of the human good that rests on preservation of a person's physical and mental integrity.

This composite professional view expresses a standard response to a request for amputation on demand. The normative force of this view can be morally and ethically justified through Immanuel Kant, who in his *Lectures on Ethics* argues that we have duties toward our own body. Fully to appreciate a Kantian response to the ethical problem posed by the treatment of self-demand amputees, we first need to understand the "internal goods" of Kant's own arguments vis-à-vis duty to ourselves as embodied beings.[4]

Kant's theory is deeply embedded in a strong moral justification of what we ought to do, rather than what is good to do or what it is good to be. The theory, then, aims to account for the obligations that we hold. Kant's notion of self-regarding duties toward self and the body, that could justify the normative view expressed above, is no exception. Indeed, in *Lectures on Ethics* he clearly states that our duty toward ourselves is not to be understood as being motivated by prudential reasons: "the basis of such obligation is not to be found in the advantages we reap from doing our duty towards ourselves."[5] In doing so, he shuns any psychologically consequential motivating factors; in his own words "the principle of self-regarding duties is a very different one, which has no connexion with our well-being or earthly happiness."[6]

Kant's moral justification for self-regarding duty lies in his deeply held view of the intrinsic value of humanity. So, accordingly, "the man who has violated the duties to himself has no inner worth."[7] And more strongly, "Even if all his amenities of life are sacrificed, maintenance of the worth of humanity makes up for the loss of them all, and sustains approbation, and *if all else is lost we still have an inner worth* [my italics]." [8]

If Kant's justification for self-regarding duties toward oneself and the body lies in his view of the intrinsic value of humanity, what does he mean by this? There are two intimately related answers. On the one hand there are metaphysical and psychological principles that found the logic of self-regarding duty and, on the other, such reasons justify a number of applied ethical examples that Kant himself uses—for example, suicide, care of one's life, sexual propriety, and even a passing remark about selling parts of the body itself.[9]

The metaphysical principles that support his idea of self-regarding duty to the intrinsic worth of oneself and body are the categorical imperative and freedom. In *Lectures on Ethics* Kant often moves from the specific to the universal, from human worth to a respect for humanity in general. This move can only be fully understood through the claims found in the *Groundwork of the Metaphysic of Morals*, where he argues that the content of our duty is determined by the categorical imperative; for example, we should always treat humanity, whether in our own person or in that of another, as an end, and never as a means only.[10] This implies a fundamental symmetry of moral recognition—because we recognize the intrinsic ideal of human worth in ourselves, we have obligations to ourselves *qua* humanity. In other words, what is intrinsically degrading to us is also intrinsically degrading to humanity.

The primacy of freedom is another metaphysical principle that Kant mobilizes to show up the illogicality of both the mind-body problem and the contradiction of human worth in any act that is intrinsically degrading. This is nicely illustrated in Kant's invective against suicide:

> The body is the total condition of life … and since the use of our freedom is only possible through the body, we see that the body constitutes part of our self. So far, then, as anyone destroys his body, and thereby takes his own life, he has employed his choice to destroy the power of choosing itself …. If freedom is the condition of life, it cannot be employed to abolish life.[11]

As well as providing metaphysical reasons for respecting human worth for itself, he gives both positive and negative psychological reasons for why we should value this. A positive reason for preserving human worth is that it leads to self-esteem, rather than happiness and well-being. Again, according to Kant "the *principium* of self-regarding duties does not consist in self-favor, but in self-esteem."[12] If a positive reason for maintaining human worth is self-esteem, then a negative psychological reason for not wanting to see it degraded and violated are the reactions it brings up in us; suicide overwhelms us with "horror," while sexual improprieties prompt a visceral "disgust" response.[13]

Having provided some of Kant's foundations to self-regarding duties toward ourselves, in which the body is an indivisible part, I critically examine how this may be extended to a line of argument as regards the treatment of self-demand amputees. From here on in I shall use the following abbreviations: SDAmp refers to self-demand amputation; SDA refers to self-demand amputee; SDAs/SDA's/SDAs' will refer to self-demand amputees/self-demand amputee's/self-demand amputees'.

It is fair to say that Kant, and most Kantians, would probably refuse SDAs the treatment they ask for, on principle. This is because amputating an organically healthy limb violates a self-regarding duty toward our self and our body. Since self-regarding duties involve a preservation of an intrinsic human worth, an amputation of this sort would be intrinsically degrading to human worth. A Kantian could elaborate what preserving human worth means in relation to our corporeality. This may be achieved by accepting Rom Harré's "organic integrity" amendment, in which he further specifies what preserving human worth is in relation to our embodiment.[14] Even so, given this further Kantian gloss, SDAs would still be refused amputations, on the grounds that such a desire clearly contravenes any ideally oriented sense of what it might be to preserve a human organic integrity.

If pushed for further justification, there are two main arguments that a Kantian might use to deny SDAmp. While one argument is purely philosophical, preserving organic integrity, and the other is quasi-psychological, preserving human worth, both rely on a strong rational justification of a human ideal. I outline both arguments respectively.

If one accepts a human ideal of organic integrity, then violating this is clearly not rational in the terms of Kant's categorical imperative. That is, the personal desire to have a leg amputated is not sufficient for it to be universalized as a good human end in itself. This resonates with a practical worry: if SDAs are aware that choosing to have a healthy limb off is not an ideal end in itself for humankind, how could they sanction their non-rational desire for an amputation without acknowledging that it might be a *mere* means to further non-rational desires, say, having another leg off (this is one of the worries professionals that sanction such amputations share)?

Another argument inspired by Kant, where one might infer his implicit disapproval of amputation on demand (if he had encountered it), rests on his remarks in "Of Suicide," in which he provides an important caveat for amputations that preserve life and organic integrity. Kant employs an implicit and indirect notion of harm when he says: "thus, a man can have his foot amputated, for example, in so far as it impedes him in life."[15] Given the context of his remarks here, it is fair to say that what he probably means by "impedes him in life" is either that it impedes him in life *per se*, perhaps directly threatening life, or that it impedes him in the course of his life. If this is what he means, then, in both senses, amputation on demand is wrong. First, because amputations of this kind are not at all necessary operations to preserve life—it is a psychological harm that *may* only indirectly lead to physical self-harm. Second, it does not impede the course of life. Indeed, quite the reverse: it would have probably appalled Kant as SDAmp is tantamount to voluntarily choosing disablement! Further, if medical professionals felt psychologically compelled by SDAs who threaten to self-harm, this could reasonably be construed as constraint on professional autonomy, upon which basis authentic ethical choice to offer a medical resolution rests.

There is a further illogicality that a Kantian may draw upon to justify a refusal to treat SDAs. Since Kant states in "Of Suicide" that the body represents the embodied possibility of freedom, its destruction is illogical because it violates this very possibility. Although this is clearly evident through a suicidal act, it is an argument that could be extended to an SDA urge for elective disablement. That is, while voluntary disablement obviously does not threaten the very potentiality of freedom, it severely hampers human freedom as a capacity for living a fully active physical life. Whereas, for a Kantian, this would offer a compelling reason not to consider amputation on demand, this sort of reasoning also plays a part for those medical professionals who might consider such an operation. Not least, because it involves professional complicity in performing an arguably non-necessary operation, on a patient who has voluntarily elected to have a limb or limbs removed.

As well as mobilizing philosophical arguments for the non-rationality of amputation on demand, Kantians might also draw on psychological reasons: arguments that cast doubt on the psychological rationality of the desire to have organically healthy limbs amputated. For Kantians amputation on demand is a violation of human worth and dignity. It is an act that shows little respect for an ideal human worth and as such provokes strong negative emotional responses, characterized by Kant as disgust. Interestingly, this disgust reaction is mirrored in many people who first come across the condition because it violates their own taken for granted sense of bodily integrity. Even professionals who choose to treat SDAs sometimes refer to the desire with pejoratives such as "mutilation" to convey their implicit personal feelings of disgust.

Again, if further psychological justification were necessary, a Kantian could respond by saying that SDAmp is wrong because rather than frustrating a consequentially driven notion of well-being it damages self-esteem operating at the heart of our internally driven sense to preserve human worth. From a Kantian perspective, then, SDAmp is prompted by a lack of self-esteem in integrity of human worth, which is ultimately an affront to the dignity of humanity *qua* respect for the moral law.

Having looked at some Kantian responses to SDAmp, I would like to turn now to some of the taken for granted normative assumptions—which I will refer to as the natural attitude—that pervade this perspective. I will critically assess whether or not the natural attitude is sufficiently sensitive to the ethical phenomena that arise from the lived world of SDAs. Before moving beyond the natural attitude of the Kantian response to the SDA problem by exposing conceptual assumptions about embodiment and human worth, I would first like to outline the advantages for a strong professional justification denying treatment.

Because Kantian approaches to duty regarding the body rely on an *ideal* view of embodiment (a normalized view of organic integrity and intrinsic human worth) any *deliberate* failure to respect this can be shown to be a non-rational desire. Moreover, such an argument is based on a very deep and intuitive sense of what it is to be *wholly* human; that is, to elect to have a leg off is not only morally reprehensible in a rational sense because of its very incomprehensibility and illogicality, it is also counter-intuitive in a deep emotional sense—self-mutilation fills most people with a powerful feeling of disgust. While disgust may, on the surface, seem a simple negative emotion, it is a deeply Janus-faced form of emotional recognition; the visceral disapproval projected toward the other is only possible through an introjection of sympathy toward a sense of organic integrity experienced at the heart of the self.

Summing up, any Kantian added ethical justification for why voluntary amputation is wrong simply supports the natural attitude that able-bodied organic integrity represents. There are, of course, a number of important caveats that, once again, fit comfortably with the natural attitude: amputations are sometimes necessary to save life and preserve organic integrity. Notwithstanding the Kantian precedent to approve of life-saving and life-preserving operations, no other precedents exist in the Kantian canon to justify elective amputation. Such views are aligned with common sense, and they are also enshrined in a very strong reading of medical professionals' interpretation of the Hippocratic Oath. Thus doing "no harm" can be understood as preserving the *overall* organic integrity and human worth that is psychologically entangled with this material ideal. In conclusion, the common sense view is premised on an ideal view of the preservation of the organic integrity of human beings, which because of its strong medical and ethical justifiability, understandably leads the majority of medical professionals to refuse treatment.

The problem with the Kantian view is that it cannot account for embodied difference—a view of embodiment that significantly deviates from what we normally consider to be constitutive of organic integrity and human worth. This is because Kantians have already assumed that all human beings naturally conform to certain identity norms, whether this is expressed physically, in terms of self-regarding duties toward preserving life and body, or psychologically, in terms of how the preservation of such norms should makes us feel in ourselves. While this seems eminently sensible for most people who are oriented to this unspoken human ideal, it denies the very possibility of SDAs and their lived experience of not existentially belonging to an able-bodied norm. Kantians have no way of understanding authentic embodied difference, other than through moral disapproval. Since they assume organic identity and human worth must conform to a stereotypically ideal type, Kantians have no way of dealing with SDAs who might just express human worth and integrity in a completely alternative way:

> Inside I feel that my legs don't belong to me ... I don't want to die, but there are times that I don't want to keep living in a body that doesn't feel like mine .... My legs are extraneous. They shouldn't be there; it doesn't feel right that they extend beyond where I feel my body should end.[16]

> The desire that I have is for an amputation of above the knee of the right leg .... It's still the reality that it seems like my body stops at mid-thigh my right leg. It's the rest of not me.[17]

In my view such expressions of embodied difference have to be treated seriously, because if SDAs *really need* amputations to regain a sense of belonging to and in themselves, then the act of sanctioning and performing surgery is justifiable on perfectly rational grounds of restoring their own sense of organic integrity and human worth. This cannot easily be dismissed, if there really are a plurality of body-images and identities that defy a common sense view of the human ideal. So, if we accept there may be another way of understanding organic integrity that leads to a plurality of body identities then it may be justifiable to treat SDAs. This is a view understood by a consultant surgeon and psychiatrist (respectively) who have freely chosen to operate on such patients:

> It is quite a difficult change of view on my part really—to remove a healthy limb is anathema to a surgeon, but I've become convinced over the years that there is a small group of patients who genuinely feel that their body is incomplete with the normal four complement of limbs.[18]

> He's going to be a whole man, paradoxically, ironically, without that leg.[19]

In sum, if we suspend the natural attitude about what ought to be constitutive of organic integrity—an argument strongly justified by Kantians who can rule out SDAmp on principle—then it might be possible to find other forms of medico-ethical justification, perhaps utilitarian ones, to provide professionally defensible reasons for treatment. It is to a utilitarian ethical justification that I turn next.

3. A Medium-Strong Utilitarian Justification for Amputation on Demand and its Partial Refutation

There are a small number of SDAs who genuinely feel incomplete with the usual complement of two arms and two legs. It is my belief that by carefully distinguishing between those who are *bona fide* SDA patients

> and those who are not, we, as professionals, are in a position to offer the treatment they need. We have to review such decisions, on a case by case basis, making sure that the benefits of carrying out such operations outweigh the harms.

This composite view represents that of a small minority of medical professionals who believe there is a case to be made for amputation on demand. The normative force of this view can be morally and ethically justified through an understanding of contemporary utilitarianism, in which both the classical doctrine and its modern restatements have been significantly revised in a quest for a universal altruism. Again, fully to appreciate contemporary utilitarian responses to the ethical problem posed by the treatment of self-demand amputees, we first need to understand the "internal goods" of such arguments.

Universal altruism, in its very simplest form, is based on the belief in an impartial concern for all sentient beings, always balancing good over perceived harm to effect maximum satisfaction of overall good. This involves universalizing what is good as opposed to what is harmful, rationally discriminating between ethical priorities as well as ensuring equality either on the basis of interests (interest utilitarianism) or on the grounds of perceived duties toward different categories of moral subject (liberal utilitarianism).[20] There are at least three core utilitarian tenets operating at the heart of universal altruism. The first concerns utility, the aggregative rule of satisfying interests or needs—interest utilitarianism requires the greatest satisfaction of interests, while liberal utilitarianism operates on a need-satisfaction principle.[21] The second involves a balancing of priorities—prioritizing major interests over minor interests in the case of interest utilitarianism or defending a principle of hierarchical needs in the case of liberal utilitarianism.[22] The third implies an important difference in understanding altruistic priorities—interest utilitarianism is based on a radical form of equality while liberal utilitarians are more concerned with a principle of autonomy that discriminates between beings on the basis of moral standing.[23]

While on the surface there are some significant similarities in the first two tenets, there is a crucial difference most clearly expressed in the third core idea. If one is an interest utilitarian, like Peter Singer, the primary motivating principle, equal consideration of interests, has its roots in the classical utilitarianism of Jeremy Bentham,[24] whereas if one is a liberal utilitarian, like Matti Häyry, then a working out of a need satisfaction principle is going to depend on a liberal interpretation of duty (see J. S. Mill for example).[25] This has important consequences for practical approaches to universal altruism. While interest utilitarians prize egalitarian reasoning over everything else, rallying against illogicality of perceived differences implicit in gender differences, racism, and speciesism, liberal utilitarians offer fine distinctions between sentient beings and their perceived levels of awareness and autonomy upon which they base a graded system of moral obligation vis-à-vis a defense of duties and rights. As a consequence, liberal utilitarians found a stronger ethical justification than interest utilitarians by concentrating on the notion of needs and liberal interpretations of duty.

To avoid confusion between the two theories, I will only provide a finer distinction when assessing *further* justifications of SDAmp where the differences between applied ethical outcomes are more evident. In providing further justification I consider a liberal utilitarian argument. In the meantime, I will give a more general interpretation in the next section of how SDAmp may be defended from a utilitarian perspective of universal altruism. So, having provided a very brief sketch of some contemporary utilitarian foundations to universal altruism, I critically examine whether this helps us to decide whether or not the treatment of self-demand amputees is ethically justifiable.

One major practical advantage a contemporary utilitarian defense of universal altruism has over a Kantian approach in its applicability to SDAmp is that it does not, automatically, as a matter of principle, rule out the possibility of such amputations. This is because there are no ideal presuppositions about human worth and organic integrity that prejudice medical professionals of a utilitarian persuasion from taking on any such unusual cases of amputation. For utilitarian universal altruists ideal presuppositions about human worth and organic integrity do not play a prominent role in ethical decision-making about amputations, because amputation is a decision that has to accord with the first utilitarian tenet, utility and the aggregative satisfaction of interests or needs. In medical terms this may translate as a decision to minimize overall harm, where *overall* harm is a contextually significant judgment about how best to satisfy a patient's interests or needs in any given situation.

At first glance this may provide a basis upon which to justify the more controversial forms of amputation required by SDAs. To understand this within the parameters of minimizing overall harm, it is useful to provide an example:

> Terry, a self-demand amputee, is given a single above the right knee amputation, on the judgment of medical experts who believe it will restore his sense of self and bodily integrity, quelling the considerable psychological harm of having an amputee identity disorder. An amputation of an organically healthy limb totally alleviates the psychological harm, restoring his sense of self and bodily integrity, giving him a renewed sense of meaning and purpose to his life, while vanquishing any potentially life-threatening urges Terry had about self-harming and forcing surgeons to treat a traumatic injury that may have led to death rather than the desired amputation. Unfortunately Terry is now an amputee, leaving him physically harmed and permanently disabled.

While we might say that the surgery did Terry *some* harm, in the sense that he has elected to become disabled, we could also logically argue that the amputation did him no *overall* harm. This is because we are using the notion of harm in different senses. In the first sense of harm, *some* harm, we are implicitly appealing to an ideal state. Obviously Terry is harmed in some way, because *ideally* it would be better if he were not an amputee at all. Arguably, this option is not available to SDAs, because their obsession to become amputees and realize their alternative body identity is not preventable by any other form of medical treatment. Provided this is a fact, we may more usefully employ this second sense of harm, *overall* harm, to understand Terry's case—harm in this sense being a way of satisfying overall interests or needs of a patient in any given medical situation. It is not the case, therefore, that Terry is any worse off than he otherwise would have been had he not had the amputation; indeed, Terry is cured of his psychological obsessive compulsion without suffering severe disablement (a bilateral amputation). His urge possibly to self-harm and to become a potential danger to himself has been quelled.

From this perspective the utilitarian altruist seems more sensitive to the normative *context* of SDAs, attending to the possible reality of a radical embodied difference where an *ideal* of organic integrity or intrinsic human worth does not become the limiting criterion to refuse treatment. Predictably, however, there are a number of further explicit and implicit principles that such an approach relies upon in order to justify controversial amputations of this sort. I call these natural attitudes, because while they offer further explicit ethical justification, they also present limits to understanding, the roots of which are taken for granted and insufficiently explored. It is to these further justifications and natural attitudes that I now turn. Here any further utilitarian justifications are grounded in liberal utilitarianism. Any apparent claim to produce the greatest satisfaction of needs, upon which an overall conception of harm can be understood, relies on a series of further professional procedures that ensure medical and ethical best practice.

Given that a liberal utilitarian could possibly countenance the possibility of this very controversial and unusual form of amputation, the greatest challenge for professionals of this persuasion is to assess and justify whether their patients *really need* this operation. This is, I believe, where the difficult challenge exists for the liberal utilitarian. There are at least two major obstacles. The first involves a possible confusion that may exist between *perceived* and *actual* harm. To put it bluntly, what an SDA says about what they need cannot be taken as the primary form of justification for amputation, without making expert professional judgment obsolete (other than in the technical sense of carrying out a successful amputation). If this were the case anybody proclaiming an urge to have a limb off could demand that a professional satisfy his or her desire. This sense of desire, desire as consumer demand, is blatantly absurd, not least because performing such operations would potentially leave permanently disabled a number of people who say they are SDAs, but actually are not. This could open the way for serious accusations of professional negligence through wrong diagnosis and treatment, either leaving mentally competent patients regretful about acting from wrong desire having had an elective amputation and changing their mind, or by encouraging mentally incompetent patients in their delusion to identify with amputees by becoming one themselves. So, professionals who are courageous enough to accept the possibility that this might be the right course of action in a select number of cases need a rigorous medical and ethical defense to support a rationale to justify amputation on demand.

Part of the judgment of someone's *really needing* a voluntary amputation has to rely on sound diagnosis. Until quite recently in the United Kingdom, when few such operations were sanctioned at Falkirk Royal Infirmary, the diagnosis of SDA involved having enough discriminative understanding to recognize it as a genuine medical condition that left professionals with limited medical options. In the words of a consultant psychiatrist:

> I think in this sense it is a psychological obsession. These people are not mentally ill .... They're not hearing voices, they're not deluded. It's not as if some force is telling them to have their limb off and following their paranoid delusion to do that. If that were the case then they would be psychotic ... neither is the cause of the problem neurosis, depression, or sexual fetish .... When a person wanting an amputation comes to a psychiatrist the options are fairly limited. On the one hand you could give them drugs to see if that cheers them up, or they're psychotic, give them an anti-psychotic. As we've said, they're not psychotic so that's not going to be of any use. Counseling, psychotherapy, cognitive behavioral therapy helps them focus on the positive things in life and get away and forget about the negative things, the wanting to have an amputation. Unfortunately talking treatments don't make a scrap of difference in these people. They are so fixed ... in a sense so locked in to what they want for themselves that you can talk till the cows come home and it won't make a scrap of difference. They're still going to want the amputation and I know for a fact, certainly in the case of Gregg.[26]

A competent medical diagnosis has a number of important ethical implications that further justify the case for amputation on demand. Minimally speaking assessing mental competency has implications for a principle of autonomy (see liberal utilitarianism).[27] In other words by pronouncing an SDA mentally fit enough, professionals are in effect identifying them as autonomous persons who are aware of their own capacity to make ethical judgments and moral choices. In practice this means that their needs to have their limb(s) amputated must be taken much more seriously, more so in fact, than someone who is mentally ill, not least because if they are psychotically deluded this would not be what they really needed.

Paradoxically their obsessive nature about what they need in combination with their *de facto* psychiatric mental competence makes them curiously well-informed when it comes to signing the informed consent form. In the words of an experienced general consultant surgeon who has taken on SDAs:

> The patients that I've seen, I've had psychiatric reports on them and the psychiatrists have indicated that these patients perfectly understand the consequences of what they're requesting. They are probably the best informed patients that I have ever had to deal with.[28]

Bona fide SDAs who have had amputations all report that they feel considerably better for having elective surgery to remove an organically healthy limb—ironically because the amputation restores *their* sense of organic integrity and human worth. Given this fact and their awareness of what it is they need, there are still serious problems in justifying such operations. Oddly enough the reason lies at the very heart of medical practice which assumes that "doctor knows best." There is this paternalistic assumption behind informed consent. Informed consent assumes that the doctor fully understands the condition of her patient and this understanding once communicated and understood by the patient leads him or her freely to give consent to whatever medical procedure is deemed necessary. Not only does it imply an "expert-lay divide" where the doctor always knows more than the patient about his or her condition, it also assumes a "deficit model of understanding" where the doctor simply informs the patient until he or she freely gives consent.[29] In effect SDAs reverse the principle of informed consent, by "demanding" that medical professionals satisfy *their* needs, based on their "superior" subjective first-person perspective of what is wrong with them. In this way the subjective interiority of the patients' own lived world and understanding of their own condition throws into stark relief the lack of available objective understanding of what this medical condition actually is. Not only does this reverse the implicit "expert-lay divide" which is normally operative in the doctor-patient relationship, it also fails to acknowledge where the deficit of understanding actually originates—lack of understanding comes from the doctor, and not from the patient.

Understanding runs deeper than a mere objective diagnosis, since subsequent treatment recommendations require medical doctors to recognize, at a very deep personal level, that the desire to have a limb or limbs off is a rational desire for a human being to have. This poses a problem for more unusual medical treatments like SDAmp. The inability to recognize the significance of a patient's problem can either lead to a downgrading of the significance of operations and their prioritization (as is the case for scheduling gender reassignment for transsexuals in amongst other National Health Service procedures), or to doctors doubting the worth of any objective medical judgment whatsoever in the even more controversial case of SDAmp. Whereas the latter provides a good reason to refuse SDAs any treatment, lack of understanding remains a key issue for those willing to recommend treatment. In a consultant psychiatrist's words:

> When I met Gregg it was very clear that he was very sane and there was absolutely no question that he was thought disordered in any way or mentally ill or sexually bizarre. He wasn't, he was an ordinary, nice man who wanted his limb off. It seemed to me at the time that that was incongruous for a nice, rational man to want his limb off. It seemed very strange. I, couldn't, I couldn't quite, to be honest, I couldn't quite understand it.[30]

In a strong justificatory sense, someone's needing to have such a radical operation can only be grounded in this deeper form of understanding where diagnosis conforms to some sort of empathetic recognition of what it is to be *wholly* human, with desires that we share with other human beings. Now, if it proves difficult to comprehend from the perspective of consultant psychiatrists and surgeons who have some understanding and sympathy for the plight of such unusual patients, one can better understand why professionals unfamiliar with this condition will respond negatively, refusing treatment by upholding the natural attitude. The heart of the matter lies prior to ethical justification; it is, first and foremost, an issue of recognition, a recognition that depends on *some* understanding of *what it is like to be a self-demand amputee*. It is from understanding as recognition, misrecognition, and non-recognition that further ethical justification arises.

The ticklish issue of recognition also arises in assessing the treatment options for such patients where a hierarchy of need satisfaction might discriminate who may and who may not be treated, the recognition of a more basic need satisfaction taking priority over a less basic need satisfaction. For example, one consultant psychiatrist who had approved an amputation of a right leg above the knee on one SDA, had refused to approve a double above knee amputation on another SDA on the grounds that the request was too extreme. In his words: "To be rid of one leg is, you know, O.K. To be rid of two is a disaster."[31]

While this may seem a plain contradiction when both patients had been correctly diagnosed as being *bona fide* SDAs, it can *plausibly* (although *not necessarily*), provide professionals of a liberal-utilitarian persuasion an opportunity to introduce a hierarchical needs-satisfaction principle as a basis to discriminate between single and bilateral amputations. In other words, the need to satisfy amputation on the grounds of the psychological trauma that a patient experiences by not feeling that they belong in their body, outweighs the need satisfaction of remaining able-bodied, *unless it involves a double amputation that leads to severe physical disability*. This is clear from a further explanation provided by the consultant surgeon:

> Physically it's perfectly feasible to do bilateral amputations, but I think from a surgeon's point of view it's really asking a bit much to expect us to take this on. I agree there is an irrepressible logic that if you're prepared to remove one leg why shouldn't you be prepared to remove two legs if the patient has this particular problem, but to a surgeon that's a very difficult concept to take on board.[32]

In practice it seems that while amputation may be considered for one limb—the psychological need for amputation taking priority over the physical need to be able-bodied—this hierarchy of need reverses when a double amputation is requested. Although this may seem intelligible to a liberal utilitarian, the reason given not to offer a bilateral amputation is based on a refusal to recognize the SDA's need, because it contravenes the recalcitrant professional identity of a surgeon who must draw a definite line concerning what is and is not acceptable in the balance of minimizing overall harm. In some ways this justification, almost definitely based on a liberal interpretation of the Hippocratic Oath, is not altogether different from that of a more conservative surgeon who refuses SDA treatment on principle. However, unlike the Kantian who offers an ethical justification for *non-recognition*, the utilitarian brought to the brink of his or her professional "comfort zone" where justification runs out, *refuses* to recognize the SDA once they ask too much. *Prima facie*, while the utilitarian argument is more sensitive to some kinds of amputation on demand, it eventually fails once recognition can no longer be squared with the ethical justification that professional identity demands.

This kind of reasoning shows up the limits of the professional identity and the ethical justification needed to secure it. Is there any way to progress beyond giving a complete medical and ethical justification for self-demand amputation? Before answering this question I want to reprise arguments given.

4. Reprise

I have critically examined two normative ethical justifications for the treatment of SDAs. The first justification is Kantian, and refuses treatment *per se*, on the grounds that SDA intrinsically degrades any ideal of human worth through compromising any recognizable sense of organic integrity. While this understandable reaction is perfectly justifiable within its own ideally oriented terms of reference, it discounts the contextual evidence that SDAs may possess an altogether different sense of human worth and organic integrity. Kantian ethics cannot, it seems, deal with embodied difference. The Kantian argument for not treating SDAs is ultimately a justification for the *non-recognition* of embodied difference.

The second justification is a utilitarian defense of universal altruism. While this seems much more promising than Kantian arguments in dealing with the practical context of embodied difference, it is much more difficult to justify whether or not SDAmp is ethically legitimate. To be more precise, while it delivers a medium-strong ethical justification for such amputation through principles such as greatest-need satisfaction, hierarchical needs, and autonomy, it raises a number of deeper questions about the limits of professional justification. Utilitarian justifications eventually fail once the recognition of the extremity of the demand outstrips the ethical justification that the professional identity demands. This leads to *refusal* of recognition.

What the utilitarian ethical argument shares with Kant is that it cannot square justification with recognition. In other words, there is a tension between ethical justification—which cannot completely escape the need to couple an ethical ideal with what the human form ought to represent—and recognition that may be more accepting of embodied difference for what it is. The questions that now arise are: is recognition of embodied difference possible without ethical justification? And, is recognition without normative ethics a possible alternative in maintaining a professional identity when treating SDAs?

5. Recognition Without Ethical Justification?

The failure for complete ethical justification lays in the struggle for recognition, an ultimately hopeless struggle where doctor and SDA cannot wholly escape what Hegel has called the master-slave relation.[33] The professional doctor-SDA relation is like Hegel's master-slave relation precisely because the master (doctor) refuses fully to recognize the slave (patient), denying him or her the affirmation of his or her full humanity.[34] So, the doctor ultimately refuses to acknowledge the slave's perceptions (of his or her own embodied difference) by forcing her own view of the world on the other (her view of what normal embodiment ultimately represents). Hence recognition is achieved through a "violent" struggle that fails to have any convincing justificatory validity. As Alexandre Kojève puts it:

> The relation between Master and Slave … *is not recognition properly so called* …. The Master is not the only one to consider himself the Master. The Slave also considers him as such. Hence, he is recognized in his human reality and dignity. But this recognition is one-sided, for he does

> not recognize in turn the Slave's human reality and dignity. Hence, he is recognized by someone whom he does not recognize. And this is what is insufficient—what is tragic—in his situation .... For he can be satisfied only by recognition *from one who he recognizes as worthy of recognizing him* [my italics].[35]

To make the parallel with the dilemma of non-recognition or misrecognition, let me juxtapose and analyze a quote from an SDA:

> The desire that I have is for an amputation of above the knee on my right leg. Now that's very specific and I have no way to understand it, comprehend it or to explain it to anybody in the world. Let alone explain it to myself and you sitting out there think it is nuts, I'm sitting in here thinking it is nuts, but I can't help it.[36]

As in the master-slave dialectic, recognition mutually reinforces a normal and deviant identity here. By recognizing the normality of wanting to be able-bodied, Gregg is reinforcing what is normal at the expense of what is not—projecting the reality of what is normal and what is not, the domain where the doctor (master) has ultimate control, while at the same time introjecting the abnormality of his subjective interiority. The real tragedy here is that the recognition is not reciprocated; either not at all by doctors who refuse treatment (non-recognition), or only partially, by doctors who will only reluctantly consider single limb as opposed to bilateral limb amputations (limited recognition).

The problem of recognition is twofold. It is first a problem of diagnosis and perceived harm. Professionals only have a moral obligation to treat SDAs if they recognize SDAmp as being a legitimate procedure to minimize *overall* harm. This rests on harm being an evaluative (rather than a naturalistic) concept; embodied difference of an SDA is not in dialectical opposition to normality, but in *relation* to its classifiable difference. The evaluation of classifiable difference from a human norm or ideal involves a deeper form of recognition still—the partial recognition of *what it is like to be an SDA* and whether or not it is possible to imagine radical difference as an elective amputation. It is this kind of hermeneutic recognition that precedes normative ethical justification. Understanding in the act of normative justification is actually a defense of our own reality and its congruence with a projected human ideal. Its rationality lies in the symmetry of recognition, where normality and ideality reflect one another in what we share with countless others. By contrast the origin of hermeneutical engagement entails an asymmetry of recognition where we have to project into a world of meanings outside our own immediate subjective sphere of reality.[37]

Hermeneutic understanding presupposes another's alternative reality, which must be something unknowable from the vantage point of subjective interiority. A hermeneutic engagement, or hermeneutics of recognition as I call it, requires attentiveness to alterity, or as Gadamer so beautifully puts it, "coming to an understanding … presupposes that the partners are ready for it and that they allow for the validity of what is alien and contrary to themselves."[38] Such understanding is difficult, but possible through our shared soma, where, for example, corporeal identification is grasped indirectly through other more socially identifiable and less alien conditions. For instance, that which prepares one consultant psychiatrist "to extend to that, which is more alien and contrary to him" is a prior recognition posed by transsexuals, providing the all important lateral bridge to be ready to understand the more alien urge for SDAmp. In his words,

> Certainly when I first heard of people wanting these amputations it seemed bizarre in the extreme but then I thought well, I see transsexuals and transsexuals want healthy parts of their body removed in order to adjust to their idealized body-image and so I think that was the connection for me.[39]

Interestingly the recognition of some sense of shared humanity, no matter how different, spurs on the search for ethical justification. The real dilemma bites when the recognition of authentic embodied difference eventually outstrips the normative justifications that professional ethics needs. Since normative explanatory justification remains the benchmark of professional identity, any serious transgression is not practically possible without leaving medical professionals open to accusations of unprofessionalism. Those who are willing to "push the envelope" of professionalism are still limited by the desire to maintain a credible professional identity. So, even though there is a form of hermeneutic recognition before ethical justification—that could be defended in a revival of moral intuitionism—professionalism tends to err on the side of being ethically normative and conservative. This does not mean that the right thing to do can always be justified, let alone completely, in the way that maintaining a professional identity demands.

NOTES

1. Gregg M. Furth and Robert Smith, *Amputee Identity Disorder: Information, Questions, Answers and Recommendations about Self-Demand Amputation* (Bloomington, IN: Authorhouse, 2002), p. 5.

2. Edmund Husserl, *Cartesian Meditations*, transl. W. R. Boyce Gibson (London: Allen and Unwin, 1931).

3. Axel Honneth, *The Struggle for Recognition: The Moral Grammar of Social Conflicts* (Cambridge: Polity Press, 1996).

4. Alasdair MacIntyre, *After Virtue: A Study in Moral Theory* (London: Duckworth, 1987).

5. Immanuel Kant, *Lectures on Ethics*, transl. Louis Infield (New York: Harper Row, 1963), p. 121.

6. *Ibid.*, p. 117.

7. Immanuel Kant, *Lectures on Ethics*, eds. Peter Heath and J. B. Schneewind, transl. Peter Heath (Cambridge: Cambridge University Press, 1997), p. 123.

8. *Ibid.*, p. 125.

9. See, e.g., Kant, *Lectures on Ethics*, pp. 122–222.

10. Immanuel Kant, *The Moral Law: Groundwork of the Metaphysic of Morals*, transl. H. J. Paton (London: Hutchinson, 1948), p. 91.

11. See, e.g., Kant, *Lectures on Ethics*, p. 144.

12. See, e.g., *ibid.*, p. 127.

13. See, e.g., *ibid.*

14. Rom Harré, "Body Obligations," *Cogito* 1 (1987), pp. 15–19.

15. See, e.g., Kant, *Lectures on Ethics*, p. 145.

16. "Complete Obsession," a *Horizon* documentary transcript, BBC2 (17 February 2000), http://www.bbc.co.uk/science/horizon/1999/obsession_script.shtml.

17. *Ibid.*

18. *Ibid.*

19. *Ibid.*

20. For interest utilitarianism see, e.g., Peter Singer, *Practical Ethics* (Cambridge: Cambridge University Press, 1987); for liberal utilitarianism see, e.g., Matti Häyry, *Liberal Utilitarianism* (London and New York: Routledge, 1994).

21. See, e.g., Singer, *Practical Ethics*, pp. 19–23; and Häyry, *Liberal Utilitarianism*, p. 124.

22. See, e.g., Singer, *Practical Ethics*, p. 55; and Häyry, *Liberal Utilitarianism*, p. 124.

23. See, e.g., Singer, *Practical Ethics*, pp. 14–47; and Häyry, *Liberal Utilitarianism*, pp. 142–145.

24. See, e.g., Jeremy Bentham, *Utilitarianism and Other Essays*, ed. Alan Ryan (Harmondsworth, Middlesex: Penguin Books, 1987).

25. See, e.g., John Stuart Mill, "On Liberty," *Three Essays*, ed. Richard Wollheim (Oxford and New York: Oxford University Press, 1975).

26. "Complete Obsession."

27. Häyry, *Liberal Utilitarianism*, p. 125.

28. "Complete Obsession."

29. See, e.g., Brian Wynne, "Misunderstood Misunderstandings: Social Identities and Public Uptake of Science," *Misunderstanding Science*, ed. A. Irwin and B. Wynne (Cambridge: Cambridge University Press, 1996).

30. "Complete Obsession."

31. *Ibid.*

32. *Ibid.*

33. Georg Willhelm Friedrich Hegel, *Phenomenology of Spirit*, transl. A. V. Miller (Oxford: Oxford University Press, 1977).

34. Ibid., pp. 116–117.

35. Alexandre Kojève, *Introduction to the Reading of Hegel*, transl. James H. Nichols (New York: Basic Books, 1969), p. 19.

36. "Complete Obsession."

37. Josef Bleicher, *Contemporary Hermeneutics* (London: Routledge, 1990), p. 57.

38. Hans-Georg Gadamer, *Truth and Method*, transl. Joel Weinsheimer and Donald G. Marshal (New York: Seabury Press, 1975), p. 348.

39. "Complete Obsession."

Seventeen

ENZYME REPLACEMENT THERAPY AND THE RULE OF RESCUE

Mark Sheehan

1. Enzyme Replacement Therapies

Enzyme replacement therapies are extremely expensive but also very effective. Despite the fact that the conditions treated by these therapies are rare, the drain on resources, particularly in socialized healthcare systems, is very obvious. With the prospect of more of these drugs in the future, the need for a properly thought-out position is pressing.

Conditions such as Gaucher's, Fabry's, and MPS1 (mucopolysaccharidosis type 1) are instances of a group of conditions known as lysosomal storage disorders. Many of these disorders result from an improperly functioning enzyme. In the case of Gaucher's disease the deficient enzyme, glucocerebrosidase, has been taken and modified from the human placenta.

These three conditions are rare but in their most severe forms are devastating. It is estimated that, in the United Kingdom, about 200 people suffer from Gaucher's disease, between 80 and 200 from Fabry's disease, and about 100 from MPS1.[1] According to the Gaucher's Association:

> Symptoms [of Gaucher's disease] range from mild to severe and can appear at any age. They include anaemia, fatigue, easy bruising and bleeding. An enlarged spleen and liver with a protruding stomach occur as well as bone pain, demineralization and fractures. In some cases it can be life-threatening and in many cases severely disabling. This describes Type 1. Types 2 and 3 Gaucher's disease include neurological symptoms as well as the above. Type 2 causes fatality within a year or two of birth while Type 3 causes a variety of neurological symptoms which range from mild to causing fatality.[2]

The evidence to date suggests that the enzyme replacement therapies for these conditions are very effective with patients who begin with little or no life expectancy. Such patients can go on to lead full and productive lives. However, the treatments are very expensive. The average cost per patient per annum for the treatment for Gaucher's (type 1) is £104,000, for Fabry's is £141,000, and for MPS1 is £335,000 (£125,000 for a child). It is important that these costs are per year and are required over a lifetime. It is estimated that costs will regularly be in the order of £2-6 million per person. By way of comparison, the National Health Service (NHS) will spend approximately £40,000 on the majority of people over their lifetime (75 years).[3]

The overall question that is faced by "resource allocators" then is whether these treatments should be funded in a socialized healthcare system like the NHS? For many (if not most) resource-allocation approaches the answer is "No." The so-called Rule of Rescue is one exception. It is this exception that is the focus of this paper.

In what follows I will consider the nature of the Rule of Rescue and its moral justification. The latter involves consideration of the distinction between agent-relative and agent-neutral obligations. If the Rule of Rescue is to be justified, it is plausible to think that it will be in the context of agent-relative obligations. Two problems with this suggestion are considered: the role of identifiability in the Rule of Rescue and the extent to which policy makers in a socialized healthcare system can be taken to have such obligations. It is argued that in both cases these problems can be overcome and hence that there is a *prima facie* obligation to follow the Rule of Rescue.

2. The Rule of Rescue

The Rule of Rescue is related particularly closely to a number of paradigm cases: the round-the-world yachtsman who becomes stranded at sea, or miners trapped in a collapsed mineshaft. In each case rescue operations costing large sums of money and possibly endangering large numbers of rescuers are mounted to save the very few who are in danger. Various attempts have been made to say what the Rule of Rescue amounts to. Among those attempts are the following:

> Any plan to distribute healthcare services must take human nature into account if the plan is to be acceptable to society. In this regard there is a fact about the human psyche that will inevitably trump the utilitarian rationality that is implicit in cost-effectiveness analysis: people cannot stand idly by when an identified person's life is visibly threatened if rescue measures are available.[4]

> Perhaps the most conspicuous feature of the RR then is the tendency to disregard opportunity costs when the life of an identifiable individual is visibly threatened. There is a tendency to "act first and ask questions later." Considerations about costs are pushed into the background. A lifesaving intervention takes on added value—or people act as though a lifesaving intervention takes on added value—if it benefits this person,

> where the demonstrative "this" refers to an individual who is, to those in a position to assist, present and identifiable.[5]

> Typically, when the RR is invoked to explain behaviour, one individual (or small group of individuals) is shocked by the desperate circumstances of another individual (or small group of individuals). Often situations evoking the RR response are unexpected and dramatic: they might involve miners trapped after an explosion, a child who has fallen down a well, or even a patient in cardiac arrest in the emergency ward. Such situations are likely to produce shock and horror in witnesses, or at the very least a sense of urgency.[6]

> The powerful human proclivity to rescue a single identified endangered life, regardless of cost, at the expense of many nameless faces who will therefore be denied healthcare.[7]

There are three important themes running through each of these accounts. The Rule of Rescue is (1) an imperative, (2) a (natural) human tendency, and (3) involves the rescue of identifiable individuals. We will examine each of these below.

3. The Status of the Rule of Rescue

An initial impediment to understanding the Rule of Rescue is its status. Is it a moral rule or an empirical fact? If it is a moral rule, what is its justification? Why think that it is something that we should obey? If it is an empirical fact then why think that it is relevant to moral deliberation? It may well be a human tendency but that, by itself, does not affect whether following this tendency is right or wrong.

This confusion is illustrated by examining the first two of the three common components in the above accounts and by the potential contradiction implied by classifying the Rule of Rescue as having both properties. Rules and imperatives are normally things that we *should* obey rather than *do* (as a matter of course) obey: they are generally prescriptive rather than descriptive. Natural human tendencies on the other hand are not things that we should "obey" but involve behavior that it is sometimes hard for us to resist. An account of human tendencies is a description of the way in which we tend to behave. For the most part then, something like the Rule of Rescue will either describe what we do or prescribe what we should do. It cannot do both.

If we suppose that the Rule of Rescue is descriptive and perhaps more aptly named the "Identifiable Victim Effect,"[8] then it is a mistake to speak of the Rule of Rescue as an imperative (unless it is clear that it is an imperative of nature). Of course, this does not mean that it has no role to play in moral reasoning, or as we shall see, that it cannot support a moral principle in some way.

If the Rule of Rescue is taken to be an empirical fact there remains a serious question about how it should feature in decisions about the distribution of resources. It is not clear whether it is something that we need to resist and work against or if it should be embraced. To see this point an analogous example is useful. We might plausibly suggest the Rule of Hate—that it is a natural human tendency to hate those who are different because of our fear of the unknown. This kind of fact clearly "mirrors" the fact encapsulated in the Rule of Rescue but we are presumably tempted in a different way in this case. More argument is needed if we are to construe the Rule of Rescue in a favorable moral light. It is worth pointing out how awkward it is to call the Rule of Hate an "imperative," thereby illustrating the moral connotation of the word "imperative."

If the Rule of Rescue as a general empirical fact does feature in our moral reasoning, it will need to be supplemented with an evaluative premise which applies a positive value to the key features of the Rule of Rescue. So, what we are interested in here are reasons for thinking that the following is true:

> People tend to be prepared to spend large sums of money rescuing seriously endangered, identifiable individuals *and this is a good thing*.

If we take the Rule of Rescue to be an established empirical fact, then it is mostly the italicized part of the statement that is of interest. The question then is: ought we to spend large sums of money rescuing identifiable individuals?

4. Moral Arguments Surrounding the Rule of Rescue

In his paper, "Rationing and Life-Saving Treatments: Should Identifiable Patients have Higher Priority?" Tony Hope considers six reasons for spending disproportionate amounts of money on identifiable individuals:[9]

1. Skepticism about the effectiveness of preventive treatment.
2. "A life in the hand is worth two in the bush."
3. Rescue is rare so we can always afford it.
4. Rescue has more effect on quality of life than prevention.
5. It is good to care about identifiable individuals.
6. A very small decrease in the chance of death is of only small benefit.

Of these it is the fifth that I will concentrate on here. It is more important than Hope allows and warrants some consideration.

The key issue involved in whether or not it is good to care about identifiable individuals is the moral status of being identifiable. We might initially be torn by two considerations. First, an uncomfortable feature of the Rule of Rescue is the role that publicity and lobbying play in its operation. If someone can interest the press in his or her story there is a good chance that the Rule of Rescue will come into play. There is something deeply objectionable about this. The thought here is that if I can make my own plight heard or visible then I will be rescued. This is worrying because it seems to be a matter of luck or whether I know how to get my voice heard that determines whether I am rescued or not. We quickly think of the individual who does not publicize her own plight or who is not fortunate enough to find the public's gaze.

On the other hand, the prospect of refusing those who do happen to be identified is not a happy one. A society that failed to rescue one of its members from serious and immediate peril might well be judged to be callous and uncaring.

In his discussion of this issue, Hope gives three sets of considerations that might be taken as support for the claim that we should care about identifiable individuals. Very roughly these considerations are: (1) individual morality; (2) consequentialist or contractualist grounds; and, (3) the "argument from callousness." It is (1) that warrants the most attention here. The other two are ably dealt with by Hope.

The key thought behind this consideration is that in our "personal morality" we tend to take our obligations toward those with whom we have relationships, those who are close to us and perhaps those who, for one reason or another, are identifiable as more pressing than our obligations to those who fall outside of these categories.

5. Agent-Neutral and Agent-Relative Obligations

We often take ourselves to have special obligations because those in question are near to us in one way or another. Often these obligations are the result of a relationship of a particular sort. Patients, clients, family members, and friends all stand in particular relationships to us that we would normally understand to generate obligations. This set of obligations has been called agent-relative obligations. An agent-relative obligation is an obligation that can only be understood in terms of the agent for whom it is an obligation.[10] So, part of my obligation to look after my son will depend on his being my son—at least part of why I ought to take care of him is because of the relationship in which I stand to him. In addition to relationships, special circumstances can give rise to agent-relative obligations. The fact that I alone am in a position to help save the drowning child places a special, agent-relative obligation upon me—

dependent upon the fact that I am in the position that I am with the knowledge and skills that I have.

On the other hand, an agent-neutral obligation is an obligation that does not ultimately refer to the agent for whom it is an obligation. Instead, such obligations may, as the name suggests, apply neutrally across all agents. So we may think that I have obligations to look after other people's children by virtue of my being a human being (agent, person, and so on). Importantly this obligation is distinct from the obligation that I owe to my son.

Perhaps the best way to illustrate the distinction is to use an example where we would normally take the agent-relative obligation to take precedence over an agent-neutral one—I should teach my child to read even if someone else's child could benefit more from my teaching. The thought here is that even though teaching someone else's child to read can do more good, I still have a more pressing obligation to my son. There are many other examples of this that we could cite—lawyer-client and doctor-patient relationships provide particularly apt cases.

It is important that the distinction between agent-relative and agent-neutral obligations is understood to be an explanation of our obligations—of the kinds of obligations that we have. The idea is that it registers a significant distinction within the ordinary obligations that we take ourselves to have. If this is a good explanation of our obligations then we can understand ourselves to have obligations of this kind.

The significance of this for the Rule of Rescue is that the general empirical fact about our human proclivities looks as though it is indicative of an agent-relative kind of obligation. That is, the fact that we are strongly inclined to expend large amounts of resources (or otherwise risk great cost to ourselves) in order to save an identifiable individual suggests that we have an agent-relative obligation to those in need of rescue. Importantly, in some cases this obligation overrides our agent-neutral obligations to do the most good with the resources we have. The thought is that we stand in a special relationship, perhaps a relationship of circumstance, to those in need of rescue and as such have an obligation to save them. Since this obligation looks to be an agent-relative obligation, it is capable of being more pressing than an agent-neutral obligation, say, to use resources to do the most good.

It is crucial to notice that nothing in this is meant to imply that the agent-relative obligation is always an overriding obligation. There may well be times when the agent-neutral obligation is more pressing than the agent-relative one—the distinction is intended to make room for agent relativity, not to argue for its dominance.

6. Problems with the Rule of Rescue: (1) Identifiability

The first set of doubts that arise about the Rule of Rescue's applicability do so from the idea of "identifiability." How are we to understand "identifiability" in the Rule of Rescue? There are three sets of considerations here:

A. Identifiability Does not Seem to Be a Morally Relevant Property

Lobbying, publicity campaigns, or preferential treatment all seem to be cases where the involvement of identifiability seems objectionable. The lesson from this is not necessarily that the Rule of Rescue is objectionable but that some ways of becoming identified are objectionable. It might be that expressing the Rule of Rescue in terms of identifiability limits the way in which the obligation involved is to be understood. We need an account of what it is to be identifiable in the right way.

B. Identifiability as a Relative Concept

Being identifiable (or identified) looks to be a matter of degree. Whether an individual or group is identifiable will depend on the "background" level of identifiability, or that compared to which it is identifiable. So, for example, a drowning child is more identifiable than one of the ten trapped miners. One of the ten trapped miners is more identifiable than one of the 25 people who will die at a particular road intersection this year. The 25 people who will die at a particular road intersection this year are more identifiable than the 25 people throughout the UK who will die this year of a particularly rare disease. There are many and varied groups against which someone can be identified. Someone can be identified relative to future or potential beneficiaries, to the masses, or to those who do not have a particular condition. Quite clearly the Rule of Rescue will have the "biggest effect" when the "rescued" is highly identifiable relative to the others for whom the resources would be used.

C. Identifiability Looks to Be a Vague, Catchall Term

Rather than just one concept, "identifiability" as it features in the Rule of Rescue involves a whole spectrum of concepts. We might mean something like "acquaintance" and include the various degrees and ways of knowing the person or people in question. Here, we might feel the pressure to rescue someone who we have seen or met before. Second, we might take identifiability to be something akin to statistical likelihood (or statistical "identifiability")—we might feel that we ought to help those who are more likely to suffer from a particular disease. Third, we might take it to mean proximity, physical, social, or cultural—we might feel more pressure to assist people from our neighborhood or our community. And finally we might think that someone is identifiable when we have a special relationship, or relationship of circumstance, with them—we might take ourselves to have a greater obligation to children or to the "vulnerable."

These three points taken together make it clear that the concept of identifiability as it appears in the Rule of Rescue is inadequate. We can readily imagine examples where each of the concepts mentioned above applies more readily and more satisfactorily than identifiability. The distinction between agent-relative and agent-neutral obligations is of some help here. Being identifiable to us is one kind of relationship that a person might have to us. Being near us is another. In both cases these relationships can be understood as giving rise to agent-relative obligations. It is not identifiability that matters in the Rule of Rescue but the way in which things like identifiability contribute to our agent-relative obligations.

7. Problems with the Rule of Rescue: (2) The Obligations of Policy Makers

It might be suggested that those making policy or resource-allocation decisions are in a different moral position than "ordinary" moral agents. The agent-relative–agent-neutral distinction is derived from reflections on our "personal morality." The obligations of the policy maker, we might think, are different from those of the ordinary person. Two reasons for thinking that policy makers do not have agent-relative obligations are (1) that making policy requires being impartial and (2) that unlike the ordinary person the policy maker has an obligation to the population as a whole.

Neither of these is acceptable. In the first case, the response begs the question. We are interested in reasons for thinking that policy makers have only agent-neutral obligations. One feature of agent-neutral obligations is that they are impartial. So, the claim that policy makers should be impartial is a restatement of the claim that they do not have agent-relative obligations.

The second reason suffers the same problem. It is certainly true that the policy maker has an obligation to the population. What is less clear, and is the question at issue, is whether this obligation is to be taken as applying only to the whole or to the individual members as well. That is, our question is whether policy makers have obligations to the population as a whole as well as to individual members of the population—this again is the agent-relative–agent-neutral distinction. Asserting that policy makers (only) have an obligation to the population as a whole is a restatement of the claim and not a reason for thinking it true.

The key question here though is why should we think that policy makers do have agent-relative obligations? There are two answers that might be given here. First, we might think that justice and goodness are to be distinguished—

that the obligations of justice are not only obligations of good-maximizing.[11] As it stands this is not an argument in favor. Like the arguments above, it simply reasserts the claim. In essence this point is a restatement of the complaint made by the non-consequentialist about the consequentialist: when we are considering what is just, this will sometimes involve not doing what is best for the population as a whole and instead might require rescuing an individual or group. So, in order to act justly the policy maker will sometimes be required to forego the interests of the population as a whole in favor of the interests of a particular member.

Second, we might suggest that the differences between "personal morality" and the policy maker's obligations are not as great as they might at first appear. It may well be very difficult to distinguish between personal and "professional" morality—it is after all the same person who must decide what ought to be done.

But the similarities might be more entrenched than this. The head of a household, a father say, can certainly be taken to have agent-relative obligations to his "constituents," his children. As in the example above, he ought to teach them to read because they are his children. However this father is also required to make resource-allocation decisions—he must make decisions based both on what is best for the family as a whole and on what is best for the individual members of the family. So there is nothing special about this kind of decision. At the next level up, the scout troop leader undoubtedly has obligations to each member of the troop—among others, to protect their welfare. But here also, the scout troop leader has obligations to the group as a whole and is similarly required to make resource allocation decisions. The scout troop leader has both agent-relative and agent-neutral obligations.

The idea here is to suggest that we can increase the numbers for whom the "policy maker" is responsible without thereby losing the agent-relative obligations. It is not the number of people involved that makes the difference. Naturally the relationship between the policy maker and the population changes as the numbers increase. The father knows his children in a way that the troop leader does not. But this is a shift in the way in which the individual can be identifiable to the policy maker, not a change in the kind of obligation involved.

There is a second more important shift in these examples—the scout leader has the obligations he does because of the role that he plays, because of what it is to be a scout leader. Our next example could be the owner of a business or corporation or it might be a vicar or a Member of Parliament. We might suspect that the obligations of the businessman are different from those of the scout troop leader and indeed of the vicar or the MP. In each case the differences in obligation depend on what we take the responsibilities or role of the particular position to be. The role of the businessman is primarily to ensure that the business turns a profit. The role of the vicar is to look after the parish—notably both the parish as a whole and the individual members. Arguably the role of the MP is to represent his constituents, again both as a whole and individually. These different roles nicely reflect the agent-relative–agent-neutral distinction. Because the businessman is primarily required to act for the benefit of the company, cost-effectiveness is the main consideration. The vicar or the MP, like the father and the scout troop leader, are plausibly understood to have both agent-relative and agent-neutral obligations—that is, obligations to particular "constituents" and obligations to the constituency as a whole.

When we turn to the policy maker in healthcare these considerations are telling. Healthcare is not a business—or better, it is not simply a business. As such those making policy decisions in healthcare can be taken to have obligations both to the population as a whole and to particular individuals—they have agent-relative and agent-neutral obligations. This is not to say that one always trumps the other. Nor is it to say that the decision between them is always straightforward. But it is to claim that an account of policymaking in healthcare which omits agent-relative obligations is an impoverished one.

8. Conclusions

While the so-called Rule of Rescue is not itself a moral principle, it does point to a particular way of thinking about our obligations. It was suggested that people's willingness to go to great lengths to save a few is an example of an agent-relative obligation. Agent-relative obligations are obligations that we have because of a particular relationship or set of circumstances. They are to be contrasted with agent-neutral obligations—obligations that apply to all independently of particular circumstance or relationship. Do healthcare policy makers have agent-relative obligations? It is plausible to think that they do, but the argument given depends on thinking that healthcare policy making is not simply like managing a business.

Overall the arguments are balanced. This means that neither the Rule of Rescue nor considerations of cost-effectiveness can be given up altogether. Not to fund enzyme replacement therapies at all would be to focus on the cost-effectiveness approach exclusively and to ignore the agent-relative obligations of policy makers. Fully funding enzyme replacement therapies would be to ignore the obligation of policy makers to use resources effectively. The more balanced these two considerations can be the better.

NOTES

1. National Horizon Scanning Centre Report on Enzyme Replacement Therapies in *Enzyme Replacement Therapy: A document prepared for West Midlands Primary Care trusts to support the development of a commissioning policy for the treatment of Gaucher's Disease, Fabrys Disease and Mucopolysaccharidosis Type 1*. NHS West Midlands Specialised Services Agency, March 2004, pp. 35–43.

2. Gaucher's Association Response in *Enzyme Replacement Therapy*, pp. 100–102.

3. *Enzyme Replacement Therapy*, pp. 14–31.

4. David C. Hadorn, "Setting Healthcare Priorities in Oregon: Cost-Effectiveness Meets the Rule of Rescue," *Journal of the American Medical Association*, 265:17 (1 May 1991), pp. 2218–2225, at p. 2219.

5. John McKie and Jeff Richardson, "The Rule of Rescue," *Social Science and Medicine*, 56:12 (June 2003), pp. 2407–2419, at p. 2408.

6. *Ibid.*, p. 2409.

7. Molly Osborne and Timothy W. Evans, "Allocation of Resources in Intensive Care: A Transatlantic Perspective," *The Lancet*, 343 (1994), pp. 778–780, at p. 779.

8. Karen E. Jenni and George Loewenstein, "Explaining the 'Identifiable Victim Effect,'" *Journal of Risk and Uncertainty*, 14:3 (19 May 1997), pp. 235–257.

9. Tony Hope, "Rationing and Life-saving Treatments: Should Identifiable Patients have Higher Priority?" *Journal of Medical Ethics*, 27:3 (1 June 2001), pp. 179–185.

10. David McNaughton and Piers Rawlings, "Agent-Relativity and the Doing-Happening Distinction," *Philosophical Studies*, 63:2 (1991), pp. 167–185; David McNaughton and Piers Rawlings, "On Defending Deontology," *Ratio (New Series)*, 11:1 (1 April 1998), pp. 37–54.

11. John Broome, "Good, Fairness, and QALYs," *Philosophy and Medical Welfare*, eds. J. M. Bell and Susan Mendus (Cambridge: Cambridge University Press, 1988); John Broome, "Fairness," *Proceedings of the Aristotelian Society*, 91:1 (1990), pp. 87–102; John Broome, "Fairness versus Doing the Most Good," *Hastings Center Report* 24:4 (1994), pp. 36–39.

Eighteen

IS "THERAPEUTIC RESEARCH" A MISNOMER?

Peter Lucas

1. Introduction

The distinction between therapeutic and non-therapeutic research is a familiar one in research ethics. This chapter argues that the term "therapeutic research" is a misnomer. I consider two broad types of ostensibly therapeutic research: controlled trials, and innovative/experimental treatments. I argue that in the former case the term therapeutic research is a misnomer because no reasonable researcher can expect patients/subjects to derive any therapeutic advantage from being entered into an ethically conducted controlled trial. In the latter case, while accepting that there may well be a reasonable expectation of therapeutic benefit from innovative treatments, I argue that the decision whether it is in the interests of a given patient to receive a given treatment is properly made on purely clinical grounds. There is no special feature of the research situation, in either of these types of case, which serves to ensure that participation, *qua* research subject, is in a patient's interests.

2. "Therapeutic" and "Non-Therapeutic" Research

The distinction between "therapeutic" and "non-therapeutic" research is a notable feature of versions of the Helsinki Declaration of the World Medical Association, which sets out an ethical framework for the regulation of medical research involving human subjects, from the original 1964 version of the declaration, up to and including the 1989 revision. The 1989 version of the declaration refers to a "fundamental" distinction between

> medical research, in which the aim is essentially diagnostic or therapeutic for a patient, and medical research, the essential object of which is purely scientific and without implying direct diagnostic or therapeutic value to the person subjected to the research.[1]

Some searching questions could be asked about the therapeutic–non-therapeutic distinction drawn here. We might for example question the assumptions apparently embodied in this statement concerning the relationship between diagnostic procedures and research. Are we to consider all diagnostic procedures to be forms of research (despite the fact that, standardly, diagnosis applies, but does not yield, generalizable knowledge)? No doubt the case for such a view could be argued. But if it were ever to become a generally accepted view, the implications for clinical practice would be radical—since clinical diagnostic procedures would then fall under the particularly stringent ethical frameworks developed for research.

We could also question the particularist emphasis in the above quotation, suggested by the phrase "diagnostic or therapeutic *for a patient*" (my emphasis). Are we to take it that therapeutic research necessarily, or even typically, has as its essential aim the production of direct therapeutic benefit for particular patients? And if so, how is this to be squared with the more familiar view that the essential aim of research is the generation of *generalizable* knowledge?

Notwithstanding the above worries, the distinction between therapeutic and non-therapeutic research has attained considerable currency. Most introductory medical ethics textbooks, if they deal with research ethics at all, will at least mention the distinction, which is typically explicated with reference to the intentions of the researcher.[2] This approach is given canonical form in Ian Kennedy and Andrew Grubb's *Principles of Medical Law*, where therapeutic research is said to be characterized by a "dual intention" on the part of the researcher.[3] In therapeutic research there is an intention on the part of the researcher "both to seek to benefit the patient who is the research subject, *and* to gather data of a generalizable nature." In non-therapeutic research, by contrast, there is "only a single intention: to gather data."[4]

This reference to the researcher's intentions does not seem an altogether happy one, in that it seems to involve an implicit appeal to what we might call a "reasonable researcher" standard, which would be much better made explicit. In order to rule out examples of irresponsible experimentation, based on unreasonable expectations of therapeutic benefit, from qualifying as therapeutic research, the Kennedy and Grubb characterization of therapeutic research would be better reformulated as "research intended to produce generalizable data, and to benefit the patient/subject of the research, *where the relevant research procedure could reasonably be expected to deliver such a result.*"

Reformulated in this way, however, the Kennedy and Grubb interpretation suggests that there exists a distinctive form of medical research in which the twin goals of delivering therapeutic benefits to patients/subjects, and of generating generalizable data, are intrinsically linked. In this chapter, my central focus will be the concept of therapeutic research, understood in this way. I will argue that, when it is so understood, the term "therapeutic research" is a misnomer. No ethically conducted program of medical research can construct the sort of essential link between the therapeutic goal and the scientific goal, which the above characterization implies. After considering and dismissing two different broad types of research which might (erroneously, in my view) be termed "therapeutic," I will close with some thoughts on why the point is an important one, and on what would be a more appropriate label for so-called therapeutic research.

3. Controlled Trials

To begin however, let us consider some salient features of the general ethical context within which biomedical research is pursued. The principle that a doctor is obliged to treat her patients according to the best proven diagnostic or therapeutic method is a well-established principle of biomedical ethics.[5] This principle is for example enshrined in successive versions of the Helsinki Declaration.[6] And yet there is an evident tension between adherence to *this* principle, and the involvement of *patients* in any form of medical research.

Unless the research in which the patient is involved bears no relation to her condition at all (in which case, for all but the most trivial complaints, their involvement as research subjects is questionable in itself), the patient/subject will be likely to be the recipient of an unproven treatment. Where this treatment is given as an alternative to the established best standard treatment for the condition the patient clearly does not receive the best *proven* treatment for his/her condition, for the simple reason that both the efficacy of the treatment in question, and the severity of any associated risks, are not yet proven. In a case in which the treatment given is in addition to the established standard treatment the patient/subject may well receive the benefits of both treatments. But she will also be exposed to the risks associated with both. These may well be compounded, and in the case of the non-standard treatment will be, again, unproven.

This tension between the principle that patients are entitled to the best proven treatment for their condition, and the involvement of patients in research, is implicitly acknowledged in the 2000 version of the Helsinki Declaration, which requires that when research is combined with clinical care, patients/subjects should be assured of the best proven treatment at the *conclusion* of the study.[7] Of course, the requirement that patients are given access to the best proven treatment at the conclusion of a study does not necessarily preclude their having access to that same treatment at an earlier stage. But in many research contexts, and most clearly in controlled clinical trials, some patients at least will not receive the best *proven* treatment during the course of the study (namely, those receiving the experimental treatment); nor will all patients necessarily receive the best proven treatment at the conclusion of the study—for example if their treatment regime remains unchanged, and the new "best proven" treatment is the former experimental treatment.

In order to evade some of the ethical difficulties associated with administering unproven treatments to patients in research contexts, it is standard, in research, to apply a negative version of the principle that patients should receive the best proven treatment: no patient should receive a known inferior treatment.[8] So in a controlled clinical trial, whether randomized or not, and whether placebo-controlled or not, the researcher proceeds ethically if and only if she remains in a state of *equipoise* between the different arms of the trial.[9] From the point at which it becomes clear that one of the arms of the trial is receiving markedly inferior treatment it is unethical to continue with the trial.[10]

It is an interesting question whether this entails that it is unethical to demand very rigorous standards of proof in controlled trials. It may well be clear to the researcher that one or other arm of the trial has a therapeutic advantage some time before fully statistically significant results have emerged. But at the point at which the researcher can reasonably be said to "know" that one arm of the trial is subject to a therapeutic disadvantage it seems unethical, by the above principle, to continue with the trial, regardless of whether fully conclusive results have yet been obtained.[11] For our purposes however, the more relevant implication of the principle of equipoise is that there can be no reasonable expectation of therapeutic advantage to a patient from being entered into an ethically conducted controlled trial. In an ethically conducted placebo-controlled trial there can be no good reason to think that the active treatment is superior to the placebo. If there is good reason to think the active treatment is superior then the trial is unethical, since equipoise is lacking; and if there is no good reason to think that the active treatment is therapeutically superior (or inferior) to the placebo, there is no good reason to think that there will be any therapeutic advantage whatever to the patient from being entered into the trial. Whatever the researcher's intentions may or may not be then, ethically conducted placebo-controlled trials cannot reasonably be characterized as "therapeutic" research, since no reasonable researcher could expect any therapeutic advantage to accrue to the patient from being entered into the trial.

Suppose however that the trial is not placebo-controlled, and the control is the established standard treatment. In this case adhering to the principle of equipoise requires that there should be no good reason to think, either prior to or during the trial, that the standard treatment is either superior to or inferior to the treatment(s) under test. From the point at which it is established that either the new treatment or the control is markedly superior it becomes unethical to continue the trial. Again then, in an ethically conducted trial, there can be no reasonable expectation of therapeutic advantage to the patient from being entered into the trial—assuming that the alternative for the patient is that of receiving the standard treatment.

So much then for the idea that controlled clinical trials represent a form of essentially therapeutic research. There can be no reasonable expectation of therapeutic advantage from being entered into such a trial; and no reasonable researcher, advising a potential research subject on whether to participate in an ethically conducted controlled trial, is in a position to claim that therapeutic considerations have any bearing on the patient/subject's decision. From the point of view of the patient/subject the only relevant question is whether she wishes to contribute to the furtherance of the scientific goal, with the inconvenience and risks this may entail.

4. Innovative Treatments

I want now to consider those forms of research which can reasonably be termed "innovative" or "experimental" treatments, that is, forms of biomedical research involving patient/subjects which either involve no comparison with a formal control, but only informal comparison with existing treatments, or no "comparison" at all, where there is no established treatment for the patient's condition. It turns out that these types of case also fail to merit the "therapeutic research" label, though for different reasons.

I have said that so-called therapeutic research is standardly characterized with reference to the dual therapeutic and research goals of the researcher. In turning to consider innovative treatments, it is reasonable to ask about the relationship between these two goals; and in particular whether they are ever essentially linked, such that the therapeutic goal is fulfilled by a process that simultaneously and necessarily involves the fulfilment of the research goal. (To clarify: if it were to be decided, as mentioned earlier, that diagnosis constitutes a form of research, this would qualify as a case in which the research goal and the therapeutic goal were essentially linked.) Raanan Gillon suggests that research and therapy are never linked in such a way when he remarks:

> so-called therapeutic research always has two components: a component of pure research intended to produce generalizable medical knowledge, and a component of therapy, where the intention is to benefit the particular patient.[12]

This way of putting the point suggests that the "therapeutic research" label might be seriously misleading: there is in fact no distinct type of research which is inherently therapeutic, as the "therapeutic research" label suggests. Rather, therapeutic and research goals can sometimes be achieved through what is, essentially, one and the same process—though it is a contingent matter that this ever happens in practice. To appreciate the full significance of this point, we need to step outside the narrow perspective of the researcher, which has, up to this point, been our preferred mode of access to "therapeutic" research, and consider the decision whether to participate in research paying close attention to the interests of the potential research participant.

Suppose we are dealing with an innovative/experimental treatment, in a case in which there is no established treatment for a patient's condition. The new treatment will have been subject to extensive laboratory-based testing prior to being available for use in a clinical context, and from this testing a reasonably clear picture of the likely risks and benefits of the treatment will have emerged. The decision to utilize this new treatment in a given case will, from the researcher's standpoint, have two motives: the motive of producing therapeutic benefit, and the motive of procuring generalizable knowledge. However, a consideration of the interests of the individual patient suggests that it is only the aim of producing therapeutic benefit that is relevant when deciding whether to consent to the new treatment. If, on balance, and bearing in mind the relative paucity of evidence, there seems to be a reasonable likelihood of therapeutic benefit to a given patient, then we may judge that the experimental treatment is clinically indicated in her case.

What kind of net benefit we need look for, and how much likelihood of producing it is required, will depend upon a host of other factors, not least amongst which are the severity of the patient's condition, and the severity of anticipated side effects. The associated question of how much risk-taking on the part of the doctor and the patient respectively is permissible, or required, is also relevant here. One area in which the label "therapeutic research" might be thought to have important application is in relation to experimental treatments for AIDS and related conditions. Controversy in these sorts of cases has tended to cluster around the issue of access to experimental treatments, and the rights of sufferers, particularly terminally ill sufferers, to expose themselves to potentially very high risks. In particular, the issue has been medical paternalism, and whether the medical profession has the right to prevent patients who wish to take risks from doing so. Nothing I say here should be taken to imply that patients should not be allowed to expose themselves to risks as research subjects. Rather, my concern is whether there is a branch of research with respect to which participation *qua* research subject can reasonably be expected to confer therapeutic benefit.

A patient considering an experimental treatment, where there is no established standard treatment, will certainly be hoping for therapeutic benefit. But the patient's motives are not the most important thing here. Even in the more common case of a placebo-controlled trial the patient will no doubt be hoping to have been included in the active arm of the trial, and will be hoping that the active treatment is therapeutically effective. Nevertheless, from the research ethics standpoint, the important question in such a case is whether we have something approaching proof that the treatment under test is likely to be therapeutically beneficial. If we have, then the trial is unethical—since the placebo arm will then be receiving a known inferior treatment. If there is no good reason to expect therapeutic benefit from the treatment under test the trial is ethical, but the patient's hope is (so far as we know) a mere hope. Similarly, in the innovative treatment case, it is not the patient's hopes but the researcher's reasonable expectations which are of prime importance.

However, because in the case of innovative/experimental treatment we are not dealing with a formal trial, in which one or other arm of the trial stands to be therapeutically disadvantaged, the decision to administer the treatment comes down to this: is this particular innovative treatment clinically indicated? The answer to this question will either be "Yes" or "No"; and only if there is reasonable expectation of therapeutic benefit to the patient will the answer be "Yes." In this latter case then, unlike those of non-therapeutic research, and controlled trials, there may be a reasonable expectation of therapeutic advantage to the patient. Indeed the ethical acceptability of the treatment regime *qua* treatment regime will hinge on this. But despite the fact that, in this type of case, the patient in question may be said to have an interest in receiving the innovative treatment, and despite the hope shared by all concerned that the innovative treatment will turn out to be effective against her condition, she cannot be said to have an interest in serving as a research subject that is in any way parallel to that in which she has an interest in receiving the innovative treatment. It may well be that it is in our patient's interests that the research be carried out. But it does not follow that she has an interest in serving as a research subject, exposing herself to the associated inconveniences, and risks. We can certainly talk of patients benefiting from research through an improved understanding of their condition, and potential treatments. But from the fact that we can say with confidence that an improved understanding of my condition will result from my participation as a research subject, *it does not follow that this benefit to me accrues to me conditionally upon my participation in the research.* Any benefit to me that accrues from a given study accrues on the condition that the study is carried out, not on the condition that I participate in it. (And my participation in the study is not, except possibly in highly unusual circumstances, a condition for the study to be carried out.) From the fact that I will benefit from the study then, it does *not*, in general, follow that it is in my interests to participate—for the benefit to me will accrue whether I participate or not.

This is not to suggest that the patient cannot share the researcher's dual goal of the production of therapeutic benefit and the furtherance of biomedical knowledge. The point is simply that only one of these intentions is relevant when considering a given patient's receipt of an innovative treatment, under the heading of "therapeutic research." That the innovative treatment is clinically indicated is both a necessary and a sufficient ethical precondition for administering it in a given case. That administering the innovative treatment will also contribute to the acquisition of generalizable knowledge is neither a necessary nor a sufficient ethical precondition for administering it in a given case. (Not necessary because a patient should not be denied access to a clinically indicated treatment just because administering the treatment in this case would be valueless in research terms; not sufficient because while knowledge might be gained even where the treatment is not clinically indicated, it would be wrong to administer the treatment where there was no expectation of therapeutic benefit—bear in mind that we are dealing here with patients, not with healthy volunteers).

So although the innovative/experimental treatment case does look to be one in which it is possible to proceed ethically while fulfilling the dual goal which we have seen is characteristic of so-called therapeutic research, closer inspection reveals that the question whether the innovative treatment is clinically indicated is the only one that really matters in a given case. So, as Jonathan Montgomery points out, the decision whether to proceed with an innovative treatment is best viewed as a matter of clinical ethics, rather than of research ethics.[13] There is no essential link between fulfilling the research intention and acting in the interests of a particular patient.

To return to Gillon's characterization of therapeutic research then, everything, I have suggested, hinges on quite how the two components he distinguishes are taken to be related. If they are understood to be essentially linked, such that, so far as we know, subjects could not receive such and such a therapeutic benefit without participating in a study designed to produce generalizable knowledge, then the established idea of therapeutic research would retain some validity. However, none of the forms of research we have considered manage to forge an essential link between participation as a research subject and anticipated therapeutic benefit. In the case of an ethically conducted controlled trial, considerations of therapeutic advantage do not enter in. In the case of innovative/experimental treatment, with no formal control, the therapeutic intention is the only relevant intention when we are considering whether it is in the interests of a given patient to participate. In both types of case it looks as if the two components, of therapy, and of the generation of generalizable knowledge, are only accidentally related.

The final type of case I want to consider is that in which participation in research is a precondition for receiving treatment—patients are effectively denied treatment unless they participate. Here, it seems to me, the patient's situation is in certain respects similar to that of the subjects of an innovative treatment. The decision whether to participate, where made with the patient's interests at heart, must rest exclusively on the potential therapeutic benefit—any anticipated research payoff is not to enter into the calculation, since this cannot be legitimately cited as a reason why *this* patient should participate in *this* study. Where the two cases do differ markedly, of course, is in the element of effective coercion. While we have no reason to think that innovative/experimental treatments are, in general, ethically suspect, the effective coercion of research subjects *is* ethically unacceptable. It follows that this sort of case cannot be cited as an example of the existence of a form of ethically acceptable research properly characterized as "therapeutic." On the basis of the above examples then, we may conclude that the idea that there is a specific form of research in which the pursuit of the research goal and that of the therapeutic goal go hand in hand is an illusion.

5. Some Implications of the Above, and a Suggestion

The above considerations suggest that the "therapeutic research" label is a misleading misnomer. Why, particularly, does this matter? The upshot of the points I have been considering is that participation *qua research subject* is always fundamentally an altruistic act. This is of particular relevance to research with vulnerable groups. When considering non-therapeutic research with competent non-vulnerable adults we accept that, because participation as a subject is a significantly altruistic act, their consent is essential. Participants are inconvenienced, and may be exposed to significant risks, for no benefit to themselves. For these reasons we are normally hesitant about asking members of vulnerable groups to participate in non-therapeutic research. The potential for exploitation when working with such groups is increased, not least because it may be difficult or even impossible to obtain informed consent from them. In the case of therapeutic research on the other hand, it may be tempting to follow the route which is standard in clinical ethics and, where informed consent is unobtainable, allow ourselves to be guided by the patient's best interests, rather than by their choices. As long as we hold to the worryingly widespread myth that participation in "therapeutic" research is beneficial to the subjects of that research then, we may think we see a way open to relaxing consent requirements for so-called therapeutic research with vulnerable groups. Indeed, this is precisely what we find in current guidance on research with children. Non-therapeutic research on children is currently discouraged, unless the research in question would be virtually risk-free. The Medical Research Council, for example, suggests that only negligible-risk, non-therapeutic studies involving children are acceptable.[14] The reason for this, as Jonathan Montgomery reminds us, is that "in non-therapeutic studies there is no obvious benefit to be gained and it can be suggested that children are being put at risk for no possible gain."[15]

When we turn to the guidance concerning "therapeutic" research however, we find that here "higher risks may be acceptable," since in this case "it is hoped the child will benefit."[16] (Indeed it seems that legally it may be permissible to proceed with "therapeutic" research against the express wishes of the child concerned, provided the parents' consent has been obtained.[17]) On this basis it is held that where valid parental consent is indeed forthcoming, "it is easy to justify [children's] involvement in therapeutic studies".[18] As I have argued at length above however, participation in so-called therapeutic research cannot reasonably be held to carry any benefits for research participants. If I am right, we should not be prepared to relax consent requirements for therapeutic research involving children in any such way. Proceeding with more than minimal-risk research with children, will, even given parental consent, be no more acceptable in the "therapeutic" case than in the "non-therapeutic" case. Moreover, since participants in so-called therapeutic research will necessarily be patients, and since patients as such can reasonably be said to represent a vulnerable group, there may well be grounds for imposing more stringent consent requirements for *all* such research.

If research involving patients is not to be termed "therapeutic," what should we call it? My suggestion would be: "Medical research combined with medical care." This is the formula employed in the 2000 version of the Helsinki Declaration, and it has the merit of explicitly directing our attention to the fact that the subjects of such research are simultaneously subjects of medical care. Instead of being a case in which it is appropriate to relax the stringent ethical safeguards governing medical research, and fall back on the standard clinical framework, which permits a good deal of risk-taking, based on an estimation of the patient's interests, this formula suggests that, *prima facie* at least, the "therapeutic" research context is one in which the requirements of *both* clinical and research ethics frameworks apply. The declaration does not speak of a relaxing of consent requirements when medical research is combined with medical care, but on the contrary counsels: "when medical research is combined with medical care, *additional standards* apply to protect the patients who are research subjects [my emphasis]."[19]

NOTES

1. WMA Declaration of Helsinki (1989), quoted in British Medical Association, *Medical Ethics Today: Its Theory and Practice* (London: BMA publishing, 1993), p. 198.

2. Alastair Campbell, Grant Gillett, and Gareth Jones, *Medical Ethics* (Oxford: Oxford University Press, 1997), pp. 171–172.

3. Ian Kennedy and Andrew Grubb, *Principles of Medical Law* (Oxford: Oxford University Press, 1998), p. 716.

4. *Ibid.*

5. Sophie Botros, "Equipoise, Consent, and the Ethics of Randomised Clinical Trials," *Ethics and Law in Health Care and Research*, ed. Peter Byrne (London: John Wiley and Sons, 1990), p. 9.

6. World Medical Association, Declaration of Helsinki (1989), para. II.3, http://www.augsburg.edu/irb/helsinki.html; World Medical Association, Declaration of Helsinki (2000), para. 30, http://www.wma.net/e/policy/b3.htm.

7. *Ibid.*

8. Botros, "Equipoise, Consent, and the Ethics of Randomised Clinical Trials," p. 18.

9. Baruch A. Brody, *The Ethics of Biomedical Research: An International Perspective* (Oxford: Oxford University Press, 1998), ch. 7.

10. See Ian Kennedy, "The Law and Ethics of Informed Consent and Randomized Controlled Trials," Ian Kennedy, *Treat Me Right* (Oxfőrd: Clarendon, 1991).

11. *Ibid.*, p. 219.

12. Raanan Gillon, "'Fully' Informed Consent, Clinical Trials, and the Boundaries of Therapeutic Discretion," *Informed Consent in Medical Research*, eds. Len Doyal and Geoffrey Tobias (London: BMJ Books, 2001), p. 263.

13. Jonathan Montgomery, "Informed Consent and Clinical Research with Children," *Informed Consent in Medical Research*, eds. Doyal and Tobias, p. 174.

14. Medical Research Council, *Issues in Research with Children* (London: MRC, 1991).

15. Jonathan Montgomery, "Informed Consent and Clinical Research with Children," p. 179.

16. *Ibid.*, p. 173.

17. *Ibid.*, p. 177.

18. *Ibid.*, p. 179.

19. Declaration of Helsinki, para. 28.

Nineteen

CAN THE SUBJECT-OF-A-LIFE CRITERION HELP GRANT RIGHTS TO NON-PERSONS?

Lisa Bortolotti

1. Introduction

In ethics we often implicitly correlate what an individual is entitled to from a moral point of view with the complexity of the mental life of that individual. This correlation gains center-stage in many attempts to answer the question whether we should accord rights or moral status to those individuals that lack the capacities required for personhood, such as the capacity for rational deliberation and self-consciousness.[1] I use the term "capacity" here and in the rest of the chapter to refer to powers that individuals might have and that they exercise when they engage in reasoning and gain awareness of their mental life. This is the established usage in the discussion on the conditions for personhood and the possible rights of different kinds of beings.

The formulation of a subject-of-a-life criterion for basic rights offers one possible account of the correlation between the entitlement to moral consideration and mental capacities.[2] Tom Regan's argument for according rights to some non-human animals and some human non-persons is based on the notion of "subject of a life," which raises some concerns. I argue in this chapter that the case for according rights or moral status to non-persons can be much more persuasive if rights or moral status are accorded to all and only those individuals that are intentional agents.

Why can we not work with a criterion that is already available in the applied ethics literature, such as sentience? Sentience is not adequate as a criterion for basic rights or moral status, according to Regan, because sentient individuals do not have all they need to obtain moral status. Basic rights or moral status should be granted for Regan to those individuals who have interests and autonomy (in a sense that I elucidate in the next section). Sentient individuals might be able to feel pain and pleasure, but they might not have beliefs, desires, and preferences. An individual's possession of these intentional states is necessary to show that the individual has interests and autonomy in the relevant sense.

Here I discuss the relation between interests, autonomy, and rights (or moral status) and conclude that the possession of intentional states and the capacity to initiate actions on the basis of those states are necessary conditions for having rights (or moral status).

2. The Justification of the Subject-of-a-Life Criterion

Regan recognizes that the best way to argue that some animals and human non-persons have rights is to show that they have morally relevant interests that need to be safeguarded. In other words, they are subjects of a life.

> Individuals are subjects-of-a-life if they have beliefs and desires; perception, memory, and a sense of the future, including their own future; an emotional life together with feelings of pleasure and pain; preference- and welfare interests; the ability to initiate action in pursuit of their desires and goals; a psycho-physical identity over time; and an individual welfare in the sense that their experiential life fares well or ill for them, logically independently of their utility for others and logically independently of their being the object of anyone else's interests.[3]

One can justify the requirements that individuals must satisfy in order to be granted basic rights or moral status on the basis of the relation between rights, interests, and autonomy. Subjects of a life are sentient, as they are able to feel pleasure and pain, but also have other capacities. They have intentional states such as beliefs, desires, emotions, and preferences, and they have the capacity to initiate action on the basis of those intentional states. These two elements, the possession of intentional states and the capacity for intentional action, seem to be the most relevant to the entitlement to basic rights, because they ground the ascription of what Regan calls "preference autonomy" and "preference interests."

Regan follows Immanuel Kant in according rights to those individuals who are autonomous agents, but he thinks that the relevant notion of autonomy does not include the capacity for rational deliberation. All that is required is preference autonomy. A dog and a very young child are preference-autonomous, as they have beliefs and desires and act in order to satisfy their desires on the basis of their beliefs. Moral agents are autonomous in a richer sense, as they can abstract from their desires and deliberate on what they ought to do. They can also act against some of their desires in conformity with a law or principle that has normative force on them. *All* subjects of a life are preference-autonomous in the sense in which the dog and the child are. They have preferences and act on those preferences. *Some* subjects of a life also have the capacity for reflection and rational deliberation and qualify as persons, but Regan believes that this richer notion of autonomy is not required for being accorded rights.

Regan distinguishes between preference interests and welfare interests.[4] Preference interests refer to those things we are actually interested in, whereas welfare interests concern those things that are good for us, whether or not we have an interest in them. It might be in my best interests to go to bed early tonight as tomorrow I have an important meeting (welfare interest), but I do not have an interest in going to bed early tonight unless I have the right combination of beliefs and desires, like the belief that an early night would do me good and the desire to be in good shape tomorrow (preference interest). It is evident that the possession of intentional states and the capacity to initiate action on the basis of those intentional states are required for individuals to have preference interests.

The notions of preference autonomy and preference interests help justify the subject-of-a-life criterion as the criterion for the attribution of basic rights. Only beings with preference interests can have rights, because only beings with interests can be benefited or harmed.[5] We can assume that having preference interests requires having beliefs, desires, and other intentional states and being able to act purposefully, but the possession of welfare interests should not appear in the list of conditions that individuals need to meet in order to be subjects of a life. Here we come to the first problem with the subject-of-a-life criterion.

All individuals with preference interests have their own welfare, but as Raymond Frey also observed, ants or plants can have their own welfare and welfare interests without having preference interests.[6] Individuals do not need to be sentient or to have beliefs and desires in order to have their own welfare. It might be in the interests of the ants inhabiting my front garden that I put off mowing the grass. But that does not require them to have any intentional state or tendency to preference-autonomous action.

By regarding the possession of welfare interests as one of the criteria for basic rights or moral status, the ground shifts without justification from the capacities one must have in order to be the subject of a life to metaphysical considerations about what kind of an individual one is. Subjects of a life are described by Regan both in terms of the capacities they must have in order to have inherent value (for example possession of intentional states) and in terms of the kind of entities they are (for example possession of a psychophysical identity and an independent welfare).

A formulation based on cognitive capacities is useful in discriminating between individuals that are entitled to basic rights and individuals that are not, since the possession of such capacities has behavioral manifestations that can be observed and tested. Instead, it is difficult to establish what would count as evidence for the metaphysical status of some non-human animals as individuals with a psychophysical identity and an independent welfare. So, some of the requirements of the subject-of-a-life criterion are unhelpful for the practical purposes of identifying subjects of a life in controversial cases and difficult to justify from a moral point of view.

3. Empirical Questions about the Subject-of-a-Life Criterion

Regan states that subjects of a life have memory, a sense of their own future, intentional states about themselves, and self-consciousness.[7] How plausible is it that non-human animals and severely impaired humans can satisfy these requirements?

Mammalian animals perceive and to some extent represent their environment,[8] but no conclusive evidence has been gathered for the claim that even great apes can remember specific events in their past experience. For years, the accepted view in comparative psychology has been that animals lack the kind of episodic memory that humans have. They retain the skills they have acquired, but they do not remember episodes as they happened to them.[9] This view has recently been challenged by studies conducted on birds,[10] great apes, and other primates.[11] The studies are aimed at showing that some animals can engage in "mental time travel," that is, they can go back to a past event with their minds.

It is probably early days for a verdict on whether there are any animals with episodic memory, and comparative psychologists still debate the issue. Whether animals have a sense of their own future seems to be even more difficult to establish. Reiss has claimed that the bottlenose dolphin exhibits "anticipatory behavior, an awareness of the contingencies of their past actions, and an awareness of the contingencies of future acts."[12] Evidence for these cognitive achievements emerged in the context of "bubble ring" play in pools by captive dolphins.

Even the scientists advancing new hypotheses on episodic memory in great apes and a sense of the future in bottlenose dolphins and those who have argued for years in favor of animal consciousness are cautious in drawing conclusions about animal *self*-consciousness.[13] And those philosophers who are happy to ascribe intentional states to animals on the basis of their manifest behavior are not at all sure that it makes sense to talk about animal consciousness as if each animal were the unified subject of different experiences.[14]

For these reasons, the addition of memory and a sense of one's own future to the list of those cognitive capacities that characterize subjects of a life is strategically surprising. Regan is not going to be able to achieve the dialectical goal of expanding the class of rights holders to include human non-persons and mammalian animals by requiring that subjects of a life have a memory of their past experiences and a sense of their own future. In the literature on moral status, awareness of one's own past and future has always been regarded as a mark of personhood.[15]

Subjects of a life are not persons because they do not need to be able to engage in rational deliberation and because they are not expected to exhibit moral agency. But self-consciousness and rational deliberation, two capacities that are conceptually distinct, might not be found independently of one another. One speculative but plausible idea is that part of what it is to have a notion of oneself as a unique individual is to feel on oneself the normative force of standards of rationality for thought or action. Some argue that in young children self-consciousness emerges approximately when they start using self-referring concepts of shame that might be seen as signs of incipient moral agency.[16]

4. Subjects of a Life or Intentional Agents?

Regan's contribution to the debate is significant no matter how we conceive our obligations to non-human animals and human non-persons. He aims at justifying the common intuition that we have direct moral obligations to non-persons. And he seems to be right in claiming that sentience alone is not quite enough for the possession of those preference autonomy and preference interests which are a prerequisite for the entitlement to basic rights or direct moral consideration. Regan's approach is promising, but the notion of "subjects of a life" does not seem to be what he needs to achieve the goal of providing a justification for according basic rights or moral status to non-persons.

As we saw in the first section, the possession of preference interests and the capacity for initiating action are plausible prerequisites for having basic rights or moral status. In reformulating the criterion, we should focus on the cognitive capacities required for the possession of interests, such as the possession of beliefs, desires, emotional states, and preferences, and the capacity to initiate action on the basis of those intentional states. All that would be necessary to revise Regan's position is a shift from subjects of a life to intentional agents.

What is an intentional agent? An intentional agent is any system whose behavior we can predict via the ascription of beliefs, desires, and other intentional states. An intentional agent typically acts on the basis of its beliefs and desires and can adapt to its environment by revising such beliefs and desires. In the literature on intentionality many authors (for example Donald Davidson, Daniel Dennett, and Jane Heal) assume that intentional agents need to be, to some extent, rational deliberators. If that were the case, my appeal to intentional agents would not fare much better than Regan's notion of "subject-of-a-life." It would be almost indistinguishable from personhood.

But intentionality and rationality are not necessarily linked. The only sense in which an intentional agent needs to be rational is the sense in which at least some of its actions can be *rationalized*, that is, they can be seen as done for a reason. Suppose I saw a big black dog barking furiously on the pavement on my way to work this morning and I crossed the road to avoid him. Why did I cross the road? Not randomly, nor as a consequence of a spasm. I crossed the road because by doing so I was hoping to avoid the dog I was afraid of. My intention to avoid the dog was the reason for my action and my action can be rationalized by my intention. That does not mean that crossing the road was *the rational thing to do*, or that my thoughts and actions need to satisfy any standards of rationality before I can be regarded as an intentional agent.[17]

Whereas persons need to be sensitive to the normative force of standards of rationality, and on occasion respond to them, intentional agents do not. Whereas persons need to be able to have beliefs and desires about themselves as individuals, in order to deliberate morally and to assess blame, praise, and responsibility, intentional agents do not need to have a sense of themselves. They just need to have basic beliefs about their surrounding environment and to respond to the stimuli they are subject to with a view to satisfying their desires given their beliefs. Some intentional agents will also be persons, others will not. And that is why the introduction of the intentional-agent criterion seems to be perfectly suitable for the inclusion of some non-human animals and marginal humans in the class of rights holders. Those individuals that have intentional states such as beliefs and desires and have the capacity to act on their beliefs and desires, have also preference interests which contribute to their own welfare. By according to them basic rights or moral status we safeguard their morally relevant interests.

Let me consider another objection to the adoption of the intentional-agent criterion. Some philosophers talk about the intentional stance in purely instrumental terms. The idea is that any system (plants and simple artifacts included) whose behavior we could predict by using belief-and-desire talk is an intentional agent for the purposes of the prediction of its behavior, even if the system probably does not have any intentional states. In other words, the intentional stance would be just a matter of speech.[18] For instance, I could talk about my plant *wanting* water without really believing that my plant has any desires. If the intentional stance is used in this instrumental way, then the risk of adopting the intentional-agent criterion is that legitimate rights holders might multiply.

But the intentional stance is successful and really useful as a predictive strategy only when the behavior of the system we want to predict is complex enough to support the ascription of beliefs and desires. In the field of cognitive ethology and comparative psychology there have been fascinating attempts to devise tests to discriminate between situations in which a non-human animal acts on a belief with a determinate content and situations in which the ascription of the belief to that animal is unjustified. The difficulty in establishing what content to ascribe to the intentional states of a non-human, an infant, or a human adult affected by dementia, can be explained by reference to how mind-reading works. We are generally good at ascribing beliefs and desires to other humans very much like ourselves because our mind-reading capacities depend on context-dependent heuristics. These heuristics are simple strategies, usually fast and accurate, that humans use to get by in a complex environment. For instance, we would not ascribe highly theoretical thoughts to young children, because we do not expect them to have a wide range of conceptually sophisticated background beliefs. The better we know the circumstances in which agents operate, the better we can read their minds. The fact that we encounter difficulties in ascribing intentional states with a determinate content to non-persons might be due to our limitations as interpreters and not to their inability to form intentional states. Our struggles do not rule out that non-persons can exhibit a behavior of the right complexity to justify the ascription of some intentional states. Where our natural talents as mind-readers fail, science can help. A more careful observation of the behavioral responses of non-human animals in some contexts can contribute to refining our attempt to ascribe preferences to them.

5. Conclusion

In this chapter I have discussed the question whether non-persons should be accorded basic rights or moral status. After assessing Regan's subject-of-a-life criterion and finding it wanting, I have suggested that we use a simpler and more adequate criterion, the intentional-agent criterion. Intentional agents do not need sophisticated cognitive capacities over and beyond the possession of intentional states and the capacity to initiate action, which are the basic requirements for preference autonomy and preference interests.

NOTES

1. Lisa Bortolotti and John Harris, "Stem Cell Research, Personhood, and Sentience," *Reproductive Biomedicine Online, Special Issue: Ethics, Science and Moral Philosophy of Assisted Human Reproduction*, 10 (2005), suppl. 1, pp. 68–74; Jon Wetlesen, "The Moral Status of Beings Who Are not Persons: A Casuistic Argument," *Environmental Values*, 8:3 (August 1999), pp. 287–323.

2. Tom Regan, *The Case for Animal Rights* (Berkeley: University of California Press, 1983); Tom Regan, "Ill-Gotten Gains," *The Great Ape Project*, eds. Paola Cavalieri and Peter Singer (New York: St. Martin's Griffin, 1993), pp. 194–205.

3. Regan, *The Case for Animal Rights*, p. 243.

4. *Ibid.*, p. 87.

5. Joel Feinberg, "The Rights of Animals and Unborn Generations," *Philosophy and Environmental Crisis*, ed. William T. Blackstone (Athens, GA: University of Georgia Press, 1974).

6. Raymond Frey, *Interests and Rights: The Case against Animals* (Oxford: Clarendon Press, 1980).

7. Regan, *The Case for Animal Rights*, ch. 2.

8. Daniel Povinelli, *Folk Physics for Apes. The Chimpanzee's Theory of How the World Works* (Oxford: Oxford University Press, 2000).

9. Endel Tulving, *Elements of Episodic Memory* (Oxford: Clarendon Press, 1983).

10. Dan Griffiths, Anthony Dickinson, and Nicola Clayton, "Declarative and Episodic Memory: What Can Animals Remember about Their Past?" *Trends in Cognitive Science*, 3:2 (1 February 1999), pp. 74–80.

11. Bennett Schwartz and Siân Evans, "Episodic Memory in Primates," *American Journal of Primatology*, 55:2 (6 September 2001), pp. 71–85.

12. Diana Reiss, "Cognition and Communication in Dolphins: A Question of Consciousness," *Toward a Science of Consciousness II: The Second Tucson Discussions and Debates*, eds. Stuart. R. Hameroff, Alfred W. Kaszniak, and Alwyn C. Scott (Cambridge, MA: MIT Press, 1998), pp. 551–560, at p. 557.

13. Donald Griffin, *Animal Minds: Beyond Cognition to Consciousness* (Chicago: University of Chicago Press, 2001).

14. Daniel Dennett, *Kinds of Minds: Towards an Understanding of Consciousness* (New York: Basic Books, 1997).

15. John Locke, *An Essay Concerning Human Understanding* (1689) (London: William Tegg, 1860), ch. XXVII; John Harris, *The Value of Life* (London: Routledge and Kegan Paul, 1985).

16. Jerome Kagan, *The Second Year* (Cambridge, MA: Harvard University Press, 1981).

17. Lisa Bortolotti, "Can We Interpret Irrational Behavior?" *Behavior and Philosophy*, 32:2 (2004), pp. 359–370.

18. E.g. Donald Davidson, "Rational Animals," Donald Davidson, *Subjective, Intersubjective, Objective* (Oxford: Oxford University Press, 2001), pp. 95–106.

Twenty

DETERMINING THE LIMITS OF JUSTIFIED PATERNALISM: IS MAXIMIZING AUTONOMY THE KEY?

Jane Wilson

1. Introduction

In a perceptive and broad-ranging paper entitled "Paternalistic Solicitude and Paternalistic Behavior: Appropriate Contexts and Moral Justifications,"[1] Tziporah Kasachkoff criticizes many of the modern, liberal rights-based discussions of paternalism, which, she says, tend not just to dominate the literature on paternalism, but also to obscure analysis of the subject itself.[2] This, she argues, is due to a number of features of these discussions, including their tendency to depict all paternalism narrowly, as coercive or restrictive; to make inferences from legal and political paternalism to paternalism of other kinds, which may not share the same features; to ignore the nature and relationship of the parties involved in paternalistic acts; and to assume that paternalism is necessarily at odds with individual autonomy rights and so morally reprehensible. Kasachkoff sums up her position as follows:

> The nature of paternalism and its putative justifying principles will inevitably remain confused unless discussion concerning these issues (1) ceases to give exclusive attention to cases of paternalism which are coercive and restrictive; (2) stops focusing exclusively on political and legal contexts for the construction of arguments whose conclusions are then applied to other areas; (3) includes some account of the nature and purview of those institutions which figure as parties to the paternalistic activity; and (4) makes it clear what it is about paternalism that demands some moral accounting.[3]

In this chapter, I will consider an analysis of paternalism and its maximization specifically within the medical domain, which, though published six years prior to Kasachkoff's paper, seems at first blush to avoid the problems of narrowness, over-generalization, and obscurity which Kasachkoff finds prevalent in much of the literature. The analysis in question is offered by Mark S. Komrad in his paper, "A Defence of Medical Paternalism: 'Maximizing Patients' Autonomy."[4] My purpose in examining Komrad's analysis will be to consider why, despite its comparative merits, it seems unsatisfactory. I will question Komrad's preferred definition of paternalism, the inference he draws from John Stuart Mill's exception to voluntary slavery contracts in *On Liberty*, and his distinctive theory of illness and medicine. I will structure my essay by drawing upon, though changing the order of, the four issues raised by Kasachkoff (above) and by examining the extent to which Komrad's paper may be interpreted as "responding" successfully to these. I will not subject Kasachkoff's paper itself to critical review, but will simply make the assertion that I am in broad agreement with its substance, hence my use of it here as the starting point and framework for my paper.

2. Broadening the Concept of Paternalism

> It is a mistake to take ... coercive or restrictive cases of paternalism as exhaustive.[5]

In examining the concept of paternalism at the beginning of his paper, Komrad, like Kasachkoff, is critical of the tendency of philosophers to depict all paternalism as necessarily coercive. Indeed, he notes that some commentators perceive in paternalism themes of superiority, domination, oppression, and dogmatism. But Komrad suggests that when characterized in this way, paternalism is more properly called "authoritarianism." He continues, "paternalism is not just coercive behaviour; there is another side to it that connotes the concern, care, and self-sacrifice of the paternalistic agent,"[6] and with this in mind, he opts for what he believes is a more temperate view of paternalism—one which he claims to find in the definition offered by Bernard Gert and Charles M. Culver, and which he cites in full as follows:

> A is acting paternalistically toward S if and only if A's behavior (correctly) indicates that A *believes* that:
>
> (1) his action is for S's good;
> (2) he is qualified to act on S's behalf;
> (3) his action involves violating a moral rule (or will require him to do so) with regard to S;
> (4) S's good justifies him in acting on S's behalf independently of S's past, present, or immediately forthcoming (free, informed) consent; and
> (5) S believes (perhaps falsely) that he (S) generally knows what is for his own good.[7]

Komrad commends this definition as "compelling," since he says that rather than assume that paternalism necessarily violates liberty of action, it makes the more general claim that paternalism violates "moral rules," only a small subset of which are concerned with liberty. The rest are concerned with such things as deception, causing pain, and cheating. Komrad is further impressed by the definition's emphasis on what he describes as the "purely fiduciary motives" inherent in paternalism. And he describes as "crucial" and "unique" condition (4), which indicates that an act is only paternalistic if the paternalistic agent, A, believes that he is acting independently of the subject S's past, present, or immediately forthcoming consent.

However, Gert and Culver's definition of paternalism is not without problems, and Komrad's relatively uncritical adoption of it suggests that he is unaware of its potential implications for the coherence of his position. For instance, their definition is underpinned by Gert's moral system: a system which treats as primary the imperative of obeying "moral rules" prohibiting actions which cause harm to others, but as only secondary (even optional) the pursuit of "moral ideals" encouraging actions which prevent harm.[8] Gert claims that this system constitutes an explication of our (near) universal common moral reasoning. But, as Dan Brock notes, on most people's moral views there is a moral requirement *actively to prevent* serious injury or loss of life to another, particularly when we can do so at little or no cost to ourselves.[9] Without this requirement, Gert's system therefore seems incomplete, a factor which in turn seems to undermine his claim of its (near) universality. Komrad does not express explicit endorsement of Gert's moral system. Indeed, he later dismisses Gert and Culver's method for establishing the justification of paternalism, based on what they believe all rational persons would do, describing it as "a presumptuous generalisation of their own morality as a canon of validity."[10] But since this method of justification is integral to Gert's system of morality, and since Gert's system of morality is fundamental to Gert and Culver's analysis of paternalism, it is questionable whether Komrad can subscribe to their definition of paternalism without subscribing to the moral system which underpins it, or, alternatively, providing us with a different account of the "moral rules" (which he does not do). Komrad's position would therefore appear to be without foundations.

Gert and Culver's specification of conditions (3) and (4) as necessary conditions of paternalism is another difficult feature of their definition of which Komrad seems unaware, since it entails that (according to them) all paternalistic acts are characterized by the violation of a "moral rule" *and* by absence of the subject's consent. The implication of this is that, on their definition, all paternalism is morally suspect on two counts: first, on the basis of Gert's moral system and, second, on the basis of the subject's right to determine her own good without interference. But it is by no means certain that Komrad is committed to this position, since he later summarizes paternalism simply as acting in another's interest in the absence of his or her immediate consent, and he makes little further mention of the role of "moral rules" in his paper. It is therefore tempting to conclude that Komrad is superficially impressed by Gert and Culver's definition of paternalism, since it appears to succeed in broadening the concept beyond that of the purely coercive, but that, as before, he remains oblivious to the implications of the means by which they attempt to achieve this: Gert's "moral rules." Certainly, it is the subject's lack of consent (rather than the paternalist's violation of "moral rules") which Komrad seems to imply is the area of potential moral concern in paternalism. This is a move that points to the subject's autonomy as key, and which take us into the general area of individual rights.

3. Paternalism and Autonomy—Are They Naturally at Odds?

> The typical explanation for paternalism's bad moral reputation is that paternalistic acts constitute a problem in the general area of rights because they (apparently) violate a subject's right to non-interference. But this claim merely begs the question.[11]

In addition to criticizing authors of the dominant liberal analyses of paternalism for their propensity to portray paternalism as coercive or restrictive of liberty, Kasachkoff also criticizes them for their associated assumption that the right to non-interference and paternalism are naturally at odds. Kasachkoff attributes this to their tendency to deal summarily with the right to non-interference, by reference to some principle of individual liberty or autonomy (derived from Mill),[12] or respect for persons (derived from Immanuel Kant),[13] and then to conclude that all paternalism must compromise this right. But, she protests, interfering with another for the sake of her welfare is surely not treating her as a means to some end other than herself, nor is it necessarily a violation of her rights. So she concludes that such approaches leave unanswered various questions that she would like to see addressed, such as "Why is 'going against' a person's own desires morally objectionable?"; "Do all forms of dependence on others compromise autonomy?"; and "Are all compromises of autonomy morally reprehensible?"[14]

Komrad does not, at first, appear to make much progress in responding to issues such as these in his paper. On the contrary, he too derives a general notion of a principle of autonomy from Kant and Mill as both a self-determined organization of the will and a right to pursue one's self-regarding choice of action (in so far as this does not harm others). And, while he notes that this principle does not confer on us all an absolute right to have our autonomy respected, since autonomy is something that admits of degrees, he seems to imply that mature individuals with sufficient capacity *do* have a right to have their choices respected. When this is combined with his view that (by definition) all paternalism is performed without the subject's consent, it suggests that Komrad also holds that all paternalism conflicts with the right to autonomy, since failure to obtain the subject's consent may be construed as failure to respect her autonomous choice. Thus Komrad's approach seems to typify those liberal analyses of paternalism of which Kasachkoff is critical. However, rather than conclude that all paternalism is therefore morally wrong on autonomy-violating grounds, Komrad goes on to flesh out his account of autonomy further, noting that Kant holds that we are compelled to be autonomous, since autonomy is the basis of all other moral behavior;[15] and that Mill holds that we are obligated to fulfill our potential for autonomy, since "the principle of freedom cannot require that [a person] should be free not to be free."[16]

Now it should be noted here that Mill makes this last remark in *On Liberty*, when condemning the practice of voluntary slavery contracts; and it marks a significant exception to his defense of liberty, since it provides the basis for his claim that it is *permissible* to interfere paternalistically with an individual in order to prevent him from irreversibly sacrificing his duty (and hence capacity) to exercise his liberty in the future. On closer analysis, therefore, Mill's broad defense of the principle of liberty seems to give priority to what Isaiah Berlin terms "positive liberty" (construed as the exercise of one's capacity for liberty, or autonomy) over "negative liberty" (construed as the right to non-interference by others),[17] and so to authorize acts of paternalism, if they are performed with a view to preserving, or even enforcing, the former. Mill's reasoning seems particularly influential on Komrad's thinking, since Komrad proceeds to modify his position to claim that autonomy is not so much a *right* to be respected as it is a *duty* to pursue, according to one's capabilities, and that, as such, it should be preserved at all costs. So Komrad concludes, like Mill, that sometimes it may be morally justified to go against a person's current desires (and so fail to respect his right to non-interference) in order to promote his capacity to exercise his autonomy in future. This, then, seems to constitute the making of a possible response to some of the questions posed by Kasachkoff, since it implies that in certain circumstances paternalistically motivated interferences in autonomy are indeed morally permissible.

4. State Paternalism Versus Medical Paternalism

> What Mill says concerning the state and the use he makes of what he says in his arguments against paternalism *by the state* cannot be transferred, without qualification, to other areas of possible paternalistic action.[18]

Despite appearing to respond to certain of Kasachkoff's questions, however, Komrad's account seems vulnerable to some of her charges. For instance, it reduces the moral debate on paternalism to just two main protagonists: autonomy and paternalism; it deals summarily with the issue of what autonomy consists in; and it shows a tendency to use what Mill says in *On Liberty* concerning paternalism by the State (in which particularized knowledge of individuals is not possible), in order to apply it elsewhere. But whereas many liberal critics adopt Mill's conclusions about the importance of the principle of autonomy and the presumed injustice of State paternalism in order to argue *against* paternalism in both this and other contexts, Komrad can now be seen to be taking a very different approach, by adopting the inference to be drawn from Mill's *exception* to these conclusions, in order to develop an argument *for* paternalism, with a view to applying it to the medical setting.

The implications of this approach begin to become apparent as Komrad develops his analysis of the relationship between paternalism and autonomy further, arguing that, rather than function as an inevitable negation of autonomy rights, paternalism can be seen to serve as an appropriate response to incapacity, so that when autonomy recedes (and with it the individual's capacity to protect her own good), paternalism advances, and *vice versa.* So he maintains that paternalism and autonomy are not so much "contrapositives" as they are "two inversely varying parameters along a spectrum of independence,"[19] both committed to the good of the same person. Komrad then combines this analysis with the inference he draws from Mill's exception to voluntary slavery—that the good of a person, which should be preserved at all costs, is his capacity to exercise his autonomy—as he turns to a consideration of the consequences of this move, within the specific context of medical practice.

5. Medical Practice, Medical Paternalism, and the Maximization of Patients' Autonomy

> Whether or not medical paternalism is in fact justified and if it is, to what extent and on what grounds, must be determined by the correct conception of the moral relation between the parties involved. But this, in turn, is determined by what is judged to be the correct view of medicine itself.... What we need, then, is some *theory* of medicine, i.e., some view as to what we are to see medicine *as*.[20]

Komrad's approach to his discussion of medical paternalism may, in certain respects, seem exemplary of the type of approach Kasachkoff urges critics to adopt. For he begins by noting the knowledge gap that is a recognized feature of the doctor-patient relationship, and the tensions that emerge as a result of societal and legal pressure on doctors to curtail their paternalistic tendencies, when many patients still desire to be treated paternalistically. And, from this, he concludes that "a formula for medical paternalism cannot be dogmatic and unconditional."[21] Reminding us of his earlier finding that paternalism is an appropriate response to take when autonomy is reduced, he then asserts that the most striking examples of lessened autonomy are in cases of illness and disease, such as schizophrenia, stroke, or tuberculosis. He continues:

> In fact, I maintain that *all illness represents a state of diminished autonomy*. The ill are dependent on others such as physicians, if not for their outright therapeutic ministrations then for their expert legitimation of their illness.[22]

The idea that conditions of ill health can serve to diminish individual autonomy is not without precedent, and Komrad cites several thinkers, including Leon Kass and Edmund Pellegrino, who argue that the ontological assault of illness impinges upon our capacity for autonomy in a distinctive way.[23] So, according to such thinkers, it is not just ignorance of our illness that diminishes our autonomy, but it is the presence and nature of the illness itself which renders us vulnerable, even child-like, and so dependent upon the doctor. Nevertheless, Komrad's claim that *all* illness constitutes an attenuation of autonomy—and not just *some*—seems bold and sweeping. And in the light of his preceding argument, it leads him to draw an equally radical conclusion about the legitimate role of the doctor in the therapeutic encounter. His conclusion is that, due to the nature of the sick role and the appropriateness of paternalism as a response to diminished autonomy, some degree of paternalism is not simply justified but is *required* of the doctor in *all* therapeutic relationships. So it is not respect for the patient's autonomy, but respect for the patient's *future potential* for autonomy, by means of paternalistic intervention to *maximize* that potential, that Komrad claims is key. Accordingly, he proposes expanding condition (1) of Gert and Culver's definition of paternalism, to reflect what he describes as "the only type of paternalism that is appropriate to the clinical setting," by adding the following:

> (1a) S's good is *solely* the *maximisation* of his capacity to be autonomous.[24]

I have noted that Komrad seems to develop his defense of justified medical paternalism along lines similar to those recommended by Kasachkoff, by expounding a theory of medical practice and illness, and examining the nature of the therapeutic relationship. Nevertheless, some of the assumptions that he makes and the conclusions to which these lead seem highly questionable. For instance, despite citing other sources, Komrad offers no empirical evidence to support his claim that *all* illness represents a state of diminished autonomy, and he pays no attention to the implications of this claim for our understanding of such things as the purpose and validity of patient consent. But if *all* illness represents a state of diminished autonomy, the capacity of patients to give valid consent to treatment must presumably be placed in doubt. Indeed, if (as Komrad claims) paternalism is deemed the appropriate response to *all* illness and if (by definition) *all* paternalism entails intervention independently of the subject's past, present, or immediately forthcoming consent, the role of patient consent in medical practice would seem to be rendered all but redundant. Komrad might try to reply to this by arguing that medical paternalism is the only appropriate response, for example, in an emergency situation, when an unconscious patient is clearly unable to consent to treatment; and that as the patient recovers her health (and with it her autonomy), the role of paternalism toward her recedes, while that of her consent comes to the fore. Such a response is suggested by some of his claims, and it implies that the type of paternalism that his model supports is what is commonly known as "soft" paternalism, since the autonomous choice of the patient is not apparently being overridden by the paternalistic doctor.

But such a reply does not dissolve all the problems for Komrad's account. For, as we have seen, Komrad holds that the legitimate goal of all paternalism is not to respect the subject's current autonomous state and desires, but to respect her good, construed *solely* as the *maximization* of her potential capacity to be autonomous in the future. So even if a patient were sufficiently autonomous to be able to give her valid consent or refusal to treatment, it seems that her doctor need not respect her decision, if to do so would be counter-productive to maximizing her autonomy. Put differently, if the patient's autonomous choice were for a course of treatment that might not maximize her autonomy—or, perhaps more significantly, for no treatment whatsoever—it seems that, on Komrad's account, her doctor would be morally justified in ignoring her wishes and paternalistically imposing treatment upon her in order to maximize her autonomy (presumably by means of optimizing her recovery from illness). This, then, would constitute what is commonly known as "hard" paternalism, since the paternalistic doctor's intervention would override the patient's autonomous choice. Once again, Komrad might try to reply to this criticism by arguing that if a patient were to refuse treatment to maximize her future autonomy, it would cast doubt upon her current level of competence and so justify paternalism towards her. But this response is not really available to him, by virtue of his own argument. For it might be quite possible to produce evidence of the patient's wishes about her treatment, prior to the time when her autonomy was diminished by illness (for instance, in the form of an advance directive), and there is nothing in Komrad's argument to suggest that these earlier autonomous wishes should be respected, if they do not contain a request by the patient to have her future capacity for autonomy maximized by means of medical treatment.

Yet another problem with Komrad's account is that it makes the implicit assumption that both the (paternalistic) doctor and the patient (presumably when she is "maximally autonomous") share the same view that the sole good of the patient is maximization of her autonomy, and that therefore paternalism directed to this end on the patient's behalf is justified. This is apparent when, having summarized paternalism as "acting in another's interest in the absence of his or her immediate consent," Komrad adds "although with the expectation of eventual consent."[25] But just as Komrad produces no empirical evidence to support his claim that *all* illness represents a diminished state of autonomy, so he produces no evidence to support this implicit claim that *all* patients regard maximization of their autonomy as the primary aim of the therapeutic encounter. Presumably Komrad makes reference to the "eventual consent" of the patient as a means of demonstrating that the patient's right to have her autonomy respected has not been entirely disrespected by the doctor's paternalistic intervention, it being a (mis)conception of critics who employ the concept of "subsequent consent" that such "consent" can serve to authorize paternalism retroactively. However, the inability of this approach to undo the presumed wrong of paternalism on autonomy-respecting grounds is well documented.[26] And given that Komrad has already implied that the affront to autonomy with which paternalism is traditionally charged does not occur in medical paternalism since the patient's autonomy is diminished by her illness, and that he has also stipulated that maximization of autonomy is "the touchstone for evaluating paternalism,"[27] such a strategy seems entirely irrelevant to his account.

A more comprehensive assessment of Komrad's theory of medicine and of the justified limits of medical paternalism is hampered by his failure to provide some much-needed detail. For example, he does not spell out the criteria by which a doctor can know that a patient is not sufficiently autonomous to make decisions about her own care, insisting only that the patient's autonomy is "never maximal as long as [s]he is in the sick role."[28] But, while Komrad confidently concludes that the paternalism that his theory of medicine sanctions is only of a very limited type, the logic of his argument seems to point to a level of paternalism which knows no bounds, other than the goal of "maximizing autonomy"; a concept which he never explains, and which leaves us wondering what the moral benefit in pursuing it might be (or whether it is even coherent). Clearly, Komrad's intention *is* to place some sort of limits on the degree of medical paternalism that can be deemed justified. Indeed, he appears to think that he has succeeded in doing this, when he claims that maximization of the patient's autonomy is "the only legitimate interest of medical paternalism."[29] But in making this assertion, it is only the *goal* of medical paternalism that Komrad succeeds in limiting to a single (supposedly always justified) good. And in taking as his lead the idea that the duty to remain autonomous is paramount, and that the capacity for autonomy is therefore too significant to forego, and combining this with his peculiar definition of ill health, Komrad appears to be issuing a license for unchecked medical paternalism.

6. Discussion

It is apparent from Kasachkoff's criticism of the dominant liberal analyses of paternalism, that she regards their general presumption that all paternalism consists in moral wrongdoing, on the grounds that it violates individual rights, to be both poorly argued and premature. And the implication of her proposal that considerations of the morality of paternalism should be context-specific and based upon a satisfactory theory (for example, of medicine) is that, in certain circumstances and within certain relationships, some paternalistic practices *may* be justified. It is likewise apparent from Komrad's criticism of similar discussions that he too regards their approach to be inadequate as a means of establishing the limits of justified paternalism within the medical setting, and that he therefore intends his context-specific approach to serve as something of a corrective. So, as I stated in my introduction, it seems possible to read Komrad's attempt to determine the limits of justified medical paternalism as a form of "response" to Kasachkoff.

Nevertheless, on closer scrutiny, Komrad's analysis can be exposed as deeply flawed for several reasons, some more significant than others. For instance, as we have seen, his adoption of Gert and Culver's definition of paternalism is a mistaken choice—partly because theirs is a problematic definition, and partly because he does not seem genuinely committed to it. But while this renders aspects of his position difficult to decipher, it does not seem to be completely fatal to Komrad's subsequent argument. A second limitation, which seems to be more serious, is his characterization of the moral debate on paternalism in terms of just two main protagonists: paternalism and autonomy. To be sure, there are some signs that he plans to develop a more subtle and nuanced approach than many. But then Komrad squanders any advantage that such an approach might have offered by endorsing the idea (never satisfactorily defended) that the duty to exercise our autonomy should take priority over the right to non-interference, and that maximization of our capacity to perform this duty is, therefore, morally justified—if necessary—by means of paternalism. This effectively serves to bypass both the need to consider other competing goods that individuals might regard as important, and the need to explore the moral complexities of the relationship that exists between the paternalist and her subject.

Komrad's mistake here seems to be his failure to learn from the problems that Mill encounters when he attempts to apply the principles, defended in his central argument in *On Liberty*, to practical cases. For having championed the individual's right to non-interference in matters concerning only himself, Mill then seems to realize that there are some self-regarding autonomous choices, such as the choice of contracting oneself into slavery, which cannot be respected due to their irrevocable consequences; and that a policy which disallows all paternalism but paternalism toward those whose autonomy is impaired is, therefore, inherently problematic. So, it seems to me that Mill's exception to voluntary slavery marks a significant modification in his original position, since it seems to constitute an acknowledgment (albeit understated) that the right to non-interference has exceptions, and that the question of the moral limits of paternalism cannot be determined without a consideration of these. Had Komrad understood this, and drawn from it the conclusion that the approach he needed to take was a more comprehensive and balanced one, his account might have been all the better for it. Instead, however, he infers from Mill's exception that the duty to be autonomous is the primary good that we should pursue (outweighing the right to non-interference), and he runs with this idea exclusively, thereby heading down a path which is as unidirectional as that of the outright anti-paternalist who defends as absolute the right to non-interference.

When Komrad turns to the business of determining the limits of justified paternalism within the medical setting, he begins by attempting to develop a theory of illness and medicine. But he does so by means of the same reductive approach that he applies to his initial consideration of paternalism and in terms of the same two concepts: paternalism and autonomy. He also brings with him the inference he has drawn about the priority of the duty to exercise our capacity to be autonomous. Accordingly, he maintains that *all* illness represents a state of diminished capacity for autonomy, and that the purpose of *all* medical intervention (implicitly agreed upon by both the doctor and, eventually, the patient) is maximization of that capacity by means of paternalism. This analysis has the one apparent advantage of avoiding the criticism of many liberal anti-paternalists, since it appears to ensure that medical paternalism does not override the patient's occurrent autonomous choice, thereby guaranteeing that such paternalism is always "soft." Nevertheless, this advantage is bought at the price of an absolutist and improbable definition of health and an assumption that paternalism is always morally permissible if its purpose is to maximize autonomy. Thus, Komrad succeeds in producing a formula for medical paternalism which, contrary to his own professed intentions, is both "dogmatic and unconditional."

Komrad does not acknowledge any inadequacies in this reductive analysis of the justified limits of paternalism, since he does not attempt to consider possible problem cases for his theory. Concerns which spring to mind, other than those already mentioned include: "What would be the moral ground for paternalistic medical intervention when a patient's future capacity for autonomy is ruled out (for instance, as a consequence of severe brain damage)?"; "What would be deemed a morally appropriate response by a doctor to an autonomous, *well* individual who wanted to donate an organ to a sick relative, for altruistic reasons, given that in so doing she might be placing her future health and consequently (according to Komrad) her future capacity for autonomy in jeopardy?"; and "Why should a patient eventually accept maximization of her potential for autonomy as the morally legitimate grounds for paternalism by her doctor (for instance, by means of continued aggressive therapy), when her experiential knowledge of her illness and treatment side-effects far exceeds that of her doctor, and she now knows that she no longer wants further treatment?" Such questions are difficult to answer with reference to Komrad's account. However, they serve to suggest that there is far more to be considered by both parties in the therapeutic encounter than just the maximization of the patient's capacity to be autonomous, and that if a means-ends approach is the morally desirable method for proceeding, then effort should be made to incorporate these.

7. Conclusion

I have chosen to read Komrad's defense of medical paternalism anachronistically, against the backdrop of Kasachkoff's critique of the liberal rights-based approaches to paternalism which dominate the literature. In so doing, I have attempted to consider where Komrad's analysis succeeds in avoiding the shortcomings of this approach and where it fails. Komrad's mistakes have been seen to differ in detail, but they remain somewhat similar in kind. So it is worthwhile returning one last time to Kasachkoff's paper, in an effort to trace the possible source of Komrad's problem.

Kasachkoff notes in her conclusion that there is a tendency among critics to use what Joel Feinberg calls "our elementary intuitions"[30] to ground attempts to justify paternalism. But, as Kasachkoff observes, "this implies more agreement concerning putative cases of paternalism and their justifying principles than is indicated by either the professional literature or public discussion."[31] Moreover, it suggests that our intuitions are more consistent with one another than they probably are. Kasachkoff concludes that since our intuitions depend upon our prior views about the nature, aims, and proper province of such things as the State and medicine, they are not elementary in the required sense. So they are wrongly placed at the beginning rather than the end of the ethical debate. This suggests a possible diagnosis of Komrad's problem, for it is tempting to speculate that in writing his paper, Komrad takes as his starting point the intuition that some degree of medical paternalism *must* be justified. After all, as he indicates, patients sometimes seem to want it and doctors sometimes seem to want to use it. And from this starting point, he proceeds to develop a defense of the principle of autonomy and a theory of medical practice which, when combined, seem guaranteed to demonstrate that his intuition is correct. However, both these aspects of his argument are seriously flawed by the absolutism with which he charges them as a means of securing the conclusion he aims to reach. Thus, as Kasachkoff argues, and this chapter hopefully illustrates, it is necessary to attempt to provide an account of the nature of the particular context in which paternalism occurs and the moral relationships that pertain in that given context, which best captures our understanding of both; to determine precisely what it is about paternalism that stands in need of moral justification (if anything); and, I would add, to incorporate the lessons learned from the mistaken approaches of others, in order to reach a more satisfactory understanding of when paternalism is justified and when it is not. A more reductive approach would, of course, be much simpler to achieve, but as we have seen from this discussion, it would most likely fail to deliver.

NOTES

1. Tziporah Kasachkoff, "Paternalistic Solicitude and Paternalistic Behavior: Appropriate Contexts and Moral Justifications," *Freedom, Equality and Social Change*, eds. Creighton Peden and James P. Sterba (Lewiston: The Edwin Mellen Press, 1994), pp. 79–91.

2. See, e.g., Joel Feinberg, "Legal Paternalism," *Canadian Journal of Philosophy*, 1:1 (1971), pp. 105–124; Gerald Dworkin, "Paternalism," *The Monist*, 56:1 (1972), pp. 64–68; Rosemary Carter, "Justifying Paternalism," *Canadian Journal of Philosophy*, 7:1 (1977), pp. 133–145.

3. Kasachkoff, "Paternalistic Solicitude and Paternalistic Behavior," p. 88.

4. Mark S. Komrad, "A Defence of Medical Paternalism: Maximising Patients' Autonomy," *Journal of Medical Ethics*, 9 (1983), pp. 38–44.

5. Kasachkoff, "Paternalistic Solicitude and Paternalistic Behavior," p. 80.

6. Komrad, "A Defence of Medical Paternalism," p. 39.

7. Bernard Gert and Charles M. Culver, "The Justification of Paternalism," *Medical Responsibility*, eds. Wade Robinson and Michael Pritchard (New Jersey: Human Press, 1979), cited in Komrad, "A Defence of Medical Paternalism," p. 39.

8. See Bernard Gert, *The Moral Rules: A New Rational Foundation for Morality* (New York: Harper and Row, 1970).

9. Dan W. Brock, "Book Review: Bioethics: A Return to Fundamentals, by Gert, B.; Culver, C. M.; and Clouser, K. D.," *Ethics*, 110:3 (April 2000), pp. 614–617.

10. Komrad, "A Defence of Medical Paternalism," p. 43.

11. Kasachkoff, "Paternalistic Solicitude and Paternalistic Behavior," p. 85.

12. John Stuart Mill, *Utilitarianism, On Liberty, and Essay on Bentham*, ed. Mary Warnock (New York: World Publishing, 1962).

13. Immanuel Kant, *Groundwork of the Metaphysics of Morals* (New York: Harper and Row, 1958).

14. Kasachkoff, "Paternalistic Solicitude and Paternalistic Behavior," pp. 85–86.

15. Komrad, "A Defence of Medical Paternalism," p. 38.

16. Mill, *On Liberty*, p. 236, cited in Komrad, "A Defence of Medical Paternalism," p. 39.

17. Isaiah Berlin, "Two Concepts of Liberty," *Four Essays on Liberty* (Oxford: Oxford University Press, 1969).

18. Kasachkoff, "Paternalistic Solicitude and Paternalistic Behavior," p. 82.

19. Komrad, "A Defence of Medical Paternalism," p. 39.

20. Kasachkoff, "Paternalistic Solicitude and Paternalistic Behavior," pp. 83–84.

21. Komrad, "A Defence of Medical Paternalism," p. 41.

22. *Ibid.*

23. Leon Kass, "Professing Ethically: On the Place of Ethics in Defining Medicine," *The Humanities and the Profession of Medicine*, ed. Allen R. Dyer (Durham, N. C.: The National Humanities Center, 1982); Edmund Pellegrino, "Toward a Reconstruction of Medical Morality: The Primacy of the Act of Profession and the Fact of Illness," *Journal of Medicine and Philosophy*, 4 (1979), pp. 32–56.

24. Komrad, "A Defence of Medical Paternalism," p. 42, emphasis mine.

25. *Ibid.*, p. 43.

26. See, e.g., Donald VanDeVeer, *Paternalistic Intervention: The Moral Bounds of Benevolence* (Princeton, N. J.: Princeton University Press, 1986), pp. 66–70.

27. Komrad, "A Defence of Medical Paternalism," p. 42.

28. *Ibid.*

29. *Ibid.*, p. 43.

30. Joel Feinberg, "Legal Paternalism," p. 106, cited in Kasachkoff, "Paternalistic Solicitude," p. 88.

31. Kasachkoff, "Paternalistic Solicitude and Paternalistic Behavior," p. 88.

Twenty-One

THE WHO OR WHAT OF STEVE: SEVERE INTELLECTUAL IMPAIRMENT AND ITS IMPLICATIONS

Simo Vehmas

1. Introduction

People with intellectual impairments are often regarded as inherently different from the rest of us. Some would perhaps even conclude that they belong to a fundamentally different species—people with severe intellectual impairments do not share with others the essential components of humanity.[1] From the viewpoint of disability studies, these kinds of views are repugnant: *all* disabled people merit full moral and social status despite their physical or mental characteristics. However, disability theory has been constructed by and on the terms of people who are intellectually competent. I argue in this chapter that the materialist and social constructionist accounts in disability studies fail to consider properly people with (severe) intellectual impairments. Conceptualizations of disability as social oppression and as social construct have little explanatory power in relation to the disabled minority whose intellectual competence is minimal.

I will therefore demonstrate some serious weaknesses in social approaches to disability. In addition, I will address the significance and meaning of ethical theories of personhood in the case of individuals with severe intellectual impairments. I will conclude that the marginality of people with intellectual impairments is not only apparent among lay people, but also in some academic disciplines, namely moral philosophy and disability studies.

I will examine four questions. (1) Are individuals with severe intellectual impairments persons? This question arises from the several philosophical accounts in which personhood is presented as the basis of people's moral status. (2) Are individuals with severe intellectual impairments burdens to other people? It hardly surprises anyone that individuals who have limited intellectual capacities are often seen as emotional and financial burdens to other people, and to society in general. (3) Are individuals with severe intellectual impairments members of an oppressed group? According to the materialist account of disability (that is, the British social model of disability), disability is a matter of oppression and should be conceptualized and defined in terms, and as a form, of social oppression. The social model has virtually been produced by people with physical impairments, and on their terms.[2] This being the case, the obvious question is, how does the social model apply to people with intellectual impairments? (4) Are severe intellectual impairments, and the resulting disabilities (that is, functional limitations), socially constructed? Several accounts in disability studies suggest that disability, whether related to physical or mental impairments, is on the whole the result of culturally formed ideas, values, representations, and social arrangements. The social world and its different phenomena, including disability, have been produced in social and cultural interaction—they are socially constructed. Because disability is always determined by cultural and historical context, it is also possible to deconstruct or reconstruct the prevailing views and practices that sustain disability.

In order to clarify the practical implications of different theoretical accounts, I will examine the questions listed above in the light of the case of a ten-year-old boy with a severe intellectual impairment. I have named this boy "Steve." I met him a few years ago, and I will briefly describe my recollections of him.

Several terms are used in the research literature to describe people like Steve: people with intellectual disability, mental retardation, and learning difficulty, to name a few. However, I use the term "people or individuals with severe intellectual impairments." I prefer to use a term that identifies people with biomedically defined conditions, without making any assumptions about the causes of their limitations, well-being, or fair treatment.[3] I will consciously *not* use the term used in the United Kingdom, "people with learning difficulties," simply because it is completely inappropriate in the case of individuals like Steve; his difficulties are not related to learning, willingness to learn, or social barriers to learning. His limitations are inherently all-inclusive and it is questionable whether he will ever be able to learn anything at all. As for people with impairments in general, I use the term "disabled people," which in the UK is identified with the social model of disability. I do find many basic tenets of the material and social constructionist accounts in disability studies sound, but do not commit myself at this point to any of these positions as such.

2. Steve

A few years ago, I visited a school for children with intellectual impairments. I spent a day in a class with some five children who had severe intellectual impairments. My attention was caught by a ten-year-old boy sitting in a wheelchair, Steve. He was completely motionless; he did not move his legs, hands, or fingers, nor did he seem to express anything with his face. His eyes were open but he did not seem to look at anything. His mouth was open, constantly in the same position. He did not seem to respond to anything or to anyone, no matter what was done. In other words, Steve seemed totally vacant—there seemed to be nobody there.

I was told that Steve had been an ordinary healthy boy until the age of five when he fell in water and nearly drowned. He was saved and resuscitated, but sustained severe brain damage. I looked at Steve and thought how tragic his fate had been. He did not seem to suffer, but on the other hand, he did not seem to enjoy his existence either. Frankly, from my viewpoint, there did not seem to be anything going on in his mind or in his life.

After a few hours Steve was put into a piece of apparatus that looked like a large bed filled with soft plastic balls. His teacher said that Steve enjoyed lying in it and having a massage. I remember questioning in my mind the teacher's evaluation; how could she know whether Steve enjoyed it, how could she say anything at all about that boy's pleasures or sufferings, given that he did not communicate in any way with anyone? However, when he was placed in the ball bed, as it were, and when his teacher started to massage his chest and belly gently, his expression changed. Steve's face was not expressionless any more, he was smiling. And after a while, he started uttering sounds which, to me, sounded like sounds of enjoyment.

In other words, there seemed to exist a meaningful interaction between Steve and his teacher after all. It was, undoubtedly, a rudimentary interaction, but it was interaction all the same; he was able to signal at least some interests or preferences to which the teacher responded.

As I mentioned earlier, in considering the way in which ethical theories of personhood determine people's moral status and the way materialist and social constructionist accounts in disability studies define disability, a few questions come to mind when one thinks of individuals such as Steve. First, is Steve a person? Second, is Steve a burden to other people? Third, is Steve a member of an oppressed group? And fourth, is Steve's disability in any way a social construct?

To provide plausible and sound answers to these questions is an intellectually and emotionally demanding task. Some people may find merely presenting and probing such questions offensive. However, these questions have great practical relevance and they reflect, I think, a common view of people with severe intellectual impairments. Only a few would say in public that people like Steve are not persons in any relevant sense, since usually people do not even dare to raise that question (unless they are philosophers). Some questions are too painful to be asked. So, often we prefer to ignore them. But we should examine these kinds of questions simply because there are situations, for example some life and death decisions, where they inevitably arise. In these situations it is better that we rely on well-thought-out notions, however imperfect they may be, than on mere gut feelings.

Intellectual impairment is also an important condition because it challenges some basic sociological and political notions in disability studies. For example, people with intellectual impairments have virtually been ignored by the British social model of disability.[4] I think it is important, however, to pay more attention to this particular impairment in order to strengthen the theoretical and practical credibility of disability studies.

3. Is Steve a Person?

In everyday usage, "person" is usually just another term for human being, and is supposed to distinguish us from inanimate objects, machines, plants, animals, and spirits. Philosophers tend to emphasize mental traits such as consciousness and rationality as the most relevant criteria in the definition of personhood. But to most people these traits are not as important as bodily shape for identifying persons. Many animals (like dolphins, chimpanzees, pigs, and dogs) are more intelligent and self-aware than human infants or human adults with severe intellectual impairments. Nonetheless, animals, however intelligent they may be, are not considered to be persons while these humans are.[5]

Personhood is usually connected to the moral realm, with the expression "person" being taken to connote a specific moral status. A person in a moral sense is a being whose interests must be respected. When we consider what is morally acceptable or preferable, we are morally obliged to take into account what will dignify or demean, benefit or harm, satisfy or dissatisfy, and so on, any being that is a person and that is likely to be affected by our actions. In other words, a person is a being with moral rights. Moral personhood has different levels, in the sense that some beings are more persons than others. For example, we usually think that children have rights to life, against abuse, and so on, although they are denied rights to property and marriage, and to vote. Some of their rights, such as autonomy, may be less fully respected than the corresponding rights of adults. So in a moral sense, children are not full persons in comparison with adults.[6]

In philosophy (and theology), there are competing views about personhood. However, most accounts regard mental competence as a necessary condition of personhood—persons are the kind of (intersubjective) beings that are conscious of the world, think about it, and seek to understand it.[7] John Locke has set a paradigm for Western philosophy in the pursuit of understanding and theorizing the concept of person. According to Locke, a person is "a thinking intelligent Being, that has reason and reflection, and can consider it self as it self, the same thinking thing in different times and places."[8] Therefore, a person is a self-conscious mental being.

One of the most well-known contemporary practical applications of the Lockean concept of personhood is carried out by Michael Tooley, who argues that only beings who are able to value their own existence have a serious right to life.[9] Beings that are not able to value their own existence cannot be wronged by killing them, for their death deprives them of nothing they can value. In practice this means, for example, that abortion is in itself morally justified. In order to be able to value one's life, a being must be self-conscious, it must be aware that it has a life to value: "An organism possesses a serious right to life only if it possesses the concept of a self as a continuing subject of experiences and other mental states, and believes that it is itself such a continuing entity."[10]

Is Steve capable of valuing his life? If our answer to this question is founded on the Lockean conception of personhood and Tooley's application of it, the answer would probably be negative, as it would be in the case of some small children, old people, and people with different mental impairments. The answer would be different if we asked instead: Would death be an evil that *deprived* Steve of being alive, that is, of doing certain things or having certain experiences?[11] Steve is not capable of doing much of anything, but he is capable of having pleasurable experiences. And since he does not seem to suffer, death would indeed deprive him of the good things with which being alive provides him.

If personhood is the basis for people's moral status, we face an extremely difficult issue of defining the contents and limits of the mental faculties necessary for personhood. Furthermore, determining in practice who actually counts as a person is a complicated empirical issue. So perhaps it is better to base morality on some principles additional to personhood. This does not mean that the concept of personhood is totally useless and meaningless; it may well have a useful place in moral theory. But it probably should not be *the* cornerstone of our moral system and people's moral standing.[12] This being the case, to admit that some being is probably not a person (as the concept is defined in philosophy) does not mean that moral beings surrounding that being should not respect that being's interests and well-being. Our moral duties toward other beings are not determined merely on the basis of the rights of those beings.[13] For example, even though the majority of the Western population probably thinks that animals do not have moral rights, they think, at the same time, that this fact does not give us permission to be cruel to animals. Even more clearly, this certainly applies to Steve.

Thus, my tentative answer to the question "Is Steve a person?" is that perhaps he is not. However, that does not mean that we should not respect his interests and well-being as a significant other. The most crucial moral issue in this kind of case is not necessarily Steve's personhood but the moral conduct and character of people surrounding him.

4. Is Steve a Burden?

It appears that the present cultural atmosphere in Western capitalist societies is bipartite and contradictory regarding the issue of individuals such as Steve being a burden. Officially, labeling people like Steve as economic burdens is politically incorrect and inhumane discourse. On the other hand, dislike of or inconvenience associated with economically unproductive people is deep-rooted in Western culture.[14] Once again, I think it is better to acknowledge the existence of the problem and examine it than to ignore it and just hope that things will turn out for the best.

As for the issue of children with intellectual impairments being a burden to their families, the basic finding of numerous empirical studies is that the experiences of the families of children with intellectual impairments are more similar to than they are different from the experiences of families with children without impairments. Families of children with impairments do not necessarily experience any more difficulties than families with "normal" children—their problems are just different.[15] Also, social and cultural factors often contribute more to the well-being or ill-being of families than the child's impairment in itself. Families that receive support from their communities are, despite the child's impairment, likely to cope better than families that are emotionally and financially on their own. In addition, the beliefs, attitudes, and values of parents regarding disability and raising children in general have a great effect on the way in which having a child with an intellectual impairment affects their well-being.[16]

Despite the fact that these remarks are probably true, we cannot and should not deny the painful reality of parents and families of children like Steve. Parents have a good reason to mourn when their child loses his or her major faculties due to an accident. In a way, in this case the parents lost their child since Steve has been a completely different individual since the accident. Some philosophers would probably even claim that Steve ceased to exist as a person. In other words, Steve's fate must be a source of great emotional tribulation and burden to his parents.

From the parents' viewpoint, there are also exhausting practical concerns; Steve demands care 24 hours a day—he is not capable of doing anything by himself. We can hardly accuse his parents of irresponsible or bad parenting over the fact that they decided to place Steve for the most of the time into an institution. Such decisions are not easy for parents and living apart from their child can be emotionally exceptionally consuming. This does not mean that Steve could not be a source of joy to his parents, but to deny their grief over Steve's fate would be completely unfair and oppressive. I do not, however, intend to deny the fact that all people can be seen as burdens to other people in different sorts of ways. Also, people are relational beings; dependence or interdependence is consequently a distinctive characteristic of all human lives.[17] Yet, it should also be admitted that Steve's impairment makes his dependence profound and all-inclusive—arguably a completely different kind of dependence from that experienced by other people (with or without impairments).

People with severe intellectual impairments are not productive members of society. Since we live in a world with finite resources, we cannot make infinite provision for every life. However, it is hardly convincing to claim that people with intellectual impairments constitute *the* minority that makes a significant difference in the nation's economy—at least not in Western countries. Instead, the point appears to be the assumed undesirable nature of intellectual impairments and even the existence of people with them that bothers so many. To appeal to the economic interests of society is more or less an excuse for the basic desire to avoid the alleged inconvenience associated with impairments and the existence of people with impairments.[18]

The kind of thinking that emphasizes the economic burden which disabled people may cause to society, does not actually fit in with the fundamental ethos of the modern welfare society. Our societies are not based merely on the requirement of the productivity of its members. According to John Rawls, who has been the most prominent theorist of welfare liberalism, people's interests are intertwined and reciprocal; it is in the interests of us all to take into account the interests of others. Also, "society must give more attention to those with fewer native assets and to those born into less favorable social positions."[19] In the case of people like Steve, this means that his impairment is the result of contingent bad luck. Therefore, his bad luck must be compensated, if possible. The principle of looking after those who are not capable of doing it themselves, is a distinctive feature of many ethical theories other than just welfare liberalism—it appears to be one substantial premise in Western societies.[20] Accordingly, the basic principles of the welfare society and theories of justice require that we have a duty to bear a burden that someone who does not bring anything to the common table may cause us. Alasdair MacIntyre, for example, has stressed that society should take for granted

> that disability and dependence on others are something that all of us experience at certain times in our lives and this to unpredictable degrees, and that consequently our interest in how the needs of the disabled are adequately voiced and met is not a special interest, the interest of one particular group rather than of others, but the interest of the whole political society, an interest that is integral to their conception of their common good.[21]

To conclude, my answer to the question "Is Steve a burden" is "Yes and no." In either case, however, his needs should be met equally compared to those of others.

5. Is Steve a Member of an Oppressed Group?

According to the British social model of disability, people with impairments are an oppressed social group. Disability is not the same as impairment and it is not caused by impairment. Instead, disability is a matter of restricted activity caused by social barriers.[22] I will examine later the issue whether Steve's restricted activity is caused by social barriers or whether it is socially constructed. For now, I deal with the issue of oppression and whether it applies to Steve.

First, what does "oppression" mean? According to the influential contribution by Iris Marion Young, oppression takes place in different ways depending on the oppressed group.[23] Accordingly, Blacks, Jews, lesbians, and gay men, for example, are oppressed in different ways. However, in a general sense, "all oppressed people suffer some inhibition of their ability to develop and exercise their capacities and express their needs, thoughts, and feelings."[24] In addition, oppression is a condition of social groups that are not mere collections of people. Groups are based on shared identity, shared social status, and common history. They are expressions of social relations; a group exists only in relation to at least one other group.[25]

It is quite far-fetched to say, in the case of people with severe intellectual impairments, that they have a shared identity due to the characteristic features of their impairment. It is also extremely problematic to claim that people like Steve have anything more in common with, for instance, a wheelchair user than with someone without any diagnosed impairment. However, since the concept of social group is controversial, let us assume, for the sake of argument, that people with severe intellectual impairments, people like Steve that is, do form a social group. But are they an *oppressed* social group?

In Young's account, oppression consists of five different dimensions: exploitation, marginalization, powerlessness, cultural imperialism, and violence. "Exploitation" refers in this context to the Marxist theory of capitalist society and the conflict between different social classes. Capitalist society is unjust because some people exercise their capacities under the control, according to the purposes, and for the benefit, of other people.[26] Thus, some people are mere means to the aim of maximizing the profit of the owners of capital. But this does not seem to apply to Steve because he is entirely outside the capitalist system—both as a producer and a consumer. He is placed in special school and an institution owned by the government, so the education, care, and treatment that he receives is not, at least in principle, a component in a system with the aim of maximal profit. In practice, however, capitalism can plausibly be seen to pervade Western societies in a way that makes all humans means in the pursuit of maximizing profit. But this does not apply to Steve anywhere near as clearly as it does to the members of the proletariat.

The second dimension of oppression, *marginalization*, appears to apply to the lives of many disabled people—it includes their removal from useful participation in social life through their education and accommodation in segregated institutions. Under the circumstances, disabled people have been put into a dependent position in relation to bureaucratic institutions for support and services and so have often had their basic rights to privacy, respect, and individual choice suspended—although this may well be an unintended consequence of an intentional attempt to respect their rights.[27]

One of the basic functions of the modern welfare society is to support families by providing them with, for instance, decent healthcare, daycare, and educational services. If, say, medical and educational institutions do not take into account the variety in children, families, and their needs, these institutions serve only some children and families while ignoring the needs of those children and families that do not fit into culturally formed expectations. In this kind of case, society prevents the parents from ensuring the fulfillment of their child's interest and well-being. The society thus discriminates against these children and their families.[28] But does this apply to Steve and his family?

One could argue that society does indeed practice a form of oppression by not providing parents of children like Steve with sufficient support mechanisms, so that the children could live at home and go to a regular school. This would be the case if Steve actually gained from living at home and going to a regular school. However, there are factors that may support Steve's placement into an institution. For example, the medical support and healthcare that Steve needs may be easier to provide and it may be more appropriate in an institutional setting than at home. Also, my strong impression was that Steve was well taken care of, and was surrounded by people devoted to ensuring his well-being and appropriate instruction. In other words, special schools and institutions are not always oppressive; sometimes placement in such an institution can be an expedient and sensible solution. Finally, Steve has not been excluded from citizenship, and as a result made dependent and marginalized; he is dependent under any social arrangement due to his lack of intellectual or any other abilities.

The third form of oppression is *powerlessness*, and is closely related to exploitation. In Young's analysis it means the following. Educated professionals are privileged in comparison with the marginalized groups of society. Their professional status guarantees them authority, autonomy, and self-respect, all of which the powerless groups seldom have because their work, often manual rather than mental, is poorly appreciated. The powerless workforce, in other words, lacks authority, status, and a sense of self. In addition, one characteristic of the lives of the powerless, such as disabled people, is the constant unequal encounters with professionals who have the power to control their everyday lives.[29]

The idea of powerlessness, however, has precious little to do with Steve, simply because it explains the experience of people who have been made powerless, but who would not be that way if society were to grant them the power to gain authority, status, and a sense of self through professional status. People like Steve, however, are inherently powerless. This does not mean that Steve's interests should not be taken into account in any decision-making that affects his life. But Steve cannot exercise power over his life—he needs a proxy with a formal place in any life-affecting deliberation.[30]

"Cultural imperialism" refers to the idea of the universalization of a dominant group's experience and culture, and its establishment as the ultimate norm. That group's views and norms come to be taken as self-evident and natural. So, just as we know that the earth goes around the sun, so we "know" that gypsies are thieves, poets are drunkards, and women are good with children. In this way, the experiences of the marginalized groups of the world are nullified and considered to be pointless and wrong.[31] For example, deafness is generally considered to be a disability despite the fact that the Deaf people insist that they constitute a linguistic minority, not an impaired minority (this is naturally a separate and controversial issue).[32]

People usually do not like to be defined in connection to some dominant group that allegedly represents the ideal form of humanity. Women do not want to be defined in relation to men and disabled people do not want to be seen in relation to so-called able-bodied people. People want to be seen in terms of their own experience and they want their own voice to be heard and taken into account. Otherwise they feel that their subjectivity has been trampled on, which virtually would imply oppression. One example of the dominant group's overwhelming views in relation to disability is what Michael Oliver has called "the personal tragedy theory of disability"; disability is a terrible happening that occurs to unfortunate individuals.[33] It is beyond dispute that the majority of people understand disability in terms of tragedy despite the fact that disabled people themselves do not often see their impairment as in any way tragic.

Again, it is a bit difficult to apply this form of oppression to Steve since it is unclear to what extent he is a self-conscious being. Culturally formed beliefs and cultural imperialism probably affect the way in which people with severe intellectual impairments are taken into account in social arrangements and how they are taken care of. But at least from a Nordic perspective it appears that the general social atmosphere is rather favorable toward people like Steve; there is a general agreement that these people are to be treated respectfully. And I think, in general, the professionals working with them act accordingly. As for Steve's impairment and disablement being a tragedy, one can surely agree with this view without making oneself guilty of oppressing him; it is hard to see how a five-year-old boy would gain from losing basically all his physical and mental faculties. Admitting that his fate indeed is tragic does not imply cultural imperialism or oppression but, rather, sense and sensibility. Thus, on the whole, the utility value of the idea of cultural imperialism in Steve's case is feeble.

The final dimension of oppression is *violence* which is often a constant concern for many marginalized groups. Violence can mean random physical attacks, sexual assaults, intimidation, and ridicule. Violence is systematic and a form of oppression when it is directed at members of a group simply because they are members of that group.[34] Now, Steve is undoubtedly an exceptionally vulnerable individual; he is totally at the mercy of other people's good will or ill will. I may be naïve, but I find it extremely difficult to believe that there actually exist people so malevolent that they would consciously abuse Steve just because of his impairment. But then again, we do know that individuals with intellectual impairments are more likely to face abuse than others.[35] So, as far as violence is concerned, Steve probably is a member of an oppressed group.

Altogether, though, the concept and idea of oppression does not seem to be wholly appropriate to explain the experience and status of people like Steve. Carol Thomas has argued that "Disability is a form of social oppression involving the social imposition of restrictions of activity on people with impairments and the socially engendered undermining of their psycho-emotional well-being."[36] However, if disability should be understood as Thomas suggests, the concept of disability applies, if at all, only partially to Steve. His membership in the disabled minority is questionable and it is unclear whether he is a disabled individual in the first place. So, if disability is conceptualized merely in terms of oppression, the concept does not have great relevance to people like Steve.

To conclude, my answer to the question "Is Steve a member of an oppressed group?" is that in some sense, he probably is. In some other sense, he probably is not. However, arrangements and practices that clearly oppress people with intellectual impairments should certainly be abolished.

6. Is Steve's Disability a Social Construct?

In disability studies it is usually argued that disability is not a matter of an individual's physiological condition, but is instead a socially produced phenomenon. In other words, disability is a social construct.[37] It should be noted that I do not separate here *social constructionism* and *social creationism* as theoretical positions in disability studies—although this dichotomy exists especially in some social-model-based contributions.[38] The social constructionist view of disability is allegedly an *idealist* position, maintained in

America, whereas the social creationist view is *materialist* and developed in the United Kingdom. This dichotomy, however, is misleading—especially if one considers the way idealism is understood in philosophy (roughly, the view that the physical world exists only as an expression of mind). Now, there are indeed differences in emphasis, but on the whole, many supposedly social constructionist (or idealist) accounts do take into account the materialist dimensions related to disability, and the way they intertwine with language, values, and ideas.[39]

This is understandable and reasonable, because social creations and constructs are closely related to each other. For example, if society does not consider the needs of the whole population in urban design, it disables some people regarding mobility. On the other hand, the way the environment is built affects how people construct views of desirable and undesirable locomotion; since people are accustomed to stairs instead of ramps, they tend to think that individuals incapable of using stairs have a disabling condition. Material arrangements, thus, shape social constructs which reciprocally have an effect on how our environment is designed and built. Views of "normal," "species-typical," or desirable ways of moving around have formed the basis for the built environment. Social constructs in themselves may put some people in marginal and inferior social positions, but they also work as the basis for disabling material arrangements.[40] So I think it is reasonable here to understand social constructionism in a broad sense: it consists both of "idealist" (social constructions) and "material" (social creations) dimensions.

Social constructionists are usually critical of the *status quo*, and regarding disability, they tend to hold that:

(1) Disability is not the same as impairment and it cannot be understood properly on the basis of impairment. Although the notion of equating impairment with disability is deeply rooted in our culture, it is not determined by the nature of things; it is not inevitable.
(2) The Western conception of disability as an individual's biological condition is incorrect and harmful.
(3) We would be much better off if the individualistic way of thinking concerning disability were done away with, or at least radically transformed.[41]

The social constructionist view of disability implies that it is socially constructed, shaped, and produced. That means that it can be eradicated by changing the views, values, structures, and practices that sustain the limited opportunities and oppression of people with impairments. Robert Bogdan and Steve Taylor, for example, have argued that as a concept, mental retardation exists in the minds of those who use it as a term to describe the intellectual states of other people.[42] It is assumed to be a term expressing an objective, existing state of reality whereas in reality it is a socially invented category that primarily reflects the state of mind of those people who use the concept, not of those who allegedly fall under it: "It is a reification—a socially created category which is assumed to have an existence independent of its creators' minds. [...] Mental retardation is a misnomer, a myth."[43] While Bogdan and Taylor suggest that mental retardation is not real, they do not deny that there are differences among people in terms of intellectual ability. The nature and significance of these differences, however, depend on how we view and interpret them.

Now, all this is quite confusing and ambiguous. Since I am not quite sure precisely what Bogdan and Taylor are saying, I will leave them be. But their stance appears to suggest some sort of extreme social constructionism. Their idea is that the concept of intellectual disability or mental retardation is not a concept of anything real, and does not reflect Steve's state of mind but, instead, mine. The fact that our theoretical concepts and classification procedures are invented, applied, and used by people that are not labeled to have intellectual impairments, does not mean that the condition we are explaining with this concept is not real, not actually there. In other words, an extreme social constructionist view denies the relevance of physical reality and muddles up our knowledge of reality with actually existing reality. Social constructionism in its extreme form therefore equates epistemology with ontology—it suggests that what and how we construct our knowledge of what exists, is the same as what actually exists in the world. This kind of metaphysical view is possible, but whether it is plausible is a different matter.

We may well admit that our knowledge and views of Steve's condition are results of social construction. But it would be completely foolish to conclude from this fact that his disability or disablement is not real. Consequently, in my view, an extreme social constructionism does not make sense. It is not even politically useful; how would it be in Steve's interest to claim that his impairment and disability is actually in the heads of people like me? His care and treatment is based on the view that his impairment and overall incapacity is an empirical fact. If it were "a myth," we could not make any expedient plans for meeting his *actual* needs.

And finally, there is the issue of epistemological and ethical relativism. If there are no ultimate truths, only constructions, how is one to decide between alternative perspectives? According to the social model of disability, disabled people are an oppressed group. But how can we say that they are oppressed if this "group" and its "oppression" are constructs which can have no greater claim to truth than any other?[44] The proponents of social approaches to disability deny some objective ideals of humanity and their moral significance by pointing out their social constructionist nature. At the same time, however, they appeal to given moral standards, such as equality, which they regard to be objectively and universally sound. As Vivien Burr has put the matter, "without some notion of truth or reality, how can we justify advocating one view of the world over another, and one way of organizing social life over another?"[45]

To conclude, my answer to the question "Is Steve's disability a social construct?" is that, the way we see it, of course it is. But his impairment and incapacity to function is very real, very much there, no matter how we construct it, and no matter how much we eradicate social barriers. So, of course it is not.

7. Conclusion

Philosophical and sociological theories of disability have little to say about people like Steve. Usually individuals with intellectual impairments are disregarded in philosophy. However, when consistently applied, the outcome of philosophical theories of personhood is that Steve is not a person and does not merit full moral rights. Sociological accounts (either material or social constructionist) do not seem to say too much about people with intellectual impairments either. It may well be arrogant to say that Steve is not a person. But it would be equally arrogant to say to Steve or to his parents that his fate is not tragic or that his disability is merely a matter of oppression, social barriers, or social constructs.

However, issues of naming and labeling are serious. Saying that someone is not a person or that someone is a burden may have significant consequences for people's moral and social status. For instance, the Nazis referred to some people as "ballast lives" and "empty human husks," partly because such labels justified their extermination.[46] Likewise, the term "burden" in the context of people with impairments may be used inappropriately in favor of assisted suicide and mercy killing. Thus, we should be careful with these kinds of stigmatizing terms and their usage.

Some readers may consider individuals like Steve to be marginal and not properly representative of disabled people. So, some of the criticism that I have leveled at the materialist and social constructionist accounts of disability could be seen as sound with regard to individuals with severe intellectual impairments, but irrelevant with regard to disability theory in general. However, severe intellectual impairment and its implications are also relevant from the viewpoint of other disabled people, in terms of the significance of impairment in their lives. It is not just people like Steve and the characteristics of their impairments that disability theory often fails to take into account properly; this ignorance concerns most impairments and most people with them. Profound impairments often have profound consequences and minor impairments have minor consequences. However, an individual's impairment is rarely a socially insignificant factor. Personal and social dimensions in people's lives are intertwined, not isolated.

There seems to exist in disability studies a kind of linguistic attempt to challenge the reality of impairment. Phrases such as "people who are viewed by others as having some form of impairment"[47] and the placing of terms like "learning difficulties" in quotation marks,[48] seem to suggest that these conditions do not have an objective organic basis.[49] This denial is related perhaps to the idea of celebrating difference; disability is not something to be merely tolerated and accepted, it should be positively valued and celebrated.[50] This idea is probably politically useful and in line with the experiences of many disabled people. But to value positively or celebrate Steve's particular kind of difference, his history, and his impairment, would be intellectually dishonest and, quite frankly, morally repugnant.

Dan Goodley has posed a question that should be properly examined in disability studies: "Are we finally prepared, in this postmodern theoretical climate, to accept a personal tragedy perspective over a social model of disability, *in the case of certain impairments*?"[51] Undoubtedly, we should be prepared to accept this *in the case of certain impairments*. This does not mean that the basic ideas of disability as a form of social oppression, and social construction, should be abandoned, but it does mean that we should admit that the level and significance of impairments and limitations varies from the trivial to the profound.[52]

To conclude, Steve's fate, his impairment, and his disablement *are* tragedies. How society treats him tells us what kind of society we live in. And how our theories deal with him, tells in part whether they are any good—or more precisely, Steve is a serious test-case for the soundness and applicability of our theories.

NOTES

1. See, for example, James Rachels, *The End of Life: Euthanasia and Morality* (Oxford: Oxford University Press, 1986), pp. 76–77.

2. Tom Shakespeare, "Social Models of Disability and Other Life Strategies," *Scandinavian Journal of Disability Research*, 6:1 (2004), pp. 8–21; Tom Shakespeare and Nick Watson, "The Social Model of Disability: An Outdated Ideology?" *Research in Social Science and Disability*, 2:1 (2001), pp. 9–28.

3. Cf. David Wasserman, "Philosophical Issues in the Definition and Social Response to Disability," *Handbook of Disability Studies*, eds. Gary Albrecht, Katherine D. Seelman, and Michael Bury (Thousand Oaks: Sage, 2001), pp. 219–251.

4. Anne Louise Chappell, "Still Out in the Cold: People with Learning Difficulties and the Social Model of Disability," *The Disability Reader: Social Science Perspectives*, ed. Tom Shakespeare (London: Continuum, 1998), pp. 211–220.

5. Steve F. Sapontzis, *Morals, Reason, and Animals* (Philadelphia: Temple University Press, 1987), pp. 48–49.

6. *Ibid*., p. 50.

7. See *Persons and Personality: A Contemporary Inquiry*, eds. Arthur Peacocke and Grant Gillett (Oxford: Basil Blackwell, 1987).

8. John Locke, *An Essay Concerning Human Understanding* (Oxford: Clarendon Press, 1975), Bk. II, ch. 27, sec. 9.

9. Michael Tooley, "Abortion and Infanticide," *Philosophy and Public Affairs*, 2:1 (Autumn 1972), pp. 37–65; Michael Tooley, *Abortion and Infanticide* (Oxford: Clarendon Press, 1983).

10. Tooley, "Abortion and Infanticide," p. 44.

11. See Thomas Nagel, *Mortal Questions* (Cambridge: Cambridge University Press, 1979), pp. 1–10.

12. See, for example, Mary Anne Warren, *Moral Status: Obligations to Persons and Other Living Things* (Oxford: Clarendon Press, 1997).

13. See Bernard Williams, *Ethics and the Limits of Philosophy* (London: Fontana Press, 1993), pp. 174–196.

14. Paul Abberley, "The Spectre at the Feast: Disabled People and Social Theory," *The Disability Reader: Social Science Perspectives*, ed. Tom Shakespeare (London: Continuum, 1998), pp. 79–93; Paul Abberley, "Work, Disability, Disabled People, and European Social Theory," *Disability Studies Today*, eds. Colin Barnes, Mike Oliver, and Len Barton (Cambridge: Polity, 2002), pp. 120–138.; Gary L. Albrecht, *The Disability Business: Rehabilitation in America* (Newbury Park: Sage, 1992), pp. 118–119; Colin Barnes, Geof Mercer, and Tom Shakespeare, *Exploring Disability: A Sociological Introduction* (Cambridge: Polity, 1999), pp. 110–116; Stephen Baron, Sheila Riddell, and Heather Wilkinson, "The Best Burgers? The Person with Learning Difficulties as Worker," *The Disability Reader: Social Science Perspectives*, ed. Tom Shakespeare (London: Continuum, 1998), pp. 94–109.

15. Philip M. Ferguson, "A Place in the Family: An Historical Interpretation of Research on Parental Reactions to Having a Child with a Disability," *The Journal of Special Education*, 36:3 (1 October 2002), pp. 124–130; Philip M. Ferguson, Alan Gartner, and Dorothy K. Lipsky, "The Experience of Disability in Families: A Synthesis of Research and Parent Narratives," *Prenatal Testing and Disability Rights*, eds. Erik Parens and Adrienne Asch (Washington, DC: Georgetown University Press, 2000), pp. 72–94; Erik Parens and Adrienne Asch, "The Disability Rights Critique of Prenatal Genetic Testing: Reflections and Recommendations," *Hastings Center Report*, 29:5 (September–October 1999), S1-S22; Simo Vehmas, "Newborn Infants and the Moral Significance of Intellectual Disabilities," *Journal of The Association for Persons with Severe Handicaps*, 24 (1999), pp. 111–121.

16. Ferguson, "A Place in the Family"; Simo Vehmas, "Parental Responsibility and the Morality of Selective Abortion," *Ethical Theory and Moral Practice*, 5:4 (December 2002), pp. 463–484.

17. E.g., Joan C. Tronto, *Moral Boundaries: A Political Argument for an Ethic of Care* (New York: Routledge, 1993); Susan Wendell, *The Rejected Body: Feminist Philosophical Reflections on Disability* (New York: Routledge, 1996).

18. Simo Vehmas, "The Grounds for Preventing Impairments: A Critique," *Scratching the Surface of Bioethics*, eds. Matti Häyry and Tuija Takala (New York and Amsterdam: Rodopi, 2003), pp. 111–122.

19. John Rawls, *A Theory of Justice* (New York: Oxford University Press, 1972), p. 100.

20. See Alasdair MacIntyre, *After Virtue: A Study in Moral Theory* (London: Duckworth, 1985); Stephen Mulhall and Adam Swift, *Liberals and Communitarians* (Oxford: Blackwell, 1992); Joan C. Tronto, "What can Feminists Learn about Morality from Caring," *Ethics: The Big Questions*, ed. James P. Sterba (Oxford: Blackwell, 1998), pp. 346–356; Robert M. Veatch, *The Foundations of Justice: Why the Retarded and the Rest of Us Have Claims to Equality* (New York: Oxford University Press, 1986).

21. Alasdair MacIntyre, *Dependent Rational Animals: Why Human Beings Need the Virtues* (London: Duckworth, 1999), p. 130.

22. E.g., Michael Oliver, *Understanding Disability: From Theory to Practice* (Basingstoke: Macmillan, 1996); Carol Thomas, "How is Disability Understood? An Examination of Sociological Approaches," *Disability and Society*, 19:6 (2004), pp. 569–583.

23. Iris Marion Young, *Justice and the Politics of Difference* (Princeton: Princeton University Press, 1990).

24. *Ibid.*, p. 40.

25. *Ibid.*, pp. 42–44.

26. *Ibid.*, pp. 48–53.

27. *Ibid.*, pp. 53–55.

28. Vehmas, "Parental Responsibility and the Morality of Selective Abortion."

29. Young, *Justice and the Politics of Difference*, pp. 56–58.

30. See MacIntyre, *Dependent Rational Animals*, p. 130.

31. Young, *Justice and the Politics of Difference*, pp. 58–61.

32. See John Harris, "Is There a Coherent Social Conception of Disability?" *Journal of Medical Ethics*, 26:2 (April 2000), pp. 95–100; John Harris, "One Principle and Three Fallacies of Disability Studies," *Journal of Medical Ethics*, 27:6 (December 2001), pp. 383–387; Simo Vehmas and Tom Shakespeare, "Disability, Harm and the Origins of Limited Opportunities," *Life of Value: John Harris, His Arguments, and His Critics*, eds. Søren Holm, Matti Häyry and Tuija Takala (New York and Amsterdam: Rodopi, forthcoming).

33. Oliver, *Understanding Disability*, p. 32.

34. Young, *Justice and the Politics of Difference*, pp. 61–63.

35. Eileen M. Furey, "Sexual Abuse of Adults with Mental Retardation: Who and Where," *Mental Retardation*, 32:3 (June 1994), pp. 173–180; Margaret A. Nosek, Catherine Clubb Foley, Rosemary B. Hughes, and Carol A. Howland, "Vulnerabilities for Abuse Among Women with Disabilities," *Sexuality and Disability*, 19:3 (September 2001), pp. 177–189; Mark Priestley, *Disability: A Life Course Approach* (Cambridge: Polity, 2003), p. 100; Vappu Viemerö, "Violence Against Disabled Women," *Gender and Disability Research in the Nordic Countries*, eds. Kristjana Kristiansen and Rannveig Traustadóttir (Lund: Studentlitteratur, 2004), pp. 327–345.

36. Carol Thomas, *Female Forms: Experiencing and Understanding Disability* (Buckingham: Open University Press, 1999), p. 60.

37. E.g., Gary L. Albrecht, "American Pragmatism, Sociology and the Development of Disability Studies," *Disability Studies Today*, eds. Barnes, Oliver, and Barton, pp. 18–37; Barnes, Mercer, and Shakespeare, *Exploring Disability*, pp. 93-95; Simi Linton, *Claiming Disability: Knowledge and Identity* (New York: New York University Press, 1998), pp. 37–45; Steve Taylor, "Disability Studies and Mental Retardation," *Disability Studies Quarterly*, 16:3 (1996), pp. 4–13; Rosemarie Garland Thomson,

Extraordinary Bodies: Figuring Physical Disability in American Culture and Literature (New York: Columbia University Press, 1997), pp. 5–7; Wendell, *The Rejected Body: Feminist Philosophical Reflections on Disability*, pp. 35–38.

38. Brendan Gleeson, *Geographies of Disability* (London: Routledge, 1999), pp. 21–22, 24–27; Mark Priestley, "Constructions and Creations: Idealism, Materialism and Disability Theory," *Disability and Society*, 13:1 (1998), pp. 75–94.

39. E.g., Anita Silvers, "'Defective' Agents: Equality, Difference, and the Tyranny of the Normal," *Journal of Social Philosophy*, 25th Anniversary Special Issue (1994), pp. 154–175; Anita Silvers, "Reconciling Equality to Difference: Caring (f)or Justice for People with Disabilities," *Hypatia*, 10:1 (Winter 1995), pp. 30–55; Linton, *Claiming Disability*, pp. 45–51; Thomson, *Extraordinary Bodies*, p. 7; Wasserman, "Philosophical Issues in the Definition and Social Response to Disability."

40. Simo Vehmas, "Ethical Analysis of the Concept of Disability," *Mental Retardation*, 42:3 (June 2004), pp. 209–222.

41. *Cf.*, Ian Hacking, *The Social Construction of What?* (Cambridge: Harvard University Press, 1999), p. 6.

42. Robert Bogdan and Steven J. Taylor, *The Social Meaning of Mental Retardation: Two Life Stories* (New York: Teachers College Press, 1994).

43. *Ibid.*, p. 7; See also Dan Goodley, "'Learning Difficulties,' the Social Model of Disability and Impairment: Challenging Epistemologies," *Disability and Society*, 16:2 (2001), pp. 207–231.

44.Vivien Burr, "Overview: Realism, Relativism, Social Constructionism and Discourse," *Social Constructionism, Discourse and Realism*, ed. Ian Parker (London: Sage, 1998), pp. 13–25, at p. 14.

45. *Ibid.*

46. E.g., Robert Proctor, *Racial Hygiene: Medicine Under the Nazis* (Cambridge: Harvard University Press, 1988).

47. Michael Oliver, "The Social Model in Action: If I Had a Hammer", *Implementing the Social Model of Disability: Theory and Research*, eds. Colin Barnes and Geof Mercer (Leeds: The Disability Press, 2004), pp. 18–31, at p. 21.

48. Goodley, "'Learning Difficulties,' the Social Model of Disability and Impairment."

49. Tom Shakespeare, *Disability Rights and Wrongs* (London: Routledge, 2006).

50. Oliver, *Understanding Disability*, p. 89.

51. Goodley, "'Learning Difficulties,' the Social Model of Disability and Impairment," p. 211.

52. Shakespeare and Watson, "The Social Model of Disability."

ABOUT THE EDITORS AND CONTRIBUTORS

Gardar Árnason is a researcher at the Department of Social and Moral Philosophy, University of Helsinki.

Lisa Bortolotti is Lecturer in Philosophy at the University of Birmingham. Her main interests are in philosophy of psychology (especially intentionality, rationality and self-knowledge) and bioethics (especially research ethics, reproductive ethics and animal ethics).

Angus Dawson is Senior Lecturer at the Centre for Professional Ethics, Keele University, and joint editor-in-chief of the journal *Public Health Ethics*.

Simona Giordano is Senior Lecturer in Bioethics at the Centre for Social Ethics and Policy, University of Manchester.

Matti Häyry is Professor of Bioethics and Philosophy of Law at the Centre for Social Ethics and Policy, University of Manchester.

Sirkku Kristiina Hellsten is Reader in Development Ethics at the Centre for the Study of Global Ethics, University of Birmingham (on Leave of Absence); and Docent of Social and Moral Philosophy at the University of Helsinki. Currently Dr Hellsten works as Governance Counselor at the Embassy of Finland, Nairobi, Kenya.

Peter Herissone-Kelly is Lecturer in Philosophy in the International School for Communities, Rights, and Inclusion, University of Central Lancashire.

Søren Holm is Professor of Bioethics at the Centre for Social Ethics and Policy, University of Manchester. He also holds a permanent visiting Chair at the Section for Medical Ethics, University of Oslo.

Harry Lesser is Senior Lecturer in Philosophy at the University of Manchester and the author of a number of articles in ethics and bioethics. He is currently editing for this series a collection of papers entitled *Justice and the Elderly*.

Peter Lucas is Senior Lecturer in Philosophy in the International School for Communities, Rights, and Inclusion, University of Central Lancashire.

John McMillan is Associate Professor in Ethics, Law and Professionalism at Flinders University, Adelaide, Australia.

Stuart Oultram is Teaching Fellow at the Centre for Professional Ethics, Keele University.

Doris Schroeder is Professor of Moral Philosophy and Head of the Centre for Professional Ethics, University of Central Lancashire, United Kingdom, as well as Professorial Fellow at the Centre for Applied Philosophy and Public Ethics, University of Melbourne, Australia.

Cathleen Schulte works for the UK Department of Health.

Niall Scott is Lecturer in Ethics in the International School for Communities, Rights, and Inclusion, University of Central Lancashire.

Mark Sheehan is James Martin Research Fellow, The Program on the Ethics of the New Biosciences, Faculty of Philosophy and James Martin 21st Century School, University of Oxford.

Anna Smajdor is a Researcher in Medical Ethics at Imperial College, London.

Tuija Takala is Adjunct Professor of Practical Philosophy at the University of Helsinki.

Floris Tomasini is a Lecturer in Philosophy and Mental Health in the International School for Communities, Rights, and Inclusion at the University of Central Lancashire and a Research Associate at the ESRC Centre CESAGen, Lancaster University.

Simo Vehmas is Professor of Special Education at the University of Jyväskylä, Finland.

Stephen Wilkinson is Professor at the Centre for Professional Ethics, Keele University.

Jane Wilson has a combined background in philosophy and healthcare practice. She is currently completing a PhD on the subject of paternalism at the Centre for Professional Ethics, Keele University.

INDEX

Titles Published

Volumes 1 - 178 see www.rodopi.nl

179. John Ryder, Gert Rüdiger Wegmarshaus, Editors, *Education for a Democratic Society: Central European Pragmatist Forum, Volume Three.* A volume in **Studies in Pragmatism and Values**

180. Florencia Luna, *Bioethics and Vulnerability: A Latin American View.* A volume in **Values in Bioethics**

181. John Kultgen and Mary Lenzi, Editors, *Problems for Democracy.* A volume in **Philosophy of Peace**

182. David Boersema and Katy Gray Brown, Editors, *Spiritual and Political Dimensions of Nonviolence and Peace.* A volume in **Philosophy of Peace**

183. Daniel P. Thero, *Understanding Moral Weakness.* A volume in **Studies in the History of Western Philosophy**

184. Scott Gelfand and John R. Shook, Editors, *Ectogenesis: Artificial Womb Technology and the Future of Human Reproduction.* A volume in **Values in Bioethics**

185. Piotr Jaroszyński, *Science in Culture.* A volume in **Gilson Studies**

186. Matti Häyry, Tuija Takala, Peter Herissone-Kelly, Editors, *Ethics in Biomedical Research: International Perspectives.* A volume in **Values in Bioethics**

187. Michael Krausz, *Interpretation and Transformation: Explorations in Art and the Self.* A volume in **Interpretation and Translation**

188. Gail M. Presbey, Editor, *Philosophical Perspectives on the "War on Terrorism."* A volume in **Philosophy of Peace**

189. María Luisa Femenías, Amy A. Oliver, Editors, *Feminist Philosophy in Latin America and Spain.* A volume in **Philosophy in Latin America**

190. Oscar Vilarroya and Francesc Forn I Argimon, Editors, *Social Brain Matters: Stances on the Neurobiology of Social Cognition.* A volume in **Cognitive Science**

191. Eugenio Garin, *History of Italian Philosophy*. Translated from Italian and Edited by Giorgio Pinton. A volume in **Values in Italian Philosophy**

192. Michael Taylor, Helmut Schreier, and Paulo Ghiraldelli, Jr., Editors, *Pragmatism, Education, and Children: International Philosophical Perspectives*. A volume in **Pragmatism and Values**

193. Brendan Sweetman, *The Vision of Gabriel Marcel: Epistemology, Human Person, the Transcendent*. A volume in **Philosophy and Religion**

194. Danielle Poe and Eddy Souffrant, Editors, *Parceling the Globe: Philosophical Explorations in Globalization, Global Behavior, and Peace*. A volume in **Philosophy of Peace**

195. Josef Šmajs, *Evolutionary Ontology: Reclaiming the Value of Nature by Transforming Culture*. A volume in **Central-European Value Studies**

196. Giuseppe Vicari, *Beyond Conceptual Dualism: Ontology of Consciousness, Mental Causation, and Holism in John R. Searle's Philosophy of Mind*. A volume in **Cognitive Science**

197. Avi Sagi, *Tradition vs. Traditionalism: Contemporary Perspectives in Jewish Thought*. Translated from Hebrew by Batya Stein. A volume in **Philosophy and Religion**

198. Randall E. Osborne and Paul Kriese, Editors, *Global Community: Global Security*. A volume in **Studies in Jurisprudence**

199. Craig Clifford, *Learned Ignorance in the Medicine Bow Mountains: A Reflection on Intellectual Prejudice*. A volume in **Lived Values: Valued Lives**

200. Mark Letteri, *Heidegger and the Question of Psychology: Zollikon and Beyond*. A volume in **Philosophy and Psychology**

201. Carmen R. Lugo-Lugo and Mary K. Bloodsworth-Lugo, Editors, *A New Kind of Containment: "The War on Terror," Race, and Sexuality*. A volume in **Philosophy of Peace**

202. Amihud Gilead, *Necessity and Truthful Fictions: Panenmentalist Observations*. A volume in **Philosophy and Psychology**

203. Fernand Vial, *The Unconscious in Philosophy, and French and European Literature: Nineteenth and Early Twentieth Century.* A volume in **Philosophy and Psychology**

204. Adam C. Scarfe, Editor, *The Adventure of Education: Process Philosophers on Learning, Teaching, and Research.* A volume in **Philosophy of Education**

205. King-Tak Ip, Editor, *Environmental Ethics: Intercultural Perspectives.* A volume in **Studies in Applied Ethics**

206. Evgenia Cherkasova, *Dostoevsky and Kant: Dialogues on Ethics.* A volume in **Social Philosophy**

207. Alexander Kremer and John Ryder, Editors, *Self and Society: Central European Pragmatist Forum*, Volume Four. A volume in **Central European Value Studies**

208. Terence O'Connell, *Dialogue on Grief and Consolation.* A volume in **Lived Values, Valued Lives**

209. Craig Hanson, *Thinking about Addiction: Hyperbolic Discounting and Responsible Agency.* A volume in **Social Philosophy**

210. Gary G. Gallopin, *Beyond Perestroika: Axiology and the New Russian Entrepreneurs.* A volume in **Hartman Institute Axiology Studies**

211. Tuija Takala, Peter Herissone-Kelly, and Søren Holm, Editors, *Cutting Through the Surface: Philosophical Approaches to Bioethics.* A volume in **Values in Bioethics**

212. Neena Schwartz: *A Lab of My Own.* A volume in **Lived Values, Valued Lives**

213. Krzysztof Piotr Skowroński, *Values and Powers: Re-reading the Philosophical Tradition of American Pragmatism.* A volume in **Central European Value Studies**

214. Matti Häyry, Tuija Takala, Peter Herissone-Kelly and Gardar Árnason, Editors, *Arguments and Analysis in Bioethics.* A volume in **Values in Bioethics**

www.ingramcontent.com/pod-product-compliance
Lightning Source LLC
LaVergne TN
LVHW102226300926
849160LV00005B/38